Frontiers in HIV Res

Current Studies in HIV Research

(Volume 2)

Edited By

SeyedAhmad SeyedAlinaghi

Iranian Research Center for HIV/AIDS
Iranian Institute for Reduction of High Risk Behaviors
Tehran University of Medical Sciences
Iran

I0038305

Frontiers in HIV Research

Current Studies in HIV Research

Editor: SeyedAhmad SeyedAlinaghi

ISSN (Online): 2405-9889

ISSN (Print): 2405-9862

ISBN (Online): 9781681082554

ISBN (Print): 9781681082561

First published in 2016.

advertisements or ideas contained in the Work.

Limitation of Liability:

In no event will Bentham Science Publishers, its staff, editors and/or authors, be liable for any damages, including, without limitation, special, incidental and/or consequential damages and/or damages for lost data and/or profits arising out of (whether directly or indirectly) the use or inability to use the Work. The entire liability of Bentham Science Publishers shall be limited to the amount actually paid by you for the Work.

General:

1. Any dispute or claim arising out of or in connection with this License Agreement or the Work (including non-contractual disputes or claims) will be governed by and construed in accordance with the laws of the U.A.E. as applied in the Emirate of Dubai. Each party agrees that the courts of the Emirate of Dubai shall have exclusive jurisdiction to settle any dispute or claim arising out of or in connection with this License Agreement or the Work (including non-contractual disputes or claims).
2. Your rights under this License Agreement will automatically terminate without notice and without the need for a court order if at any point you breach any terms of this License Agreement. In no event will any delay or failure by Bentham Science Publishers in enforcing your compliance with this License Agreement constitute a waiver of any of its rights.
3. You acknowledge that you have read this License Agreement, and agree to be bound by its terms and conditions. To the extent that any other terms and conditions presented on any website of Bentham Science Publishers conflict with, or are inconsistent with, the terms and conditions set out in this License Agreement, you acknowledge that the terms and conditions set out in this License Agreement shall prevail.

Bentham Science Publishers Ltd.
Executive Suite Y - 2
PO Box 7917, Saif Zone
Sharjah, U.A.E.
Email: subscriptions@benthamscience.org

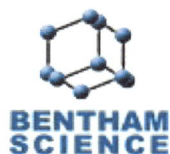

CONTENTS

FOREWORD

It is estimated that about 35 million people worldwide are currently living with HIV/AIDS and, fortunately, the number of AIDS deaths and new infections is also declining. The introduction of antiretroviral therapy for effective control and prevention has had a great role to play in reducing this infection. Further, age of HIV-infected patients have been markedly increased so that the issues related to *"HIV and aging"* are discussed in more details by many textbooks and articles. However, fundamental challenges still remain such as HIV stigma and discrimination, adherence to antiretroviral therapy, access to high-risk groups including homosexuals and vulnerable women, types of intervention and their effectiveness on high risk groups, as well as achieving commitment to agreed goals by countries.

A textbook may be required to address new developments on the HIV/AIDS from different aspects. The present book can be regarded as a useful resource on HIV for researchers, clinicians, and others dealing with HIV. It provides a review of hot topics in HIV/AIDS compiled by Iranian and foreign experts. Indeed, edited by Dr. SeyedAlinaghi, the book covers important basic, epidemiological and clinical research aspects and presents updated information to readers. It also refers to a number of new issues which have not been extensively studied.

We truly appreciate all the authors who help the editor by writing the book chapters, and hope to provide valuable information to readers and receive positive feedback for our work.

Alireza Yalda
Distinguished Professor
Tehran University of Medical Sciences
Tehran
Iran

PREFACE

The present book focus on hot topics in HIV/AIDS research and every chapter was prepared by experts in the field.

Despite a global decline in the number of new HIV infection, in some areas including the Middle East the incidence rate of HIV infection is increasing. Consequently, effective prevention strategies as well as increased access to antiretroviral therapy (ART) are needed. In fact, control efforts for HIV infection requires to achieve a 50 percent reduction of HIV transmission among people who are infected through injection drug use or sexual intercourse, and elimination of mother-to-child transmission by way of providing antiretroviral treatment to pregnant HIV-positive women with a coverage target of 90% by 2015. On the other hand, one of the main objectives of international organizations is to increase the access to ART both as a life saving medication for people living with HIV and as an effective practice to prevent the infection. Fortunately, the infection with HIV is not considered a fatal disease anymore and it turned into a chronic disease and HIV infected people may enjoy near-normal life expectancy and reach old age.

Unfortunately, HIV-related stigma and discrimination is still significant in most areas of the world. However, the integration of HIV services with Primary Health Care (PHC) has proved to be an effective measure put in place by some nations. Further, reforming current laws and regulations and the development of new anti-discrimination legislation seem to be important for effective preventive and treatment activities.

The current book does not cover all aspects of HIV/AIDS. But, it presents a brief account of major issues and developments dealing with basic, epidemiology and clinical research for medical and scientific applications in this field.

The editor appreciates the effort and patience of all authors who participated in the writing of the chapters.

Dr. SeyedAhmad SeyedAlinaghi
Iranian Research Center for HIV/AIDS
Iranian Institute for Reduction of High Risk Behaviors
Tehran University of Medical Sciences
Iran

List of Contributors

Alireza Hosseini — Iranian Research Center for HIV/AIDS, Iranian Institute for Reduction of High-Risk Behaviors, Tehran University of Medical Sciences, Tehran, Iran; Students' Scientific Research Center (SSRC), Tehran University of Medical Sciences, Tehran, Iran

Ali Teimoori — Department of virology, Jundishapur University of Medical science, Ahvaz, Iran

Amin Farzanegan — Faculty of Medical sciences, Tarbiat Modares University, Tehran, Iran

Asghar Abdoli — Department of Hepatitis and AIDS, Pasteur Institute of Iran, Tehran, Iran

Banafsheh Moradmand Badie — Discipline of Public Health, School of Medicine, Flinders University, South Australia

Behnam Farhoudi — Islamic Azad University, Tehran Medical Sciences Branch, Iran

Donald J. Hamel — Department of Immunology and Infectious Diseases, Harvard School of Public Health, Boston MA 02115 , USA

Ghobad Moradi — Social Determinants of Health Research Cente, Kurdistan University of Medical Sciences, Sanandaj, Iran

Hamid Emadi Koochak — Iranian Research Center for HIV/AIDS, Iranian Institute for Reduction of High Risk Behaviors, Tehran University of Medical Sciences, Tehran, Iran

Holly Rawizza — Brigham and Women's Hospital, Harvard Medical School, Boston, USA

Hossein Malekafzali Ardakani — Department of Epidemiology and Biostatistics, School of Public Health, Tehran University of Medical Sciences, Tehran, Iran

Katayon Tayeri — Iranian Research Center for HIV/AIDS, Iranian Institute for Reduction of High Risk Behaviors, Tehran University of Medical Sciences, Tehran, Iran

Kazem Baesi — Hepatitis and AIDS Department, Pasteur Institute of Iran, Tehran, Iran

Kenneth McIntosh — Harvard Medical School, Harvard School of Public Health Emeritus Chief, Infectious Diseases Division, Boston Children's Hospital, USA

Koosha Paydary — Iranian Research center for HIV/AIDS, Iranian Institute for Reduction of High-Risk Behaviors,Tehran University of Medical Sciences, Tehran, Iran; Students' Scientific Research Center (SSRC), Tehran University of Medical Sciences (TUMS), Tehran, Iran

Lillian Mwanri — Discipline of Public Health, School of Health Sciences, Faulty of Medicine, Nursing and Health Sciences, Flinders University, South Australia, Australia

Maryam Foroughi — Iranian Research Center for HIV/AIDS, Iranian Institute for Reduction of High Risk Behaviors, Tehran University of Medical Sciences, Tehran, Iran

May Sudhinaraset
Global Health Sciences, University of California San Francisco, San Francisco, CA, USA

Minoo Mohraz
Iranian Research Center for HIV/AIDS, Iranian Institute for Reduction of High Risk Behaviors, Tehran University of Medical Sciences, Tehran, Iran

Mohammad Reza Aghasadeghi
Department of Hepatitis and AIDS, Pasteur Institute of Iran, Tehran, Iran

Mona Mohammadi Firouzeh
Iranian Research Center for HIV/AIDS (IRCHA), Iranian Institute for Reduction of High-Risk Behaviors, Tehran University of Medical Sciences, Tehran, Iran

Omid Zamani
HIV/STI Surveillance Research Center, and WHO Collaborating Center for HIV Surveillance, Institute for Futures Studies in Health, Kerman University of Medical Sciences, Kerman, Iran

Pegah Valiollahi
Department of Clinical and Experimental Medicine of Linköping University, Linköping, Sweden

Sahra Emamzadeh-Fard
Department of Radiology, Division of Interventional Radiology, Memorial Sloan-Kettering Cancer Center, New York, USA

Sara Sardashti
Iranian Research Center for HIV/AIDS, Iranian Institute for Reduction of High-Risk Behaviors, Tehran University of Medical Sciences, Tehran, Iran

Sepideh Khodaei
Iranian Research Center for HIV/AIDS, Iranian Institute for Reduction of High-Risk Behaviors, Tehran University of Medical Sciences, Tehran, Iran

SeyedAhmad SeyedAlinaghi
Iranian Research Center for HIV/AIDS, Iranian Institute for Reduction of High-Risk Behaviors, Tehran University of Medical Sciences, Tehran, Iran

Seyed Hadi Razavi
Faculty of Medical Sciences, Tarbiat Modares University, Tehran, Iran

Seyed Ramin Radfar
University of California, Los Angeles, Integrated Substance Abuse Programs, Los Angeles, USA

Seyed Younes Hosseini
Gastroenterohepatology Research Center, Shiraz University of Medical Sciences, Shiraz, Iran

Shayan Tabe-Bordbar
Physiology Department, University of Illinois at Urbana-Champaign (UIUC), USA

Shooka Esmaeeli
Iranian Research center for HIV/AIDS, Iranian Institute for Reduction of High-Risk Behaviors, Tehran University of Medical Sciences, Tehran, Iran; Students' Scientific Research Center (SSRC), Tehran University of Medical Sciences, Tehran, Iran

Siavash Eskandari
Iranian Research center for HIV/AIDS, Iranian Institute for Reduction of High-Risk Behaviors, Tehran University of Medical Sciences, Tehran, Iran; Students' Scientific Research Center (SSRC), Tehran University of Medical Sciences, Tehran, Iran

Soda Neamatzade   Kurdistan University of Medical Sciences, Sanandaj, Iran

Zahra Goodarzi   Applied Virology Research Center, Baqyatallah University of Medical Sciences, Tehran, Iran

Zeinab Najafi   Iranian Research center for HIV/AIDS, Iranian Institute for Reduction of High-Risk Behaviors, Tehran University of Medical Sciences, Tehran, Iran; Students' Scientific Research Center (SSRC), Tehran University of Medical Science, Tehran, Iran

Frontiers in HIV Research

Current Studies in HIV Research

(Volume 2)

CHAPTER 1

Diversity and Global Epidemiology of HIV

Kazem Baesi[1,2,3,*], **Seyed Younes Hosseini**[2], **Ali Teimoori**[4] and **Mohammad Gholami**[5]

[1] *Hepatitis and AIDS Department, Pasteur Institute of Iran, Tehran, Iran*

[2] *GastroenteroHepatology Research Center, Shiraz University of Medical Sciences, Shiraz, Iran*

[3] *Shiraz HIV/AIDS Research Center, Shiraz University of Medical Sciences, Zand, Iran*

[4] *Department of virology, Jundishapur University of Medical sciences, Ahvaz, Iran*

[5] *Iranian Research Center for HIV/AIDS, Iranian Institute for Reduction of High Risk Behaviors, Tehran University of Medical Sciences, Tehran, Iran*

Abstract: HIV has probably originated from multiple zoonotic transmissions of Simian Immunodeficiency Virus (SIV) from non-human primates to humans in West and Central Africa. There are two HIV types: HIV type 1 (HIV-1) groups M, N, O and P and HIV type 2 (HIV-2) groups A–H. Within the HIV-1 group M, nine subtypes are found, designated by the letters A–D, F–H, J, and K. Within a subtype, changes in the amino acid sequence is observed in the range of 8-17%, but it can be as high as 30%, while differences between subtypes are generally found in the range of 17-35%.

In fact, when new combinations between different HIV-1 subtypes occurs, it results in different Unique Recombinant Forms (URFs), some developed into Circulating Recombinant Forms (CRFs) as propagated in three or more epidemiologically unlinked individuals. The viruses fueling these epidemics vary according to geographical regions, with clade C virus being the most prevalent worldwide, and clade B being currently the most prevalent in the United States and Europe.

Thirty years after the first description of AIDS, an estimated 35.0 million [33.2 million–37.2 million] people were living with HIV at the end of 2013. 2.1 million [1.9–2.4 million] had become newly contaminated with HIV in 2013, including 240000 children, and 1.5 million [1.4–1.7 million] HIV-infected persons died.

* **Correspondence to Kazem Baesi:** Hepatitis and AIDS Department, Pasteur Institute of Iran, Pasteur Ave., Tehran 1316943551, Tehran, Iran; Shiraz HIV/AIDS Research Center, Shiraz University of Medical Sciences, Zand, Iran; Tel/Fax: +98 (21) 66969291; E-mail: kbaesi@gmail.com.

Keywords: AIDS, CRF, Diversity, Epidemiology, HIV, Mutation, Recombination, Sequence, Subtype, URF.

1. INTRODUCTION

HIV has probably stemmed from multiple zoonotic transmissions of Simian Immunodeficiency Virus (SIV) from non-human primates to humans in West and Central Africa. Cross-species transmission appeared in the process of butchering and hunting of primates for capture and the bush meat, trade and custody of monkeys as pets [1]. More than 40 different non-human primate species harbor SIV infections, with each specie carrying a specie-specific virus [2, 3].

2. HIV GENETIC DIVERSITY

Several factors supply to the extraordinary high genetic heterogeneity of HIV-1: (a) error-prone viral DNA synthesis during reverse transcription, (b) high recombination frequencies accompanying reverse transcription, (c) the high levels of progeny virus production *in vivo*, and (d) large numbers of infected individuals [4, 5]. It has been estimated that within an HIV-1-infected person, viral genetic diversity increases by 1% every year from the founder viral strain during the early symptomatic phase of the infection [6].

There are various HIV types: HIV type 1 (HIV-1) groups M, N, O and P and HIV type 2 (HIV-2) groups A–H. The range of the epidemic caused by each group varies considerably. HIV-1 group M is liable for the global HIV pandemic (approximately 33 million contaminated individuals), group N has been found in a handful of people in Cameroon; while group O causes a few tens of thousands of infections in West–Central Africa and group P was recently identified in two individuals originating from Cameroon [7, 8]. HIV-1 groups M and N might have stem directly, but independently, from SIVcpz observed in the chimpanzee *pan troglodytes* in West–Central Africa [9, 10]. Conceivably, more HIV types in humans will be found in the future, as all HIV types may not yet have been discovered and new cross-species transmissions may happen in the future. In the HIV epidemics, the sequences of the different HIV-1 groups have further diversified in the populations, which have enhanced further classifications [3]. In the HIV-1 group M, nine subtypes are detected, selected by the letters A–D, F–H,

J, and K [11]. Within a subtype, variations at the amino acid level is in the range of 8–17%, but can be as high as 30%, while variations between subtypes are usually between 17-35% [3].

According to analyses on several genome regions and particularly full length genome sequencing, recombination is a substitution event between viral strains. Intra-subtype recombination was observed to be very general within group M subtype C [12]. In fact, recombination between different HIV-1 subtypes has developed different many Unique Recombinant Forms (URFs), several developed into Circulating Recombinant Forms (CRFs) as propagated in three or more epidemiologically unlinked individuals. To date, 68 different CRFs have been found [11]. Recombination of some CRFs with other subtypes or CRFs results in the so-called Second-Generation Recombinants (SGRs) [3].

Group O sequence shows a high diversity, leading to a classification of sequences into clades I–V and they are as genetically far-away from each other as group M subtypes. On the other hand, lower subtype-like signal in group O was obtained *versus* to group M because group O has not spread too a lot past its origin in West–Central Africa [13 - 15]. All group N viruses found in humans are narrowly associated, as the only two group P sequences reported [8].

3. GLOBAL DISTRIBUTION

In agreement with our increasing knowledge about the mechanisms of HIV transmission, this infection has decreased markedly over the past decade. The viruses fueling these epidemics vary according to geographical regions, with clade C virus being the most prevalent worldwide, and clade B being currently the most prevalent in the United States and Europe (Table **1**).

Table 1. Distribution of all HIV-1 sequences that have been included in the Los Alamos database [16].

Subtype	Number	Percentage
01_AE	28453	5.3%
02_AG	14826	2.8%
A	39389	7.4%
B	303348	56.8%

(Table 1) contd.....

Subtype	Number	Percentage
C	84723	15.9%
D	19681	3.7%
F	4867	0.9%
G	5955	1.1%
other	32881	6.2%
total	534123	100.0%

4. THE IMPACT OF HIV DIVERSITY

4.1. The Impact of HIV Diversity on Pathogenesis

The importance of the HIV biological mutability *in vivo* has been studied by many natural history researches. The pathogenesis of the two key types of HIV demonstrate significant differences, with HIV-2 being both less transmissible and less pathogenic than HIV-1 [17, 18]. The role HIV-1 biological mutability plays in pathogenesis has been studied often in the cases of HIV infection with subtype B viruses in the developed world. As found, syncytia-inducing (SI) and rapid/high biological phenotypes are typically related with late stages of immunodeficiency, while viruses without such feature are more commonly involved in with asymptomatic individuals or patients with mild symptoms [19].

4.2. The Impact of HIV Diversity on Disease Progression and Transmission

Coming into the role of HIV subtypes in disease progression as well as in transmission and viral load has been reported by cohort research carried out in areas with different subtypes co-circulate, especially Eastern Africa. Independent studies in Tanzania, Kenya and Uganda all indicate that subtype D disease is related with sooner disease progression compared to subtype A among populations where these subtypes co-circulate. The lowered survival rate was related with decreased counts of CD4 in subtype D infection *versus* to subtype A in some studies [20, 21]. In a European research, subtype D was further found to have a four-fold higher rate of CD4 count refuse, in the absence of anti-retroviral therapy, compared to other subtypes (A, B, C and CRF02_AG), even when adjusted for baseline CD4 count [22]. In terms of transmissibility, a study from

Uganda showed that subtype A shows a higher rate of heterosexual transmission compared to subtype D [22]. The studies from Kenya and Uganda revealed a significant decline in the amount of subtype D *versus* subtype A over a certain time period [22]. Such variations in the amounts of subtypes A and D are compatible with both the sooner disease progression and the lower rate of heterosexual transmission of subtype D compared to subtype A [22].

4.3. The Impact of HIV Diversity on Response to HAART and Drug Resistance

A wide range of research directed in Asian and African countries with a variety of different drug regimens in a range of settings have found similar susceptibility of different group M subtypes for currently used anti-retroviral drugs, which were originally developed based on subtype B. A big universal collaboration indicated that all of the 55 known subtype B drug-resistance mutations was seen in at least one non-B subtype. Moreover, of the 67 resistance mutations found in at least one non-B subtype, only 61 were found in subtype B isolates, meaning that numerous novel mutations take place in non-B subtypes [3, 23]. For some resistance-associated mutations, the resistance pathway is shorter in several non-B subtypes compared to subtype B [3, 23]. The decision-making about the selection of second-line regimens are affected by such variations in resistance pathways.

4.4. HIV Diversity and HIV Vaccines

A preventive vaccination will be the ideal intervention to control the HIV pandemic, because it is considered a safe, simple, highly effective and affordable intervention. However, HIV diversity is recognized, in individuals and in populations, as one of the key challenges in the development of a worldwide effective HIV vaccine. Rapid evolution and generation of escape mutants by the infecting HIV strain is an enormous challenge for the immune system to overcome, even after priming by vaccination [15].

5. THE GLOBAL EPIDEMIC AT A GLANCE

HIV-1 stay a global health problem of unpreceding dimensions. Since the begin of the epidemic, approximately 78 million [71 million–87 million] people have become infected with HIV and 39 million [35 million–43 million] people have died of AIDS-related illnesses [24].

Thirty years after the first explanation of AIDS, an estimated 35.0 million [33.2 million–37.2 million] people were living with HIV at the end of 2013. 2.1 million [1.9–2.4 million] had become newly infected with HIV in 2013, including 240000 children, and 1.5 million [1.4–1.7 million] HIV-infected persons died. Of the 35 million people, more than two-thirds are living with HIV in sub-Saharan Africa. In Asia and the Pacific, about 4.8 million people are living with HIV. About 0.8% of adults aged 15-49 years are estimated to live with HIV around the world, although the prevalence varies remarkably from country to country and regions [24, 25].

CONFLICT OF INTEREST

The authors confirm that they have no conflict of interest to declare for this publication.

ACKNOWLEDGEMENTS

Declared none.

REFERENCES

[1]   Hahn BH, Shaw GM, De Cock KM, Sharp PM. AIDS as a zoonosis: Scientific and public health implications. Science 2000; 287(5453): 607-14.
        [http://dx.doi.org/10.1126/science.287.5453.607] [PMID: 10649986]

[2]   Aghokeng AF, Ayouba A, Mpoudi-Ngole E, *et al.* Extensive survey on the prevalence and genetic diversity of SIVs in primate bushmeat provides insights into risks for potential new cross-species transmissions. Infect Genet Evol 2010; 10(3): 386-96.
        [http://dx.doi.org/10.1016/j.meegid.2009.04.014] [PMID: 19393772]

[3]   Hemelaar J. The origin and diversity of the HIV-1 pandemic. Trends Mol Med 2012; 18(3): 182-92.
        [http://dx.doi.org/10.1016/j.molmed.2011.12.001] [PMID: 22240486]

[4]   Jetzt AE, Yu H, Klarmann GJ, Ron Y, Preston BD, Dougherty JP. High rate of recombination throughout the human immunodeficiency virus type 1 genome. J Virol 2000; 74(3): 1234-40.
        [http://dx.doi.org/10.1128/JVI.74.3.1234-1240.2000] [PMID: 10627533]

[5]   Mansky LM, Temin HM. Lower *in vivo* mutation rate of human immunodeficiency virus type 1 than that predicted from the fidelity of purified reverse transcriptase. J Virol 1995; 69(8): 5087-94.
        [PMID: 7541846]

[6]   Shankarappa R, Margolick JB, Gange SJ, *et al.* Consistent viral evolutionary changes associated with the progression of human immunodeficiency virus type 1 infection. J Virol 1999; 73(12): 10489-502. [PMID: 10559367]

[7]   Plantier JC, Leoz M, Dickerson JE, *et al.* A new human immunodeficiency virus derived from gorillas. Nat Med 2009; 15(8): 871-2. [http://dx.doi.org/10.1038/nm.2016] [PMID: 19648927]

[8]   Vallari A, Holzmayer V, Harris B, *et al.* Confirmation of putative HIV-1 group P in Cameroon. J Virol 2011; 85(3): 1403-7. [http://dx.doi.org/10.1128/JVI.02005-10] [PMID: 21084486]

[9]   Gao F, Bailes E, Robertson DL, *et al.* Origin of HIV-1 in the chimpanzee Pan troglodytes troglodytes. Nature 1999; 397(6718): 436-41. [http://dx.doi.org/10.1038/17130] [PMID: 9989410]

[10]   Keele BF, Van Heuverswyn F, Li Y, *et al.* Chimpanzee reservoirs of pandemic and nonpandemic HIV-1. Science 2006; 313(5786): 523-6. [http://dx.doi.org/10.1126/science.1126531] [PMID: 16728595]

[11]   Aldric C, Hemelaar J. Global HIV-1 diversity surveillance. Trends Mol Med 2012; 18(12): 691-4. [http://dx.doi.org/10.1126/science.1126531]

[12]   Rousseau CM, Learn GH, Bhattacharya T, *et al.* Extensive intrasubtype recombination in South African human immunodeficiency virus type 1 subtype C infections. J Virol 2007; 81(9): 4492-500. [http://dx.doi.org/10.1128/JVI.02050-06] [PMID: 17314156]

[13]   Yamaguchi J, Vallari AS, Swanson P, *et al.* Evaluation of HIV type 1 group O isolates: identification of five phylogenetic clusters. AIDS Res Hum Retroviruses 2002; 18(4): 269-82. [http://dx.doi.org/10.1089/088922202753472847] [PMID: 11860674]

[14]   Yamaguchi J, Bodelle P, Vallari AS, *et al.* HIV infections in northwestern Cameroon: identification of HIV type 1 group O and dual HIV type 1 group M and group O infections. AIDS Res Hum Retroviruses 2004; 20(9): 944-57. [http://dx.doi.org/10.1089/aid.2004.20.944] [PMID: 15585082]

[15]   Paul A. Human immunodeficiency viruses and their replication Chapter 60 in the fields virology of bernard N fields. New York: Lippincott-Raven Press 2006; Vol 2.

[16]   HIV sequence database. Available at: Available from: http://www.hiv.lanl.gov/components/sequence/ HIV/geo/ geo.comp. , 2015 [Accessed on: April 2015];

[17]   Kanki PJ, Travers KU, MBoup S, *et al.* Slower heterosexual spread of HIV-2 than HIV-1. Lancet 1994; 343(8903): 943-6. [http://dx.doi.org/10.1016/S0140-6736(94)90065-5] [PMID: 7909009]

[18]   Marlink R. Lessons from the second AIDS virus, HIV-2. AIDS 1996; 10(7): 689-99. [http://dx.doi.org/10.1097/00002030-199606001-00002] [PMID: 8805859]

[19]   Expert Group of the Joint United Nations Programme on HIV/AIDS. Implications of HIV variability for transmission: scientific and policy issues. AIDS 1997; 11(4): S1-S15. [PMID: 9084818]

[20]   Kiwanuka N, Laeyendecker O, Robb M, *et al.* Effect of human immunodeficiency virus Type 1 (HIV-1) subtype on disease progression in persons from Rakai, Uganda, with incident HIV-1 infection. J Infect Dis 2008; 197(5): 707-13.
[http://dx.doi.org/10.1086/527416] [PMID: 18266607]

[21]   Baeten JM, Chohan B, Lavreys L, *et al.* HIV-1 subtype D infection is associated with faster disease progression than subtype A in spite of similar plasma HIV-1 loads. J Infect Dis 2007; 195(8): 1177-80.
[http://dx.doi.org/10.1086/512682] [PMID: 17357054]

[22]   Conroy SA, Laeyendecker O, Redd AD, *et al.* Rakai Health Sciences Program. Changes in the distribution of HIV type 1 subtypes D and A in Rakai District, Uganda between 1994 and 2002. AIDS Res Hum Retroviruses 2010; 26(10): 1087-91.
[http://dx.doi.org/10.1089/aid.2010.0054] [PMID: 20925575]

[23]   Kosakovsky Pond SL, Smith DM. Are all subtypes created equal? The effectiveness of antiretroviral therapy against non-subtype B HIV-1. Clin Infect Dis 2009; 48(9): 1306-9.
[http://dx.doi.org/10.1086/598503] [PMID: 19331584]

[24]   UNAIDS. Available from: http://www.unaids.org/en/resources/documents/2014 Access Date: [June 2015]

[25]   De Cock KM, Jaffe HW, Curran JW. The evolving epidemiology of HIV/AIDS. AIDS 2012; 26(10): 1205-13.
[http://dx.doi.org/10.1097/QAD.0b013e328354622a] [PMID: 22706007]

CHAPTER 2

HIV Transmission

Behnam Farhoudi[*]

Islamic Azad University, Tehran Medical Sciences Branch, Iran

Abstract: The risk of HIV transmission varies widely by the type of exposure. Anal intercourse for both receptive and insertive partners has a higher risk *versus* vaginal intercourse, and vaginal intercourse is a higher risk act compared to oral intercourse. Also, receptive intercourse (both vaginal and anal) has an increased risk compared to insertive intercourse. Generally, the risk of HIV transmission for receptive anal intercourse, receptive vaginal intercourse and receptive oral intercourse is 0.5%, 0.1% and 0.01% per act, respectively. However, the risk varies widely depending on differences in factors such as co-occurrence with other sexually transmitted infections (STIs), level of viral load, stage of disease, and circumcision. Plasma viral load is considered as the strongest determinant of sexual transmission of HIV.

Higher rates of infection with HIV are exhibited among injection drug users mainly because of unsafe injecting behavior. The risk of HIV transmission per each drug injection is 0.67%.

Vertical transmission may occur during pregnancy by micro-transfusion of blood across the placenta; or during labor and delivery by the exposure of neonate with maternal blood and genital tract secretions, and after the birth through breastfeeding. It is estimated that 24-45% of HIV infected mothers transmit the virus to their offspring if there is no intervention. Maternal plasma viral load, co-infection with STIs, chorioamnionitis, concurrent HCV infection or active tuberculosis, and vaginal *versus* caesarean delivery are associated with the increased risk of vertical transmission. Contributing factors to mother to child transmission include breastfeeding pattern and duration, health status of maternal breast, and high plasma or breast milk viral load.

[*] **Correspondence to Behnam Farhoudi:** Islamic Azad University, Tehran Medical Sciences Branch, Shariati Street, Gholhak, Tehran, Iran; Tel/Fax:+98 (21) 22006660-7, E-mail: b_farhoudi@yahoo.com.

SeyedAhmad SeyedAlinaghi (Ed.)

Keywords: Anal intercourse, HIV exposure, HIV sexual transmission, HIV transmission, HIV viral load, Mother to child HIV transmission, Oral intercourse, People who Inject Drugs, Risk of HIV transmission, Route of HIV transmission, Sexually Transmitted Infections, Vaginal intercourse, Vertical transmission.

1. INTRODUCTION

The HIV transmission risk varies widely by the type of exposure. Worldwide, the most common route of HIV transmission is sexual followed by drug injection and mother to child transmission [1]. The possibility of HIV acquisition varies for each type of exposure. Table **1** lists the risk of transmission for different exposures.

Some parameters may increase or decrease the risk of transmission. For example, receiving antiretroviral treatment can reduce the risk of HIV transmission from People Living with HIV (PLWH) to another by as much as 96% [2]. The use of condoms lowers the risk of HIV acquisition or transmission by about 80% [3]. On the other hand, concurrent Sexually Transmitted Infection (STIs) or a high viral load (usually in early and late-stage infection) can enhance the risk of HIV transmission. In the following sections, each three main route of transmission is discussed in more details.

Table 1. Estimated transmission risk of HIV per-act of different exposure type* [4].

Exposure route	Risk per 10,000 exposures to an infected source
Blood transfusion	9,000
Needle-sharing injection-drug use	67
Receptive anal intercourse	50
Percutaneous needle stick	30
Receptive penile-vaginal intercourse	10
Insertive anal intercourse	6.5
Insertive penile-vaginal intercourse	5
Receptive oral intercourse	1
Insertive oral intercourse	0.5

*Sexual risk of HIV transmission is estimated without condom use.

Recently reported study indicate that estimates for both receptive and insertive anal intercourse are greater than those reported in Table **1** (increased 1.8 and 0.7-fold, respectively); however, the former estimates fall within the updated CIs for these exposures. In this study, the projected per-act HIV transmission risk (all expressed as per 10000 exposures) took the highest value for blood transfusion 9250 (95% CI 8900–9610), followed by mother-to-child transmission 2255 (95% CI 1000–2990), receptive anal intercourse 138 (95% CI 102–186), needle-sharing injection drug use 63 (95% CI 41–92), and percutaneous needle stick injuries 23 (95% CI 0–46). Risk for other sexual exposures were 4 (95% CI 1–14) for insertive penile–vaginal intercourse, 8 (95% CI 6–11) for receptive penile–vaginal intercourse, and 11 (95% CI 4–28) for insertive anal intercourse. The risk of transmission for receptive and insertive oral sex is pretty low (95% CI 0-4) [5].

2. SEXUAL TRANSMISSION OF HIV

In most countries, HIV epidemic is driven sexually [1]. To HIV transmission risk quantification by each type of sex remains challenging. Ideal estimations would be result from prospective studies in serodiscordant partners for whom all sex acts and their context were recorded. But estimates often derived on longitudinal or cross-sectional research with population-based HIV prevalence estimates. Recall bias can happen in these retrospective studies. For more suitable estimations, important variables are often ignored, such as the HIV status of all sexual partners. Furthermore, people do not often engaged in only one type of sex to abstain from other types of sexual contact with a partner [5]. So concerning these restrictions, the estimates should be understood carefully [5].

Nevertheless, all studies have consistently presented that anal intercourse is a higher risk act *versus* to vaginal intercourse, which is a higher risk compared to oral intercourse. On the other hand the associated risk with receptive intercourse (both vaginal and anal) is higher compared to insertive intercourse [6, 7]. It should be noted that these estimations mainly derived from studies implemented before the availability of active antiretroviral therapy (ART) [7]. So these studies estimate the risk of HIV transmission from an untreated PLWH with unsuppressed average viral load [8].

2.1. Anal Intercourse

Anal intercourse has a greater risk of HIV transmission for both receptive and insertive intercourse compared to vaginal intercourse. Indeed, the risk of HIV transmission is 5-18 times greater for receptive anal intercourse compared to receptive vaginal intercourse [9]. This is because of nature of rectal mucosa compared with vaginal mucosa. The higher concentration of lymphoid follicles in rectal mucosa and its more vulnerability to abrasions than vaginal mucosa may contribute to this increased transmissibility [10].

The results of cohort studies and meta-analyses suggest estimated risk of transmission from receptive anal intercourse from 0.5%-3.38% per-act [6]. Most of these estimates derived from studies among Men who have Sex with Men (MSM). Nevertheless, the risk involved in anal intercourse seems to be similar in heterosexual populations [6]. Risk estimations for insertive anal intercourse range between 0.06% and 0.16% per-act [8].

2.2. Vaginal Intercourse

The risk of HIV transmission from receptive vaginal intercourse has been estimated from 0.08% to 0.19% [8]. The risk estimates for insertive vaginal intercourse is somewhat lower, ranging from 0.05% to 0.1% [8].

Many studies have evaluated sexual transmission risks among heterosexual populations, without typifying the nature of the sex acts (*i.e.*, vaginal *versus* anal intercourse). Though, the majority of the sex acts were expected to be penile-vaginal. In two meta-analyses and a recent analysis of a large cohort study, the risk of sexual transmission among heterosexuals was reported as 1-2 cases per 1000 sex acts (or roughly 0.1%) [8, 11].

Rates for male-to-female sexual transmission is higher than those for female-to-male sexual transmission and it may be due to biological mechanisms, including larger anatomical surface and /or higher numbers of susceptible cell types in the vagina compared to the penis mucosa [12]. However, it is not clear whether serodiscordant women are at higher risk than men [12]. But this association may vary in high-income countries *versus* low-income ones. Female-to-male transmission estimates were about half the male-to-female transmission estimates, while in low-income countries the estimates for female-to-male and male-to-female were comparable [13].

2.3. Oral Intercourse

It is difficult to estimate the risk of HIV transmission through oral intercourse because many people do not engage in oral sex to the exclusion of other sex acts. Clearly, there is a considerably lower risk of transmission by oral intercourse (whether penile-oral or vaginal-oral) compared to anal or vaginal intercourse (see Table **1**). The oral cavity has a thick epithelial layer, a low number of CD4 target cells, and antiviral antibodies, all of them make it fairly resistant to HIV transmission [14]. However, if oral sex occurs with high frequency which is frequently unprotected, this action may lead to HIV transmission [15].

3. FACTORS AFFECTING SEXUAL TRANSMISSIBILITY OF HIV

As mentioned before, the risk estimates of HIV transmission following sexual exposure differ extensively [5, 8, 12], probably as a result of varied extent of biological co-factors such as co-infection with other sexually transmitted infections, viral load and stage of disease, and circumcision in study populations [13].

Wide range of studies underlined the role STIs in increasing the infectiousness of HIV-positive individuals and the susceptibility of HIV-negative individuals. Although, there is a multifaceted association between STIs and HIV, and the evidence is relatively inconsistent or difficult to interpret because of the existence of confounders. Various meta-analyses and systematic reviews have tried to evaluate these issues through investigations of only those studies using a temporal relationship, objective methods of detecting STIs, and accounting potential confounders (*e.g.*, sexual behavior). Regarding these reviews, STIs was found to increase predisposition to HIV by a factor of 2 to 4. This effect has been found for both men and women, specifically for herpes simplex virus type 2, syphilis, Gonorrhoea, Clamydia, Trichomonas, and exposure categorized as "any STI," "genital ulcer disease" and "non-ulcerative STIs" [16]. A study of 4295 MSM with a median follow-up of three years found an increased risk of HIV acquisition in association with HSV-2 infection [17]. HIV acquisition was accompanied with recent incident (Hazard Ratio HR 3.6, 95% Confidence Interval CI 1.7-7.8), remote incident (HR 1.7, 95% CI 0.8-3.3), and prevalent HSV-2 infection (HR 1.5, 95% CI 1.1-2.1) compared to HSV-2 seronegative individuals. A cross-sectional surveillance survey consisting of 3280 MSM in Peru revealed a robust association between HSV-2 seropositivity and HIV infection [18]. However, equivocal results were obtained from Randomized Controlled Trials (RCTs) evaluating the effect of STI treatment on HIV transmission risk [19, 20].

Plasma viral load is the strongest determinant of sexual transmission of HIV [21]. As research confirmed, there is a dose-response association where each 10-fold increase in plasma viral load increased relative risk of transmission of 2.5 to 2.9 per sexual contact [22].

Antiretroviral therapy considerably affects transmissibility of HIV infection. Reduction of infectious HIV-1 in blood and genital secretions through provision of ART is highly effective in reducing the risk HIV transmission [23]. The outcome of successful implementation of ART on reduced probability of HIV transmission was demonstrated by observational researches [24, 25]. There were no HIV transmission events in couples treated with Highly Active Antiretroviral Therapy (HAART) with a plasma viral load of less than 400 copies/ml [24]. In 11 of 13 such studies no HIV transmission observed when the infected partner was receiving ART [23]. Cases accompanied with transmission events despite ART, the HIV-infected partners were probable not consistently adherent to ART [23].

Regular administration of oral emtricitabine/ tenofovir disoproxil fumarate as pre exposure prophylaxis declines HIV-1 transmission rate among MSM [26]. This therapy was also effective among serodiscordant heterosexual couples [27], and heterosexual adults [28]. Daily oral tenofovir alone was also effective for pre exposure prophylaxis in heterosexual couples [27].

Well-designed clinical researches of serodiscordant couples showed the high effect of continued use of latex condoms against sexually HIV transmission. Meta-analyses suggest that regular use of condoms decreases the risk of HIV acquisition by approximately 80 to 95% [29, 30]. Among 13 cohort studies reviewed in one meta-analysis, there were only 11 seroconversions among 587 couples reporting constant use [29].

It seems that HIV prevention should be considered as combination of behavioral or biomedical intervention rather than just one of them [23]. A study suggested for couples using any single prevention strategy, a substantial cumulative risk of HIV transmission remained. For a male–female couple using only condoms, estimated risk over 10 years was 11%; for a male–male couple using only condoms, estimated risk was 76%. ART use by the HIV-infected partner was the most effective single strategy in reducing risk; among male–male couples, adding consistent condom use was essential to retain the 10-year risk below 10% [31].

Substantial significant evidence demonstrates that male circumcision lessens the risk of female-to-male sexual transmission. A Cochrane systematic study of the three trials obtained a reduced risk of 54% at 21 and 24 months after circumcision [32]. The effect of circumcision of male PLWH on transmission to women has been studied just by one RCT. This trial finished early due to uselessness (*i.e.*, the likelihood of finding a treatment effect was thought to be low): after 24 months, 18% of women in the intervention group and 12% of women in the control group acquired HIV, showing a statistically non-significant difference in the rates of transmission. This trial also pointed to a potential short-term increase in HIV transmission if sex is restarted before the surgical wound is entirely cured [33]. As mathematical models stated, women would take benefits indirectly from the scale up of male circumcision due to decreased HIV transmission between probable male partners [34]. Circumcision has no significant influence on HIV transmission among MSM [35].

The distribution of the different subtypes of HIV varies worldwide [36]. Different subtypes may have diverse biological properties, which could affect the transmission rate; however, there is no evidence to specify any impact of different subtypes on HIV transmission to date [36].

4. HIV TRANSMISSION AMONG PEOPLE WHO USE DRUGS

People who Inject Drugs (PWID) exhibit higher rates of infection with HIV and other blood-borne viruses, such as hepatitis C virus (HCV), because of unsafe injecting behavior [37]. Estimates found that 15.9 million (range 11.0–21.2 million) people might inject drugs worldwide; the largest numbers of injectors were found in China, USA and Russia, where mid estimates of HIV prevalence among injectors were 12%, 16%, and 37%, respectively. The prevalence of HIV among people injecting drugs was 20–40% in five countries and over 40% in nine countries. It is estimated that, worldwide, about 3.0 million (range 0•8–6•6 million) PWID might be HIV positive [37].

4.1. Risk per Drug Injection

Few researches have been directed to examine HIV transmission risk per injection with a contaminated needle and syringe [38]. Because of difficulties to precisely quantify the number of exposure and other risk factors, such as viral load, mathematical models have been used to indirectly estimate the likelihoods of such transmission. These models stated the probability of HIV transmission per injection from a contaminated needle and syringe to be 0.67% and 0.84% [39]. These studies do not consider the potential heterogeneity in transmission risk per injection, which relies on the infectiousness of the HIV-positive person who injects and the susceptibility of the uninfected person [39].So they may be misleading.

Sharing drug preparation equipments other than needles and syringes (*e.g.,* sharing water, cooker or filter) is involved with increased risk of HIV transmission. A study stated that 10 of the 83 PWID who sero-converted shared only cotton, cookers, or water, but not needles, during the risk period before conversion [40].

Kinds of drug mostly injected play a role in risky injecting practices. Cocaine in particular has been concomitant with binge drug use [41], which typically involves erratic behaviors, resulting in an increase in the possibility of unsafe injecting practices [42]. Cross-sectional studies revealed a relationship between injecting stimulants, cocaine or crack and increasingly risky practices [43, 44].

The transmission of HIV among people using drugs through non-injecting routes is the conclusion of sexual contact. Research shows a pervasive exchange of sex for drugs and drugs for sex in this group [45]. Moreover, it seems that high rates of HIV acquisition in individuals using non-injection drugs may be the relative product of the effects of "bridging" or mixing with PWID, because of overlapping social and sexual networks [45]. Due to significant probability of overlap between their drug and sexual networks, women are extremely at risk [45]. Crack smoking has been accompanied with an increase in the numbers of sex partners [46] and unprotected sex [47]. The risk of HIV acquisition is similarly associated with consuming amphetamines because they are often used to rise sexual pleasure and lower sexual inhibitions [48].

Pre exposure prophylaxis among injection drug users may decrease HIV transmission risk by 0.52 (95% CI: 0.28-0.90) [5].

5. MOTHER-TO-CHILD TRANSMISSION OF HIV

Vertical transmission can happen through three directions: during pregnancy by micro-transfusion of maternal blood cross ways the placenta; during labor and delivery through exposure with maternal blood and genital tract secretions; and after the birth through breastfeeding [49].

For non-breastfeeding populations, about 4% of transmissions occur during the first 14 weeks of pregnancy, 16% between 14 and 36 weeks of gestation, half in the days before delivery, and additional 30% during active labor and delivery [50]. As estimated, absence of any preventive intervention is associated with 15% to 30% risk of HIV transmission during gestation and delivery [49].

5.1. Factors Affecting Mother to Child HIV Transmission

Higher maternal plasma viral load has been considerably associated with the higher risk of vertical transmission [51]. Prospective cohort studies showed transmission rates increase as maternal plasma viral loads increase [52, 53]. In a Zimbabwe study of HIV-positive women, for every 10-fold increase in maternal plasma viral load, a two-fold increase was seen in the rate of vertical transmission [52].

The quantity of virus in the genital tract has also been shown to have an effect on the risk of mother-to-child transmission. An analysis of HIV-positive women with vaginal deliveries displayed that the existence of HIV in the genital tract was associated with a three-fold increase in the risk of vertical transmission, and for each 10-fold increase in the mean titer of HIV DNA there is nearly two-fold increase in the risk of vertical transmission [54].

The influence of maternal HIV-1 subtype on the risk of vertical transmission is uncertain [55]. Coexisting STIs show an increased risk of vertical transmission. Observational studies suggest that HSV-2, syphilis and gonorrhea, increase the risk of HIV vertical transmission [56].

Chorioamnionitis (bacterial infection of the fetal membranes and amniotic fluid), caused by ascending sexually transmitted or non-sexually transmitted bacterial infections, has been associated with four to eight-times elevated risk of vertical transmission [57]. Alternatively, no change in vertical transmission rates was seen between women treated for chorioamnionitis with antibiotics and women given a placebo [58].

Additionally, co-infection with either HCV or active tuberculosis is with an increase in the risk of HIV vertical transmission [56]. The mechanism for HCV infection may be through immunosuppression [56], while active tuberculosis may be involved because of high viral loads and placental inflammation [56].

As stated by the results of a RCT and a meta-analysis, the elective caesarean section (caesarean delivery before labor and before ruptured membranes) reduces the risk of vertical transmission by 50% to 80% [59]. Nevertheless, these researches often took place before the age of widespread ART usage. Prenatal ART substantially lowers the risk of HIV transmission; studies show no additional benefits to elective caesarean section for women with low viral loads, under ART.

In addition, mother-to-child HIV transmission follows breastfeeding. The likelihood of HIV acquisition through breastfeeding ranges from 9% to 16%. Co-conditions involved in risk of transmission from breastfeeding comprise duration and pattern of breastfeeding, maternal breast wellbeing, and high plasma or breast milk viral load.

CONFLICT OF INTEREST

The author confirms that author has no conflict of interest to declare for this

publication.

ACKNOWLEDGEMENTS

Declared none.

REFERENCES

[1]   Joint United Nations Programme on HIV/AIDS (UNAIDS). Global report: UNAIDS report on the global AIDS epidemic ds 2013.

[2]   Cohen MS, Chen YQ, McCauley M, *et al.* HPTN 052 Study Team. Prevention of HIV-1 infection with early antiretroviral therapy. N Engl J Med 2011; 365(6): 493-505.
[http://dx.doi.org/10.1056/NEJMoa1105243] [PMID: 21767103]

[3]   Weller SC, Davis-Beaty K. Condom effectiveness in reducing heterosexual HIV transmission (Review) The Cochrane Collaboration. New Jersey, USA: Wiley and Sons 2011.

[4]   Smith DK, Grohskopf LA, Black RJ, *et al.* U.S. Department of Health and Human Services. Antiretroviral postexposure prophylaxis after sexual, injection-drug use, or other nonoccupational exposure to HIV in the United States: recommendations from the U.S. Department of Health and Human Services. MMWR Recomm Rep 2005; 54(RR-2): 1-20.
[PMID: 15660015]

[5]   Lasry A, Sansom SL, Wolitski RJ, *et al.* HIV sexual transmission risk among serodiscordant couples: assessing the effects of combining prevention strategies. AIDS 2014; 28(10): 1521-9.
[http://dx.doi.org/10.1097/QAD.0000000000000307] [PMID: 24804859]

[6]   Baggaley RF, White RG, Boily MC. HIV transmission risk through anal intercourse: systematic review, meta-analysis and implications for HIV prevention. Int J Epidemiol 2010; 39(4): 1048-63.
[http://dx.doi.org/10.1093/ije/dyq057] [PMID: 20406794]

[7]   Varghese B, Maher JE, Peterman TA, Branson BM, Steketee RW. Reducing the risk of sexual HIV transmission: quantifying the per-act risk for HIV on the basis of choice of partner, sex act, and condom use. Sex Transm Dis 2002; 29(1): 38-43.
[http://dx.doi.org/10.1097/00007435-200201000-00007] [PMID: 11773877]

[8]   Fox J, White PJ, Weber J, Garnett GP, Ward H, Fidler S. Quantifying sexual exposure to HIV within an HIV-serodiscordant relationship: development of an algorithm. AIDS 2011; 25(8): 1065-82.
[http://dx.doi.org/10.1097/QAD.0b013e328344fe4a] [PMID: 21537113]

[9]   Grulich AE, Zablotska I. Commentary: probability of HIV transmission through anal intercourse. Int J Epidemiol 2010; 39(4): 1064-5.
[http://dx.doi.org/10.1093/ije/dyq101] [PMID: 20511336]

[10]   Bélec L, Dupré T, Prazuck T, *et al.* Cervicovaginal overproduction of specific IgG to human immunodeficiency virus (HIV) contrasts with normal or impaired IgA local response in HIV infection. J Infect Dis 1995; 172(3): 691-7.
[http://dx.doi.org/10.1093/infdis/172.3.691] [PMID: 7658060]

[11]   Powers KA, Poole C, Pettifor AE, Cohen MS. Rethinking the heterosexual infectivity of HIV-1: a

systematic review and meta-analysis. Lancet Infect Dis 2008; 8(9): 553-63.
[http://dx.doi.org/10.1016/S1473-3099(08)70156-7] [PMID: 18684670]

[12]   Fox J, Fidler S. Sexual transmission of HIV-1. Antiviral Res 2010; 85(1): 276-85.
       [http://dx.doi.org/10.1016/j.antiviral.2009.10.012] [PMID: 19874852]

[13]   Boily MC, Baggaley RF, Wang L, *et al.* Heterosexual risk of HIV-1 infection per sexual act:
       systematic review and meta-analysis of observational studies. Lancet Infect Dis 2009; 9(2): 118-29.
       [http://dx.doi.org/10.1016/S1473-3099(09)70021-0] [PMID: 19179227]

[14]   Campo J, Perea MA, del Romero J, Cano J, Hernando V, Bascones A. Oral transmission of HIV,
       reality or fiction? An update. Oral Dis 2006; 12(3): 219-28.
       [http://dx.doi.org/10.1111/j.1601-0825.2005.01187.x] [PMID: 16700731]

[15]   Baggaley RF, White RG, Boily MC. Systematic review of orogenital HIV-1 transmission probabilities.
       Int J Epidemiol 2008; 37(6): 1255-65.
       [http://dx.doi.org/10.1093/ije/dyn151] [PMID: 18664564]

[16]   Sexton J, Garnett G, Røttingen JA. Metaanalysis and metaregression in interpreting study variability in
       the impact of sexually transmitted diseases on susceptibility to HIV infection. Sex Transm Dis 2005;
       32(6): 351-7.
       [http://dx.doi.org/10.1097/01.olq.0000154504.54686.d1] [PMID: 15912081]

[17]   Brown EL, Wald A, Hughes JP, *et al.* High risk of human immunodeficiency virus in men who have
       sex with men with herpes simplex virus type 2 in the EXPLORE study. Am J Epidemiol 2006; 164(8):
       733-41.
       [http://dx.doi.org/10.1093/aje/kwj270] [PMID: 16896053]

[18]   Lama JR, Lucchetti A, Suarez L, *et al.* Peruvian HIV Sentinel Surveillance Working Group.
       Association of herpes simplex virus type 2 infection and syphilis with human immunodeficiency virus
       infection among men who have sex with men in Peru. J Infect Dis 2006; 194(10): 1459-66.
       [http://dx.doi.org/10.1086/508548] [PMID: 17054077]

[19]   Grosskurth H, Mosha F, Todd J, *et al.* Impact of improved treatment of sexually transmitted diseases
       on HIV infection in rural Tanzania: randomised controlled trial. Lancet 1995; 346(8974): 530-6.
       [http://dx.doi.org/10.1016/S0140-6736(95)91380-7] [PMID: 7658778]

[20]   Hayes R, Watson-Jones D, Celum C, van de Wijgert J, Wasserheit J. Treatment of sexually transmitted
       infections for HIV prevention: end of the road or new beginning? AIDS 2010; 24 (Suppl. 4): S15-26.
       [http://dx.doi.org/10.1097/01.aids.0000390704.35642.47] [PMID: 21042049]

[21]   Chan DJ. Factors affecting sexual transmission of HIV-1: current evidence and implications for
       prevention. Curr HIV Res 2005; 3(3): 223-41.
       [http://dx.doi.org/10.2174/1570162054368075] [PMID: 16022655]

[22]   Quinn TC, Wawer MJ, Sewankambo N, *et al.* Rakai Project Study Group. Viral load and heterosexual
       transmission of human immunodeficiency virus type 1. N Engl J Med 2000; 342(13): 921-9.
       [http://dx.doi.org/10.1056/NEJM200003303421303] [PMID: 10738050]

[23]   Marrazzo JM, del Rio C, Holtgrave DR, *et al.* International Antiviral Society-USA Panel. HIV
       prevention in clinical care settings: 2014 recommendations of the International Antiviral Society-USA
       Panel. JAMA 2014; 312(4): 390-409.

[http://dx.doi.org/10.1001/jama.2014.7999] [PMID: 25038358]

[24]   Attia S, Egger M, Müller M, Zwahlen M, Low N. Sexual transmission of HIV according to viral load and antiretroviral therapy: systematic review and meta-analysis. AIDS 2009; 23(11): 1397-404.
[http://dx.doi.org/10.1097/QAD.0b013e32832b7dca] [PMID: 19381076]

[25]   Donnell D, Baeten JM, Kiarie J, *et al*. Partners in Prevention HSV/HIV Transmission Study Team. Heterosexual HIV-1 transmission after initiation of antiretroviral therapy: a prospective cohort analysis. Lancet 2010; 375(9731): 2092-8.
[http://dx.doi.org/10.1016/S0140-6736(10)60705-2] [PMID: 20537376]

[26]   Grant RM, Lama JR, Anderson PL, *et al*. iPrEx Study Team. Preexposure chemoprophylaxis for HIV prevention in men who have sex with men. N Engl J Med 2010; 363(27): 2587-99.
[http://dx.doi.org/10.1056/NEJMoa1011205] [PMID: 21091279]

[27]   Baeten JM, Donnell D, Ndase P, *et al*. Partners PrEP Study Team. Antiretroviral prophylaxis for HIV prevention in heterosexual men and women. N Engl J Med 2012; 367(5): 399-410.
[http://dx.doi.org/10.1056/NEJMoa1108524] [PMID: 22784037]

[28]   Thigpen MC, Kebaabetswe PM, Paxton LA, *et al*. TDF2 Study Group. Antiretroviral preexposure prophylaxis for heterosexual HIV transmission in Botswana. N Engl J Med 2012; 367(5): 423-34.
[http://dx.doi.org/10.1056/NEJMoa1110711] [PMID: 22784038]

[29]   Weller S, Davis K. Condom effectiveness in reducing heterosexual HIV transmission. Cochrane Database Syst Rev 2001; (3): CD003255.
[PMID: 11687062]

[30]   Pinkerton SD, Abramson PR. Effectiveness of condoms in preventing HIV transmission. Soc Sci Med 1997; 44(9): 1303-12.
[http://dx.doi.org/10.1016/S0277-9536(96)00258-4] [PMID: 9141163]

[31]   Lasry A, Sansom SL, Wolitski RJ, *et al*. HIV sexual transmission risk among serodiscordant couples: assessing the effects of combining prevention strategies. AIDS 2014; 28(10): 1521-9.
[http://dx.doi.org/10.1097/QAD.0000000000000307] [PMID: 24804859]

[32]   Siegfried N, Muller M, Deeks JJ, Volmink J. Male circumcision for prevention of heterosexual acquisition of HIV in men. Cochrane Database Syst Rev 2009; (2): CD003362.
[PMID: 19370585]

[33]   Wawer MJ, Makumbi F, Kigozi G, *et al*. Circumcision in HIV-infected men and its effect on HIV transmission to female partners in Rakai, Uganda: a randomised controlled trial. Lancet 2009; 374(9685): 229-37.
[http://dx.doi.org/10.1016/S0140-6736(09)60998-3] [PMID: 19616720]

[34]   Hankins C, Hargrove J, Williams B, Abu-Raddad L, Auvert B, Bollinger L, *et al*. UNAIDS/WHO/SACEMA Expert Group on Modelling the Impact and Cost of Male Circumcision for HIV Prevention. Male circumcision for HIV prevention in high HIV prevalence settings: what can mathematical modelling contribute to informed decision making? PLoS Med 2009; 6(9): e1000109.
[http://dx.doi.org/10.1371/journal.pmed.1000109] [PMID: 19901974]

[35]   Wiysonge CS, Kongnyuy EJ, Shey M, *et al*. Male circumcision for prevention of homosexual acquisition of HIV in men. Cochrane Database Syst Rev 2011; (6): CD007496.

[PMID: 21678366]

[36] Hemelaar J, Gouws E, Ghys PD, Osmanov S. Global and regional distribution of HIV-1 genetic subtypes and recombinants in 2004. AIDS 2006; 20(16): W13-23.
[http://dx.doi.org/10.1097/01.aids.0000247564.73009.bc] [PMID: 17053344]

[37] Mathers BM, Degenhardt L, Phillips B, *et al.* 2007 Reference Group to the UN on HIV and Injecting Drug Use. Global epidemiology of injecting drug use and HIV among people who inject drugs: a systematic review. Lancet 2008; 372(9651): 1733-45.
[http://dx.doi.org/10.1016/S0140-6736(08)61311-2] [PMID: 18817968]

[38] Baggaley RF, Boily MC, White RG, Alary M. Risk of HIV-1 transmission for parenteral exposure and blood transfusion: a systematic review and meta-analysis. AIDS 2006; 20(6): 805-12.
[http://dx.doi.org/10.1097/01.aids.0000218543.46963.6d] [PMID: 16549963]

[39] Hudgens MG, Longini IM Jr, Halloran ME, Choopanya K, Vanichseni S, Kitayaporn D, *et al.* Estimating the transmission probability of human immunodeficiency virus in injecting drug users in Thailand. Appl Stat 2001; 50(1): 1-14.
[http://dx.doi.org/10.1111/1467-9876.00216]

[40] Lee R. Occupational transmission of bloodborne diseases to healthcare workers in developing countries: meeting the challenges. J Hosp Infect 2009; 72(4): 285-91.
[http://dx.doi.org/10.1016/j.jhin.2009.03.016] [PMID: 19443081]

[41] Miller CL, Kerr T, Frankish JC, *et al.* Binge drug use independently predicts HIV seroconversion among injection drug users: implications for public health strategies. Subst Use Misuse 2006; 41(2): 199-210.
[http://dx.doi.org/10.1080/10826080500391795] [PMID: 16393742]

[42] Bourgois P, Bruneau J. Needle exchange, HIV infection, and the politics of science: Confronting Canada's cocaine injection epidemic with participant observation. Med Anthropol 2000; 18(4): 325-50.
[http://dx.doi.org/10.1080/01459740.2000.9966161]

[43] Booth RE, Lehman WE, Kwiatkowski CF, Brewster JT, Sinitsyna L, Dvoryak S. Stimulant injectors in Ukraine: the next wave of the epidemic? AIDS Behav 2008; 12(4): 652-61.
[http://dx.doi.org/10.1007/s10461-008-9359-3] [PMID: 18264752]

[44] Buchanan D, Tooze JA, Shaw S, Kinzly M, Heimer R, Singer M. Demographic, HIV risk behavior, and health status characteristics of "crack" cocaine injectors compared to other injection drug users in three New England cities. Drug Alcohol Depend 2006; 81(3): 221-9.
[http://dx.doi.org/10.1016/j.drugalcdep.2005.07.011] [PMID: 16171952]

[45] Strathdee SA, Stockman JK. Epidemiology of HIV among injecting and non-injecting drug users: current trends and implications for interventions. Curr HIV/AIDS Rep 2010; 7(2): 99-106.
[http://dx.doi.org/10.1007/s11904-010-0043-7] [PMID: 20425564]

[46] Longshore D, Anglin MD. Number of sex partners and crack cocaine use: Is crack an independent marker for HIV risk behavior? J Drug Issues 1995; 25(1): 1-10.
[http://dx.doi.org/10.1177/002204269502500101]

[47] Kwiatkowski CF, Booth RE. HIV-seropositive drug users and unprotected sex. AIDS Behav 1998;

2(2): 151-9.
[http://dx.doi.org/10.1023/A:1022198930699]

[48] Colfax G, Santos GM, Chu P, *et al.* Amphetamine-group substances and HIV. Lancet 2010; 376(9739): 458-74.
[http://dx.doi.org/10.1016/S0140-6736(10)60753-2] [PMID: 20650520]

[49] Lehman DA, Farquhar C. Biological mechanisms of vertical human immunodeficiency virus (HIV-1) transmission. Rev Med Virol 2007; 17(6): 381-403.
[http://dx.doi.org/10.1002/rmv.543] [PMID: 17542053]

[50] Kourtis AP, Bulterys M, Nesheim SR, Lee FK. Understanding the timing of HIV transmission from mother to infant. JAMA 2001; 285(6): 709-12.
[http://dx.doi.org/10.1001/jama.285.6.709] [PMID: 11176886]

[51] John GC, Kreiss J. Mother-to-child transmission of human immunodeficiency virus type 1. Epidemiol Rev 1996; 18(2): 149-57.
[http://dx.doi.org/10.1093/oxfordjournals.epirev.a017922] [PMID: 9021309]

[52] Katzenstein DA, Mbizvo M, Zijenah L, *et al.* Serum level of maternal human immunodeficiency virus (HIV) RNA, infant mortality, and vertical transmission of HIV in Zimbabwe. J Infect Dis 1999; 179(6): 1382-7.
[http://dx.doi.org/10.1086/314767] [PMID: 10228058]

[53] Warszawski J, Tubiana R, Le Chenadec J, *et al.* ANRS French Perinatal Cohort. Mother-to-child HIV transmission despite antiretroviral therapy in the ANRS French Perinatal Cohort. AIDS 2008; 22(2): 289-99.
[http://dx.doi.org/10.1097/QAD.0b013e3282f3d63c] [PMID: 18097232]

[54] Tuomala RE, O'Driscoll PT, Bremer JW, *et al.* Women and Infants Transmission Study. Cell-associated genital tract virus and vertical transmission of human immunodeficiency virus type 1 in antiretroviral-experienced women. J Infect Dis 2003; 187(3): 375-84.
[http://dx.doi.org/10.1086/367706] [PMID: 12552421]

[55] Hu DJ, Buvé A, Baggs J, van der Groen G, Dondero TJ. What role does HIV-1 subtype play in transmission and pathogenesis? An epidemiological perspective. AIDS 1999; 13(8): 873-81.
[http://dx.doi.org/10.1097/00002030-199905280-00002] [PMID: 10475680]

[56] Ellington SR, King CC, Kourtis AP. Host factors that influence mother-to-child transmission of HIV-1: Genetics, coinfections, behavior and nutrition. Future Virol 2011; 6(12): 1451-69.
[http://dx.doi.org/10.2217/fvl.11.119]

[57] Chi BH, Mudenda V, Levy J, Sinkala M, Goldenberg RL, Stringer JS. Acute and chronic chorioamnionitis and the risk of perinatal human immunodeficiency virus-1 transmission. Am J Obstet Gynecol 2006; 194(1): 174-81.
[http://dx.doi.org/10.1016/j.ajog.2005.06.081] [PMID: 16389028]

[58] Taha TE, Brown ER, Hoffman IF, *et al.* A phase III clinical trial of antibiotics to reduce chorioamnionitis-related perinatal HIV-1 transmission. AIDS 2006; 20(9): 1313-21.
[http://dx.doi.org/10.1097/01.aids.0000232240.05545.08] [PMID: 16816561]

[59] Dunn DT, Newell ML, Mayaux MJ, *et al.* Perinatal AIDS Collaborative Transmission Studies. Mode

of delivery and vertical transmission of HIV-1: a review of prospective studies. J Acquir Immune Defic Syndr 1994; 7(10): 1064-6.
[PMID: 8083824]

CHAPTER 3

Mother-to-Child Transmission of HIV Infection: Timing, Risk Factors and Strategies for Prevention

Kenneth McIntosh[*]

Harvard Medical School, Harvard School of Public Health Emeritus Chief, Infectious Diseases Division, Boston Children's Hospital, USA

Abstract: Mother-to-child transmission of human immunodeficiency virus type 1 (HIV) occurs during gestation, during delivery, and during breast feeding. In an unprotected mother-child pair, transmission over-all occurs in 30-40%, with about one quarter of these transmissions *in utero*, one half during delivery, and one quarter during breast feeding. Most *in utero* transmission occurs in the third trimester. There are many risk factors for transmission, but the most important are the maternal viral load and the maternal CD4 concentration. Antiretroviral treatment of the mother has a potent preventive effect but must be administered throughout the risk period (that is, from early second trimester through the end of breast feeding). For *in utero* and intrapartum transmission, treatment probably acts through two mechanisms, namely pre-exposure prophylaxis in the fetus or newborn, and reduction in maternal viral load. Adequate voluntary counseling and testing for HIV and access to antiretroviral drugs are now critical preventive issues in this important mode of transmission.

Keywords: Antiretroviral therapy, Breast feeding, CD4 concentration, Delivery, HIV, Mother-to-child transmission, Pregnancy, Viral load.

1. INTRODUCTION

The realization that an acquired immunodeficiency might be passed from mother to child during pregnancy or at delivery came before the word AIDS had been

---

[*] **Correspondence to Kenneth McIntosh:** Harvard Medical School, Division of Infectious Diseases, BCH3104, Boston Children's Hospital, 300 Longwood Ave., Boston, MA 02115, Enders Rm 861.3, USA; Tel: 617-919-2900; Fax: 617-730-0255; E-mail: kenneth.mcintosh@childrens.harvard.edu.

SeyedAhmad SeyedAlinaghi (Ed.)

coined, and before HIV had been discovered. In the early 1980's, in San Francisco, Newark, New York and Miami, pediatricians recognized infants were being born to women who used intravenous drugs (who by that time were known to be at risk of the newly described immunodeficiency then afflicting gays and drug users) or were the spouses of high-risk Haitian men, and that these infants were themselves developing a rapid-onset immunodeficiency, with severe opportunistic infections such as toxoplasmosis, pneumonia due to *Pneumocystis jirovecii* and refractory candidiasis, followed by premature death [1 - 4].

After HIV was discovered, the tests for antibody to it were made available, and methods were developed to grow it in culture, detect p24 in serum, and, finally, amplify its pro-viral or cDNA through Polymerase Chain Reaction (PCR). The picture of mother-to-child transmission of HIV was considerably clarified. It is the purpose of this chapter to review the information that has led us to our current concepts of mother-to-child transmission of HIV and the logic of our attempts to prevent it.

2. THE TIMING AND RISKS OF MOTHER-TO-CHILD HIV TRANSMISSION

2.1. HIV Transmission *In Utero*

Some of the earliest information on the timing of HIV transmission emerged from virologic studies of a second trimester abortus from a HIV-infected woman [5, 6]. Further studies from Baylor University in Houston indicated that pathologic examination of the products of conception from HIV-infected women who spontaneously aborted revealed widespread destruction of lymphoid tissue [7]. In this intriguing study, the products of conception from 14 pregnancies in HIV-infected women who spontaneously aborted throughout pregnancy (most in the 2nd or early 3rd trimester) were carefully examined. Seven of the 14 abortuses were HIV-infected with widespread destruction of the lymphatic system, indicating that the virus could be passed on to the fetus with lethal consequences in or before the 2nd trimester. Two early reports of induced abortions indicated frequent PCR positivity in fetal tissues obtained at 11-24 weeks' gestation [8, 9]. One study of 24 abortuses (one set of twins) timed from 11-24 weeks of gestation indicated that

30% had HIV nucleic acid detectable by PCR of various tissues (brain, liver, or lung), but only the one set of twins were positive by *in situ* hybridization [9]. No clinical information was presented in this publication (*i.e.* CD4 count, maternal clinical stage, maternal viral load). The other study found PCR positivity in all nine fetuses examined, but cultures and p24 assays were negative in all [8]. In this study all but a few mothers were asymptomatic at the time of the abortions. The PCR positivity rate in both studies is not compatible with subsequent information about the rate of *in utero* transmission in live-born infants (see below), so it seems likely that some contamination with maternal blood (despite attempts to avoid this) occurred, or that, for some other reason, PCR was picking up signals that did not indicate active infection of the fetus. Self-cure of the fetus cannot of course be ruled out but seems unlikely.

One important historical step in determining the timing and quantitative risk of vertical HIV transmission stemmed from the realization that the "sensitivity" of HIV culture and PCR in detecting the virus in infant blood was relatively low in samples obtained at birth in relation to samples taken at later times during the first year of life [10]. This observation was translated into a consensus definition of *in utero* infection (HIV culture or PCR positive in peripheral blood obtained at birth or within the first 48 hours) and intrapartum, or perinatal, infection (HIV culture or PCR negative on peripheral blood obtained during the first week of life, but positive later in a non-breast-fed infant) that became widely accepted [11]. Many studies from the U.S., Europe, Asia, and Africa then confirmed that the risk of infection *in utero* (without any intervention) was between 6 and 10%, and the risk of infection perinatally was about double that figure [12].

Quantitative information on the risk of infection during the various months of gestation has been, however, more difficult to determine. For example, the risk during the first trimester is unknown. The risk during the combined first and second trimesters, with survival of the fetus, is probably quite low, in the range of 1-2% or less. There is some information on this figure obtained from the trial of Lallemant and colleagues in Thailand that investigated the comparative efficacy of long maternal zidovudine (beginning at 28 weeks' gestation) *vs.* short (beginning at 36 weeks) [13]. Infection detectable in peripheral newborn blood at birth in those whose mothers received ZDV beginning at 28 weeks' gestation was

1.6%. Since protection of fetal infection through ZDV maternal prophylaxis is unlikely to be complete, and since "cure" of fetal HIV infection would appear unlikely with ZDV alone, the transmission rate before 28 weeks in this population was probably somewhat less than this figure.

In the third trimester there is more information, both conjectural and more direct. In the early 1990's French investigators, examining the evolution of neonatal and maternal band patterns on Western blots showing antibody to HIV peptides, deduced that most babies infected *in utero* were infected late in the third trimester, with the risk rising as term approached [14]. These indirect estimates were refined by the randomized, double-blind clinical trial conducted by Lallemant and colleagues mentioned in the previous paragraph [13]. This study showed a highly significant difference in PCR positivity at birth between the offspring of those mothers randomized to receive zidovudine for the entire third trimester (point estimate 1.6%) in comparison to those randomized to receive zidovudine only for the final month (point estimate 5.1%) ($P<0.001$). The implication of this trial was that some transmissions occurred in the first two months of the third trimester, and the proportion of all births where transmission occurred in this interval was 5.1 minus 1.6, or 3.5%. There was no group in this trial that received no zidovudine during pregnancy, and thus we have no information to estimate the risk of transmission during the final month of the third trimester, but it seems likely that it is about 3-5% (depending on other risk factors for transmission).

2.2. HIV Transmission During Delivery

Analogy to some other viruses such as herpes simplex and hepatitis B virus made the possibility of risk during the process of birth a significant one. Micro-transfusions from mother to infant occurring during labor are considered to be a major source of hepatitis B perinatal transmission [15]. As data emerged from studies of HIV transmission, it became clear that delivery was a time of high risk. One of the first pieces of published evidence for this was a paper summarizing the higher infection risk of the first-born twin [16]. Further studies of risk factors associated with transmission during delivery clarified the impression that it was critically important to concentrate prevention efforts on this brief interval [17].

2.3. HIV Transmission During Breast Feeding

The first direct evidence of transmission during breast feeding came from an unexpected quarter: a case report of a mother who, in 1965 before the availability of the HIV antibody test in blood donors, received an HIV-infected blood transfusion shortly after a Caesarean section birth, then breast-fed her baby for six weeks. It was discovered some months later that both she and her baby were HIV-infected, the baby presumably through the breast milk [18]. This was followed by reports of HIV in breast milk and then prospective surveys from Africa, where breast feeding was considered essential in spite of the risk of HIV transmission, showing a transmission risk of about 0.8% per month of breast feeding [19]. This risk was also found to be modulated by the pattern of breast feeding: infants who exclusively breast-fed, considered nutritionally desirable at least until 6 months of age, ran a lower risk of HIV transmission than those who ingested both breast milk and other liquids or solids. This finding, found accidentally at first, was subsequently confirmed by prospective studies [20].

3. RISK FACTORS FOR HIV TRANSMISSION FROM MOTHER TO CHILD

It stands to reason that the risk factors for mother-to-child transmission of HIV would differ, at least in part, in the three major periods of transmission – during gestation, during delivery, and during breast feeding. This has, in fact, turned out in part to be the case. Two major maternal risk factors appear to apply to all transmission periods: maternal viral load and maternal CD4 concentration. These two appear as independent risk factors in almost every study that has been done. Viral load seems intuitively obvious on a statistical basis, since higher concentrations of infectious virus (particularly concentrations that are higher by logarithmically larger factors such as 1000, 10,000, or 100,000 and more) seem more likely to penetrate natural barriers to transmission. The defensive role of maternal CD4 cells is not so obvious, although it implies that at least some of the natural barriers lie in the ability of the maternal immune system to control infected cells and cell-free virus and keep them on the maternal side of whatever physical barriers there are. Maternal disease stage, closely related to CD4 concentration, has also been a strong correlate of transmission.

There are also several risk factors whose relationship to particular phases of the exposure risk (*in utero*, peripartum, breast feeding), for various reasons, simply cannot be resolved. One of the most important of these is low birth weight/prematurity. While these two should be separable, often they are not since they co-vary in many infants. All these variables will be discussed after a presentation of those where the timing is clear.

3.1. Risk Factors for *In Utero* Transmission

Several risk factors for intrauterine transmission involve the placenta. The actual mechanism by which HIV crosses the placenta into the fetal circulation has not been elucidated, but a recent study analyzed plasma separated from blood taken at birth from an incision of the basal plate of the placenta. The placentas were from HIV-infected mothers who transmitted during gestation, at delivery, or not at all and gave birth in Malawi from 2000 to 2004 when antiretrovirals were not available. They measured the levels of 27 cytokines, chemokines, and growth factors and correlated the differences in levels in the three groups using multivariate models. The one factor that correlated strongly and independently with *in utero* HIVtransmission was CXCL10, or interferon-gamma induced protein 10 (IP10), a substance that is also correlated with higher production of infectious HIV [21]. Interestingly, efforts to reduce placental inflammation by administering antibiotics aimed at treating chorioamnionitis have failed, although this negative outcome fails to shed much light on this subject [22].

Other risk factors for *in utero* transmission of HIV (in addition to HIV RNA concentration and CD4 cell level) are maternal use of "hard drugs," maternal infection with HIV in subtype C, coincident congenital cytomegalovirus (CMV) infection and, possibly, placental malaria. Although there has been some disagreement on this issue, the most detailed study of hard drug use and HIV mother-to-child transmission, performed in the U.S. Women and Infants Transmission Study (WITS) population, showed a very clear risk of HIV transmission [23]. Placental malaria has been widely studied, but its correlation with HIV mother-to-child transmission is controversial [24].

Renjifo and colleagues, examining pregnant women in Tanzania where multiple subgroups of HIV circulate, typed isolates from 253 infected infants using the envelope sequences, and found that the ratio of *in utero* infection to intrapartum infection was significantly higher in those babies infected with subtype C than either subtype A or subtype D. This was true both before and after adjusting for other risk factors such as viral load and CD4 count [24].

Khamduang and colleagues in Chiang Mai, Thailand performed a case-control study of women participating in an early protocol of long *versus* short zidovudine for prevention of mother-to-child HIV transmission [25]. They found that congenital, that is *in utero*, CMV infection was common in those infants who were HIV-infected (14%, *versus* 3% in infants who were not HIV-infected, similar to data from several previous studies), and that it was highly correlated with *in utero* HIV infection (Odds Ratio 8.1, *P*=0.01), whereas intrapartum CMV infection was not.

3.2. Risk Factors for Peripartum Transmission

Several risk factors have been identified that increase the probability of HIV transmission during delivery. One of the earliest risk factors that were described related to birth order. Analysis of a large collection of twin births indicated that the first twin has a greater chance of infection than the second [16]. Rupture of membranes for more than four hours has been found in several studies to be a major risk factor, with the most compelling data again from the WITS population [26]. This fact, plus the suspicion that microtransfusions were occurring during labor, led to the concept that elective, pre-labor Cesarean section would evade peripartum transmission. A large meta-analysis also came to this conclusion [27] and it was essentially proven in a randomized trial conducted in Europe that showed a very low transmission rate in mothers who were receiving zidovudine and also underwent elective C-section in relation to those receiving zidovudine alone [28].

It has been suspected for many years that ulcerative genital disease would predispose to intrapartum mother-to-child transmission of HIV. Although chancroid is common in some parts of the world where HIV rates are also high, neither it nor active maternal syphilis has been statistically associated with HIV transmission. On the other hand, genital herpes simplex virus infection has, although the correlation was found with prevalent, rather than incident herpes virus type 2 (HSV-2) infection [29]. Interestingly, treatment of mothers with valacyclovir during pregnancy and breast feeding has been shown to reduce the titer of HIV in maternal plasma and also breast milk, implying that HSV-2 co-infection with HIV somehow raises the titer of the latter, perhaps leading then to increased transmission [30].

Common sense would indicate that infant skin breaks and maternal bleeding during delivery would be risk factors for transmission as well, and current recommendations include the avoidance of scalp electrodes and other invasive infant monitoring, as well as guidelines for cesarean section when maternal viral loads are over 1000 copies/ml at term [31].

3.3. Risk Factors during Breast Feeding

The major risk factors for breast milk transmission are the amount of virus in breast milk and the length of time the child breast-feeds. Maternal CD4 count is also related, as is maternal plasma viral load. The level of breast milk virus, which is closely related to plasma virus, has been divided into cell-free and cell-associated virus. Cell-associated virus is associated with transmission throughout the period of breast-feeding, whereas cell-free virus is associated with transmission after about nine months of age [32].

Besides viral load and mixed feeding, the major risk factor for transmission during breast feeding appears to be mastitis, either clinically apparent [33, 34] or subclinical [35]. Breast feeding during weaning has also been associated with transmission, and an investigation of virus in breast milk during weaning revealed that concentrations are considerably higher during and after weaning [36]. The same study showed that virus concentrations were high during intermittent breast feeding, perhaps helping to explain the apparent protective effect of exclusive breast feeding.

Several early studies of vitamin A levels in HIV-infected mothers indicated that those with low measured levels had a higher risk of mother-to-child transmission than those with normal levels [37]. These studies, not all of which showed this correlation, stimulated the construction and performance of a large randomized trial of vitamin supplementation for pregnant women who planned to breast-feed their infants in Tanzania. The major result of this study was the conclusion that vitamin A/beta carotene supplementation increased HIV transmission, and that this increase occurred during breast feeding (not during pregnancy and delivery) [38]. The likely mechanism by which this occurred was considered to be an increase in the breast milk viral load of women receiving the supplementation [39]. Interestingly, in this trial, multivitamins that did not contain vitamin A/beta carotene had no effect on HIV transmission.

3.4. Risk Factors That Have Not Been Assigned to a Particular Time of Transmission

There is one important risk factor that may be related to infection during gestation, or may be related to infection at delivery, and that may be either a cause or an effect (or both) of HIV infection: this is prematurity, and its closely linked partner, low birth weight. There are many unknowns here. Most studies of risk factors find one or the other linked to HIV infection. There are data that cite low birth weight as a risk factor for *in utero* transmission, distinguishing this from prematurity, which was associated with both *in utero* and intrapartum transmission [23]. Another study found prematurity associated only with intrapartum, and not with *in utero* transmission [40]. Many studies find the two so closely linked that they cannot be separated [25].

A number of other risk factors have simply not been studied with sufficient detail to know just what stage they function at. One such risk factor is infant Class I HLA homozygosity. In a large study in Nairobi, Kenya, Macdonald and colleagues found a quantitative association between "perinatal" transmission and the number of Class I HLA haplo-identities between mother and infant [41]. Sadly, there was no differentiation between *in utero* and intrapartum transmission in this study, but breast feeding transmission (which was common) was not correlated with HLA homozygosity. The most attractive theory for the mechanism of this kind of susceptibility/protection involves rejection of *vs.* tolerance to maternal cells that cross the placenta during labor and delivery, but this is theory has not been supported by studies that allow more precise timing of transmission.

Class I HLA types have been associated with disease progression, and maternal (but not infant) HLA types have also been associated with mother-to-child transmission, independent of maternal viral load. Maternal HLA A*2301 has been associated with transmission in a Kenyan cohort [42]. In a U.S. cohort, various maternal HLA-B alleles have been associated with increased transmission (B*3501, B*3503, B*1302, B*4402, and B*5001) or decreased transmission (B*4901 and B*5301) [43]. None of these B alleles have been associated with either slow or rapid disease progression. These associations were also independent of maternal viral load. The association of Class I HLA alleles with mother-to-child transmission independent of viral load implies mechanisms related to both the maternal adaptive and innate immune systems, but the mechanism is otherwise not clear [43]. The other genetic factor that has been studied is maternal and infant CCR5 polymorphisms. Interestingly, maternal or infant heterozygosity for CCR5 Delta 32 has never been shown to correlate with lower mother-to-child transmission of HIV, despite many efforts to show this [44].

Several other infectious diseases have been associated with HIV mother-to-child-transmission. Maternal tuberculosis was found to be associated with transmission after correcting for other risk factors, although this association was not strong (odds ratio 2.5, 95%CL 1.05-6.02, $P=0.04$) [45]. Likewise, maternal hepatitis C infection has been associated with a high rate of transmission, although correcting for hard drug use in this population almost rendered the HCV association no longer significant [46]. Epstein-Barr Virus (EBV) shedding in the saliva has been also correlated with transmission, and this correlation appears to be independent of CD4 percentage. However, the correlation was not strong (univariate $P=0.06$, multivariate $P=0.04$) [47].

4. THE IMPORTANCE OF ANTIVIRAL TREATMENT IN MOTHER-TO-CHILD TRANSMISSION OF HIV

Following completion of the landmark study of zidovudine to prevent mother-to-child transmission, ACTG-076, it became clear that maternal antiretroviral (ARV) use could enormously diminish the risk of maternal transmission of HIV [48]. As ARVs became more and more potent and as physicians learned how to combine ARVs to maximally suppress circulating virus and prevent the development of resistance, it became clear that access to ARVs and adherence to ARV treatment would have an enormous impact on the percentage of infants infected through mother-to-child transmission [49]. Antiviral drugs work in this context in two quite different ways: in the 076 trial it was clear that the major preventive effect was not through a reduction in maternal viral load, but rather through some other mechanism [50]. This mechanism is most likely true fetal pre-exposure prophylaxis, mediated through the high levels of zidovudine that crossed the placenta, entered the fetal circulation and then were converted to active drug intracellularly. All ARVs that cross the placenta readily probably have, to a greater or lesser extent, this mechanism of action. Drugs, such as most protease inhibitors, that do not cross the placenta readily, act primarily through the other mechanism, namely reduction in maternal viral load, and drugs that both reduce viral load effectively and cross the placenta in an active form probably work through both mechanisms.

Prevention to rates of 2% or less was achieved through the former mechanism in a trial in a non-breastfeeding population in Thailand that combined zidovudine mono-therapy starting at the beginning of the third trimester with single-dose nevirapine (which also crosses the placenta readily) administered during labor and in a single dose to the infant [51]. Likewise, pre-exposure prophylaxis during breast-feeding, consisting of daily nevirapine to the uninfected infant, was shown to protect the infant with great efficiency in a trial in Malawi [52]. Triple therapy ("combination antiretroviral therapy", or CART) started at the beginning of the third trimester and continuing throughout breast feeding was shown, in a trial in Botswana, to result in transmission rates around 1% over-all, demonstrating that this approach would effectively cover all phases of the birth process [53]. The large, randomized PROMISE study, performed in pregnant women with CD4 counts over 350 and completed in 2015, showed that maternal protease-based combination therapy yielded a lower transmission rate (0.6%) than zidovudine-based therapy with single-dose nevirapine (1.8%), but with a higher incidence of prematurity (20.5% *vs.* 13.1%) [54]. Current guidelines from WHO recognize that antiretroviral treatment must begin before transmission has occurred, and thus, for its fullest effect, must start either before pregnancy or at least around 14 weeks of gestation, toward the beginning of the 2nd trimester. Starting later than this leaves open the possibility of earlier (and incurable) transmission and does not result in full prevention.

Now we are in a phase of the HIV epidemic when lack of access to antiretroviral treatment during pregnancy and breast feeding has become the largest risk factor for mother-to-child transmission. All aspects of this issue are important, and all pose their own particular challenges: reaching women before or in the first trimester of pregnancy to allow the possibility of counseling and testing for HIV antibody; persuading women to return for the results of these tests and counseling them on proper infection control; consistent and dependable access to appropriate ARV drugs; availability of the necessary toxicity, viral load, CD4, and clinical monitoring; and working with the inevitable burden of stigma accompanying a positive diagnosis of HIV infection. All of these are important, and all are barriers to the 100% prevention that we should strive to achieve.

CONFLICT OF INTEREST

The author confirms that author has no conflict of interest to declare for this publication.

ACKNOWLEDGEMENTS

Declared none.

REFERENCES

[1]   Ammann AJ, Cowan MJ, Wara DW, *et al.* Acquired immunodeficiency in an infant: possible transmission by means of blood products. Lancet 1983; 1(8331): 956-8.
[http://dx.doi.org/10.1016/S0140-6736(83)92082-2] [PMID: 6132270]

[2]   Oleske J, Minnefor A, Cooper R Jr, *et al.* Immune deficiency syndrome in children. JAMA 1983; 249(17): 2345-9.
[http://dx.doi.org/10.1001/jama.1983.03330410031024] [PMID: 6834633]

[3]   Rubinstein A, Sicklick M, Gupta A, *et al.* Acquired immunodeficiency with reversed T4/T8 ratios in infants born to promiscuous and drug-addicted mothers. JAMA 1983; 249(17): 2350-6.
[http://dx.doi.org/10.1001/jama.1983.03330410036025] [PMID: 6220166]

[4]   Scott GB, Buck BE, Leterman JG, Bloom FL, Parks WP. Acquired immunodeficiency syndrome in infants. N Engl J Med 1984; 310(2): 76-81.
[http://dx.doi.org/10.1056/NEJM198401123100202] [PMID: 6606781]

[5]   Lyman WD, Kress Y, Kure K, Rashbaum WK, Rubinstein A, Soeiro R. Detection of HIV in fetal central nervous system tissue. AIDS 1990; 4(9): 917-20.

[http://dx.doi.org/10.1097/00002030-199009000-00014] [PMID: 2252565]

[6]   Sprecher S, Soumenkoff G, Puissant F, Degueldre M. Vertical transmission of HIV in 15-week fetus. Lancet 1986; 2(8501): 288-9.
       [http://dx.doi.org/10.1016/S0140-6736(86)92110-0] [PMID: 2874312]

[7]   Langston C, Lewis DE, Hammill HA, *et al.* Excess intrauterine fetal demise associated with maternal human immunodeficiency virus infection. J Infect Dis 1995; 172(6): 1451-60.
       [http://dx.doi.org/10.1093/infdis/172.6.1451] [PMID: 7594702]

[8]   Courgnaud V, Lauré F, Brossard A, *et al.* Frequent and early *in utero* HIV-1 infection. AIDS Res Hum Retroviruses 1991; 7(3): 337-41.
       [http://dx.doi.org/10.1089/aid.1991.7.337] [PMID: 2064830]

[9]   Soeiro R, Rubinstein A, Rashbaum WK, Lyman WD. Maternofetal transmission of AIDS: frequency of human immunodeficiency virus type 1 nucleic acid sequences in human fetal DNA. J Infect Dis 1992; 166(4): 699-703.
       [http://dx.doi.org/10.1093/infdis/166.4.699] [PMID: 1527405]

[10]   Rogers MF, Ou CY, Rayfield M, *et al.* New York City Collaborative Study of Maternal HIV Transmission and Montefiore Medical Center HIV Perinatal Transmission Study Group. Use of the polymerase chain reaction for early detection of the proviral sequences of human immunodeficiency virus in infants born to seropositive mothers. N Engl J Med 1989; 320(25): 1649-54.
       [http://dx.doi.org/10.1056/NEJM198906223202503] [PMID: 2725615]

[11]   Bryson YJ, Luzuriaga K, Sullivan JL, Wara DW. Proposed definitions for in utero *versus* intrapartum transmission of HIV-1. N Engl J Med 1992; 327(17): 1246-7.
       [http://dx.doi.org/10.1056/NEJM199210223271718] [PMID: 1406816]

[12]   McIntosh K, Pitt J, Brambilla D, *et al.* The Women and Infants Transmission Study Group. Blood culture in the first 6 months of life for the diagnosis of vertically transmitted human immunodeficiency virus infection. J Infect Dis 1994; 170(4): 996-1000.
       [http://dx.doi.org/10.1093/infdis/170.4.996] [PMID: 7930747]

[13]   Lallemant M, Jourdain G, Le Coeur S, *et al.* Perinatal HIV Prevention Trial (Thailand) Investigators. A trial of shortened zidovudine regimens to prevent mother-to-child transmission of human immunodeficiency virus type 1. N Engl J Med 2000; 343(14): 982-91.
       [http://dx.doi.org/10.1056/NEJM200010053431401] [PMID: 11018164]

[14]   Rouzioux C, Costagliola D, Burgard M, *et al.* The HIV Infection in Newborns French Collaborative Study Group. Estimated timing of mother-to-child human immunodeficiency virus type 1 (HIV-1) transmission by use of a Markov model. Am J Epidemiol 1995; 142(12): 1330-7.
       [PMID: 7503054]

[15]   Lin HH, Lee TY, Chen DS, *et al.* Transplacental leakage of HBeAg-positive maternal blood as the most likely route in causing intrauterine infection with hepatitis B virus. J Pediatr 1987; 111(6 Pt 1): 877-81.
       [http://dx.doi.org/10.1016/S0022-3476(87)80210-X] [PMID: 3681555]

[16]   Goedert JJ, Duliège AM, Amos CI, Felton S, Biggar RJ. High risk of HIV-1 infection for first-born twins. The International Registry of HIV-exposed Twins. Lancet 1991; 338(8781): 1471-5.
       [http://dx.doi.org/10.1016/0140-6736(91)92297-F] [PMID: 1683916]

[17]   Guay LA, Musoke P, Fleming T, *et al.* Intrapartum and neonatal single-dose nevirapine compared with zidovudine for prevention of mother-to-child transmission of HIV-1 in Kampala, Uganda: HIVNET 012 randomised trial. Lancet 1999; 354(9181): 795-802.
       [http://dx.doi.org/10.1016/S0140-6736(99)80008-7] [PMID: 10485720]

[18]   Ziegler JB, Cooper DA, Johnson RO, Gold J. Postnatal transmission of AIDS-associated retrovirus from mother to infant. Lancet 1985; 1(8434): 896-8.
       [http://dx.doi.org/10.1016/S0140-6736(85)91673-3] [PMID: 2858746]

[19]   Miotti PG, Taha TE, Kumwenda NI, *et al.* HIV transmission through breastfeeding: a study in Malawi. JAMA 1999; 282(8): 744-9.
       [http://dx.doi.org/10.1001/jama.282.8.744] [PMID: 10463709]

[20]   Iliff PJ, Piwoz EG, Tavengwa NV, *et al.* Early exclusive breastfeeding reduces the risk of postnatal HIV-1 transmission and increases HIV-free survival. AIDS 2005; 19(7): 699-708.
       [http://dx.doi.org/10.1097/01.aids.0000166093.16446.c9] [PMID: 15821396]

[21]   Kumar SB, Rice CE, Milner DA Jr, *et al.* Elevated cytokine and chemokine levels in the placenta are associated with in-utero HIV-1 mother-to-child transmission. AIDS 2012; 26(6): 685-94.
       [http://dx.doi.org/10.1097/QAD.0b013e3283519b00] [PMID: 22301415]

[22]   Taha TE, Brown ER, Hoffman IF, *et al.* A phase III clinical trial of antibiotics to reduce chorioamnionitis-related perinatal HIV-1 transmission. AIDS 2006; 20(9): 1313-21.
       [http://dx.doi.org/10.1097/01.aids.0000232240.05545.08] [PMID: 16816561]

[23]   Magder LS, Mofenson L, Paul ME, *et al.* Risk factors for in utero and intrapartum transmission of HIV. J Acquir Immune Defic Syndr 2005; 38(1): 87-95.
       [http://dx.doi.org/10.1097/00126334-200501010-00016] [PMID: 15608531]

[24]   Renjifo B, Gilbert P, Chaplin B, *et al.* Tanzanian Vitamin and HIV Study Group. Preferential in-utero transmission of HIV-1 subtype C as compared to HIV-1 subtype A or D. AIDS 2004; 18(12): 1629-36.
       [http://dx.doi.org/10.1097/01.aids.0000131392.68597.34] [PMID: 15280773]

[25]   Khamduang W, Jourdain G, Sirirungsi W, *et al.* Program for HIV Prevention and Treatment (PHPT) Study Group. The interrelated transmission of HIV-1 and cytomegalovirus during gestation and delivery in the offspring of HIV-infected mothers. J Acquir Immune Defic Syndr 2011; 58(2): 188-92.
       [PMID: 21792064]

[26]   Landesman SH, Kalish LA, Burns DN, *et al.* Obstetrical factors and the transmission of human immunodeficiency virus type 1 from mother to child. The Women and Infants Transmission Study. N Engl J Med 1996; 334(25): 1617-23.
       [http://dx.doi.org/10.1056/NEJM199606203342501] [PMID: 8628356]

[27]   The International Perinatal HIV Group. The mode of delivery and the risk of vertical transmission of human immunodeficiency virus type 1--a meta-analysis of 15 prospective cohort studies. N Engl J Med 1999; 340(13): 977-87.
       [http://dx.doi.org/10.1056/NEJM199904013401301] [PMID: 10099139]

[28]   European Mode of Delivery Collaboration. Elective caesarean-section *versus* vaginal delivery in prevention of vertical HIV-1 transmission: a randomised clinical trial. Lancet 1999; 353(9158): 1035-9.

[http://dx.doi.org/10.1016/S0140-6736(98)08084-2] [PMID: 10199349]

[29]   Cowan FM, Humphrey JH, Ntozini R, Mutasa K, Morrow R, Iliff P. Maternal Herpes simplex virus type 2 infection, syphilis and risk of intra-partum transmission of HIV-1: results of a case control study. AIDS 2008; 22(2): 193-201.
       [http://dx.doi.org/10.1097/QAD.0b013e3282f2a939] [PMID: 18097221]

[30]   Drake AL, Roxby AC, Ongecha-Owuor F, *et al.* Valacyclovir suppressive therapy reduces plasma and breast milk HIV-1 RNA levels during pregnancy and postpartum: a randomized trial. J Infect Dis 2012; 205(3): 366-75.
       [http://dx.doi.org/10.1093/infdis/jir766] [PMID: 22147786]

[31]   Panel on Treatment of HIV-Infected Pregnant Women and Prevention of Perinatal Transmission. Recommendations for Use of Antiretroviral Drugs in Pregnant HIV-1-Infected Women for Maternal Health and Interventions to Reduce Perinatal HIV Transmission in the United States 2012. Available at: http://aidsinfo.nih.gov/contentfiles/lvguidelines/PerinatalGL.pdf.

[32]   Koulinska IN, Villamor E, Chaplin B, *et al.* Transmission of cell-free and cell-associated HIV-1 through breast-feeding. J Acquir Immune Defic Syndr 2006; 41(1): 93-9.
       [http://dx.doi.org/10.1097/01.qai.0000179424.19413.24] [PMID: 16340480]

[33]   Ekpini ER, Wiktor SZ, Satten GA, *et al.* Late postnatal mother-to-child transmission of HIV-1 in Abidjan, Côte d'Ivoire. Lancet 1997; 349(9058): 1054-9.
       [http://dx.doi.org/10.1016/S0140-6736(96)06444-6] [PMID: 9107243]

[34]   Embree JE, Njenga S, Datta P, *et al.* Risk factors for postnatal mother-child transmission of HIV-1. AIDS 2000; 14(16): 2535-41.
       [http://dx.doi.org/10.1097/00002030-200011100-00016] [PMID: 11101065]

[35]   Kantarci S, Koulinska IN, Aboud S, Fawzi WW, Villamor E. Subclinical mastitis, cell-associated HIV-1 shedding in breast milk, and breast-feeding transmission of HIV-1. J Acquir Immune Defic Syndr 2007; 46(5): 651-4.
       [http://dx.doi.org/10.1097/QAI.0b013e31815b2db2] [PMID: 18043320]

[36]   Kuhn L, Kim HY, Walter J, *et al.* HIV-1 concentrations in human breast milk before and after weaning. Sci Transl Med 2013; 5(181): 181ra51.
       [http://dx.doi.org/10.1126/scitranslmed.3005113] [PMID: 23596203]

[37]   Semba RD, Miotti PG, Chiphangwi JD, *et al.* Maternal vitamin A deficiency and mother-to-child transmission of HIV-1. Lancet 1994; 343(8913): 1593-7.
       [http://dx.doi.org/10.1016/S0140-6736(94)93056-2] [PMID: 7911919]

[38]   Fawzi WW, Msamanga GI, Hunter D, *et al.* Randomized trial of vitamin supplements in relation to transmission of HIV-1 through breastfeeding and early child mortality. AIDS 2002; 16(14): 1935-44.
       [http://dx.doi.org/10.1097/00002030-200209270-00011] [PMID: 12351954]

[39]   Villamor E, Koulinska IN, Aboud S, *et al.* Effect of vitamin supplements on HIV shedding in breast milk. Am J Clin Nutr 2010; 92(4): 881-6.
       [http://dx.doi.org/10.3945/ajcn.2010.29339] [PMID: 20739426]

[40]   Kuhn L, Steketee RW, Weedon J, *et al.* Distinct risk factors for intrauterine and intrapartum human immunodeficiency virus transmission and consequences for disease progression in infected children.

Perinatal AIDS Collaborative Transmission Study. J Infect Dis 1999; 179(1): 52-8.
[http://dx.doi.org/10.1086/314551] [PMID: 9841822]

[41] MacDonald KS, Embree J, Njenga S, *et al.* Mother-child class I HLA concordance increases perinatal human immunodeficiency virus type 1 transmission. J Infect Dis 1998; 177(3): 551-6.
[http://dx.doi.org/10.1086/514243] [PMID: 9498431]

[42] Mackelprang RD, Carrington M, John-Stewart G, *et al.* Maternal human leukocyte antigen A*2301 is associated with increased mother-to-child HIV-1 transmission. J Infect Dis 2010; 202(8): 1273-7.
[http://dx.doi.org/10.1086/656318] [PMID: 20812845]

[43] Winchester R, Pitt J, Charurat M, *et al.* Mother-to-child transmission of HIV-1: strong association with certain maternal HLA-B alleles independent of viral load implicates innate immune mechanisms. J Acquir Immune Defic Syndr 2004; 36(2): 659-70.
[http://dx.doi.org/10.1097/00126334-200406010-00002] [PMID: 15167284]

[44] Matt C, Roger M. Genetic determinants of pediatric HIV-1 infection: vertical transmission and disease progression among children. Mol Med 2001; 7(9): 583-9.
[PMID: 11778647]

[45] Gupta A, Bhosale R, Kinikar A, *et al.* Six Week Extended-Dose Nevirapine (SWEN) India Study Team. Maternal tuberculosis: a risk factor for mother-to-child transmission of human immunodeficiency virus. J Infect Dis 2011; 203(3): 358-63.
[http://dx.doi.org/10.1093/jinfdis/jiq064] [PMID: 21208928]

[46] Hershow RC, Riester KA, Lew J, *et al.* Increased vertical transmission of human immunodeficiency virus from hepatitis C virus-coinfected mothers. Women and Infants Transmission Study. J Infect Dis 1997; 176(2): 414-20.
[http://dx.doi.org/10.1086/514058] [PMID: 9237706]

[47] Pitt J, Schluchter M, Jenson H, *et al.* Maternal and perinatal factors related to maternal-infant transmission of HIV-1 in the P2C2 HIV study: the role of EBV shedding. Pediatric Pulmonary and Cardiovascular Complications of Vertically Transmitted HIV-1 Infection (P2C2 HIV) Study Group. J Acquir Immune Defic Syndr Hum Retrovirol Dec 15 1998; 19(5): 462-70.

[48] Connor EM, Sperling RS, Gelber R, *et al.* Reduction of maternal-infant transmission of human immunodeficiency virus type 1 with zidovudine treatment. Pediatric AIDS Clinical Trials Group Protocol 076 Study Group. N Engl J Med 1994; 331(18): 1173-80.
[http://dx.doi.org/10.1056/NEJM199411033311801] [PMID: 7935654]

[49] Cooper ER, Charurat M, Mofenson L, *et al.* Women and Infants' Transmission Study Group. Combination antiretroviral strategies for the treatment of pregnant HIV-1-infected women and prevention of perinatal HIV-1 transmission. J Acquir Immune Defic Syndr 2002; 29(5): 484-94.
[http://dx.doi.org/10.1097/00042560-200204150-00009] [PMID: 11981365]

[50] Sperling RS, Shapiro DE, Coombs RW, *et al.* Maternal viral load, zidovudine treatment, and the risk of transmission of human immunodeficiency virus type 1 from mother to infant. Pediatric AIDS Clinical Trials Group Protocol 076 Study Group. N Engl J Med 1996; 335(22): 1621-9.
[http://dx.doi.org/10.1056/NEJM199611283352201] [PMID: 8965861]

[51] Lallemant M, Jourdain G, Le Coeur S, *et al.* Perinatal HIV Prevention Trial (Thailand) Investigators. Single-dose perinatal nevirapine plus standard zidovudine to prevent mother-to-child transmission of

HIV-1 in Thailand. N Engl J Med 2004; 351(3): 217-28.
[http://dx.doi.org/10.1056/NEJMoa033500] [PMID: 15247338]

[52] Chasela CS, Hudgens MG, Jamieson DJ, *et al.* BAN Study Group. Maternal or infant antiretroviral drugs to reduce HIV-1 transmission. N Engl J Med 2010; 362(24): 2271-81.
[http://dx.doi.org/10.1056/NEJMoa0911486] [PMID: 20554982]

[53] Shapiro RL, Hughes MD, Ogwu A, *et al.* Antiretroviral regimens in pregnancy and breast-feeding in Botswana. N Engl J Med 2010; 362(24): 2282-94.
[http://dx.doi.org/10.1056/NEJMoa0907736] [PMID: 20554983]

[54] Fowler M, Qin M, Shapiro D, Fiscus S. PROMISE: Efficacy and safety of two strategies to prevent perinatal HIV transmission. In: Abs # 31 LB. 22nd Conference on Retroviruses and Opportunistic Infections (CROI); 23–26 Feb 2015; Seattle, Washington: 2015.

CHAPTER 4

Reducing Pre-partum and Intra-partum Transmission of HIV to Infants

Banafsheh Moradmand Badie[*] and **Lillian Mwanri**

Discipline of Public Health, School of Medicine, Flinders University, South Australia, Australia

Abstract: The Acquired Immune Deficiency Syndrome (AIDS) is one of the major causes of deaths among women of reproductive age and a significant contributor to high infant mortality rates globally. Mother-to-child transmission occurs when HIV infection is transmitted from an HIV infected mother to her baby in pregnancy, labour, delivery and breastfeeding. Preventing Mother-to-Child Transmission (PMTCT) of HIV is critical to save lives and restrain the impact of the HIV epidemic. Mother-t--child transmission before, during and after delivery can be the result of HIV transmission in 30-35% of infants of HIV-positive infected mothers. In the past three decades, HIV screening and treatment for pregnant females as well as prophylaxis for perinatal HIV transmission prevention were developed. Because of prenatal HIV counselling and testing, antiretroviral prophylaxis, programmed caesarean sections and evading of breastfeeding, the amount of perinatal HIV transmission has significantly diminished in the world today. The World Health Organization's protocol recommends the increase of the eligibility of pregnant females with HIV infection to lifelong antiretroviral therapy when possible in order to achieve optimum health outcomes. The main missed opportunity in preventing perinatal HIV infection is a lack of prenatal care. Antenatal HIV counselling comprising testing of pregnant females is an efficient medical intervention that contributes to PMTCT of HIV.

Keywords: AIDS, Antiviral therapy, HIV, Mother-to-Child Transmission, PMTCT, Prenatal care, Prevention.

---

[*] **Correspondence to Banafsheh Moradmand Badie:** Discipline of Public Health, School of Medicine, Flinders University, South Australia, GPO Box 2100, Adelaide 5001, Australia; Tel: 08 (618) 82013911; Fax: 08 (618) 82012580; E-mail: mora0106@flinders.edu.au

SeyedAhmad SeyedAlinaghi (Ed.)

1. INTRODUCTION

In 1983, the first cases of AIDS in infants were reported in America [1]. Because of new therapies and better understanding of HIV infection, perinatal infection rates have remarkably declined since 1983. Despite this decline, in 2004 there were still 138 infants born with HIV infection reported in the United States [2]. An infant born with HIV represents a missed opportunity, and commonly, more than one opportunity is missed during the care for the mother-infant pair. The Centers for Disease Control and Prevention (CDC) refers to these missed opportunities as the Perinatal Prevention Cascade [3]. Prevention opportunities can take place throughout a succession of stages and include:

• primary HIV prevention for women,
• prevention of accidental pregnancies in HIV positive females,
• improve ease of access to prenatal care,
• universal prenatal testing and counseling, and
• Antiretroviral (ARV) prophylaxis and treatment for all HIV positive pregnant females and their exposed newborns [3].

2. PREVENTING MOTHER TO CHILD TRANSMISSION (PMTCT)

Preventing Mother-to-Child Transmission (PMTCT) of HIV was first proposed as a global health policy in the late1990s [4], after the earlier diagnosis of HIV infected newborns. It has been reported that HIV transmission can decrease to 1-5% by using a possible prophylactic antiretroviral treatment. In the past three decades, HIV screening and treatment for pregnant females as well as prophylaxis for prevention of perinatal transmission have been developed considerably in United States and other developed countries [5]. This development has also improved HIV management across the world including the developing countries. In fact, treatment of HIV infection in pregnancy has increased with a rising number of women taking combination antiretroviral therapy or triple antiretroviral drug prophylaxis. With the worldwide prenatal HIV counselling and testing, antiretroviral prophylaxis, programmed caesarean sections, and evading of breastfeeding, the amount of perinatal HIV transmission has significantly declined to 2% in European countries as well as the United States [5].

In some regions of the world where effective combination regimens of antiretroviral drugs are accessible, the use of these regimens has resulted in a noticeable increase of survival of HIV infected individuals; and amounts of transmission of HIV from infected mothers to their infants has been diminished to as low as 1%. On the other hand, in poorly resourced settings and where effective combination of antiretroviral regimens are not easily accessible, the use of less intensive antiretroviral regimens has resulted in lesser but still remarkable decline in the number of HIV infant cases that contracted the infection through mother to child transmission [6, 7].

In recent years, the supply of antiretroviral drugs for the prevention of mother to child HIV transmission has grown rapidly in low and middle income countries. Consequently, numbers of HIV infected pregnant females receiving antiretroviral interventions have increased from 10% to 53% (2004 - 2009) [8]. Similar to any new drug, the emergence of the utilisation of antiretroviral drugs for HIV transmission in utero poses a challenge. While the evidence on birth defects and mitochondrial toxicity remains unclear, evidence has related protease inhibitors to preterm delivery, low birth weight and transient hematologic toxicities [9].

The World Health Organization (WHO, 2013) protocol recommends the expansion of the eligibility of HIV infected pregnant females to lifelong antiretroviral therapy when possible in order to achieve optimum health outcomes. Regardless of the CD4 count and the clinical stage (stage 3 or 4), this expansion would lead to an increase in the CD4 threshold. The increase in a CD4 count is indicative of good outcomes for HIV status. For females not requiring therapy for their own health, recommendations were made for them to receive ARV treatment to prevent HIV transmission to their infants during pregnancy [10].

According to the WHO reports, the prevention of HIV infection among infants needs four strategic approaches including:

1. Primary prevention of HIV infected patients;
2. Prevention of unplanned pregnancies in HIV infected females,
3. Prevention of transmission of HIV infection from mothers to children,
4. Providing ongoing support, care, and treatment to HIV infected females and

their families.

Health care providers considering the use of ARV drugs for HIV infected females throughout the pregnancy have to take two related issues [5]:

1. ARV treatment of maternal HIV infection to reduce the maternal viral load,
2. ARV chemoprophylaxis to decrease the risk of perinatal transmission of HIV.

3. THE DIAGNOSTIC TESTS FOR HIV INFECTION IN INFANTS AND CHILDREN

The diagnosis of HIV infection in infants and children is performed by:

-Virologic tests detect HIV directly, and have to be used to diagnose HIV infection in infants younger than 18 months. Virologic diagnostic test in infants with perinatal HIV exposure is recommended at ages 14 to 21 days, 1 to 2 months, and 4 to 6 months also the test has to be considered for infants at high risk of HIV infection.

-HIV DNA polymerase chain reaction (PCR) and HIV RNA assays are recommended as preferred virologic assays.

- A positive virologic assay has to be confirmed by a virologic retesting on a second specimen.
- Definitive exclusion of HIV infection in infants who are non-breastfed should be based on two or more negative virologic tests, with one achieved at one or more than one month of age and one at four or more than four months of age, or two negative HIV antibody tests from separate specimens obtained at six or more than six months of age.
- Many experts confirm the absence of HIV infection at 12 to 18 months of age in infants with prior negative virologic tests by performing an antibody test to document loss of maternal HIV antibodies.
- HIV antibody tests alone can be used for diagnosing HIV infection in children with perinatal exposure who are eighteen months or more and also in children with non-perinatal exposure [11].

After an infant is exposed to HIV, testing is needed because infants who have

HIV infected mothers are born with transplacentally acquired maternal antibodies. As positive results with such testing-traditional serologic test- do not necessarily mean that they have acquired HIV infection, PCR assay is required to confirm their infectious status. This assay takes several days to weeks to provide results because it is conducted in sophisticated biologic containment and is labour intensive. Three successive negative PCR tests at birth time, 6 weeks and 12 weeks of age as well as negative HIV antibody at 18 months show the absence of HIV infection. Other Nucleic Acid Amplification Techniques (NAATs), directly detect amplified viral nucleic acids, and are among the most common approaches for diagnosing HIV infection in infants. Also, detecting HIV protein p24 from blood samples using a four-generation enzyme immunoassay (EIA) is an HIV diagnostic approach [12 - 14].

4. PRENATAL CARE

The main missed opportunity in preventing perinatal HIV infection is a lack of prenatal care. It is well recognised that women who are not under an appropriate prenatal care are less likely to be offered HIV testing and prophylaxis when required [15, 16].

4.1. Antiretroviral Therapy in Reducing Perinatal Transmission of HIV

The ARVs are recommended during perinatal period for HIV infected women. These prevent mother to child transmission of HIV in three ways including:

- reducing HIV RNA concentration (viral load) in maternal blood and genital secretions,
- protecting infant from infection through pre-exposure prophylaxis and providing protection for infant through post-exposure prophylaxis.

The importance of maternal viral load as a risk factor for mother to child transmission has been demonstrated [17]. For example, among females with plasma viral loads less than 1000 copies/mL, more intensive maternal antiretroviral regimens are associated with lower risks of transmission. Maternal plasma viral load at delivery and antepartum antiretroviral treatments are the most important factors for reducing the mother to child transmission of HIV infection.

The ARV drugs can diminish perinatal transmission through a number of mechanisms. Antenatal drug administration reduces maternal viral load in blood and genital secretions, which is an important mechanism of action in females with high viral loads. Among women with HIV RNA levels less than 1,000 copies/mL, ARV drugs have indicated the potential to decrease risk of transmission. Moreover, the level of HIV RNA at delivery and receipt of antenatal ARV drugs are individually associated with risk of transmission, suggesting that the reduction in viral load is not the only responsible factor for the efficacy of ARV prophylaxis. Thus, combination of antepartum, intrapartum, and infant antiretroviral prophylaxis is suggested for the protection of infant from perinatal transmission of HIV. In short, antiretroviral drugs diminish perinatal transmission through mechanisms, including:

- lowering maternal antepartum viral load,
- providing infant pre-exposure prophylaxis, and
- providing infant post-exposure prophylaxis [18].

Regardless of HIV RNA viral load and CD4 count, all HIV infected pregnant females should be made aware of the benefits of antiretroviral drugs during pregnancy for the prevention of perinatal transmission. Generally, the suggestions for the commencement of antiretroviral therapy in females of reproductive age or in pregnant women are the same as those for other HIV infected adolescents [5]. Antiretroviral therapy should be started in individuals with the following characteristics [19]:

- Presence of any opportunistic infections
- A positive history of an AIDS defining illness
- Lower CD4 counts (*i.e.* <350 cells/mm^3)
- HIV nephropathy
- Acute HIV infection
- HIV/Hepatitis B (HBV) co-infection
- HIV/Hepatitis C (HCV) co-infection
- Rapidly declining CD4 counts (*i.e.* >100 cells/mm^3 decrease per year)
- Higher viral loads (*i.e.* >100,000 copies/mL)
- Pregnancy

• Elderly HIV infected patients

A number of experts advise ARV therapy for people with a CD4 cell count between 350 and 500 cells/mm^3 [20]. When antiretroviral therapy is started, it should be utilised for life. Antiretroviral therapy is used during pregnancy and should be continued during the intra-partum period. It is also noteworthy that mode of administration of ARV varies. For instance, zidovudine is intravenously transfused during delivery while other antiretroviral drugs are administered orally. All these are suitable for administration postpartum [5, 8 - 10, 17 - 20].

The initial commencement of ARV differs from patient to patient. Often, some women start antiretroviral therapy when they decide to get pregnant, but others may start ARV therapy after conception. Normally, if antiretroviral therapy is already being administered when an HIV infected individual becomes pregnant, for effective prevention of HIV, this regimen should be continued if tolerable [21]. Efavirenz (EFV) has been recommended as the preferred choice for a non-nucleoside reverse transcriptase inhibitor in optimized first-line antiretroviral treatment. Nonetheless, concerns remain about its safety in early pregnancy. Nevirapine (NVP) containing regimen is effective in suppressing HIV and it should be continued irrespective of the CD4 cell count, if the HIV infected pregnant female is tolerating the regimen. For females who are not taking antiretroviral therapy when they become pregnant and meet the treatment criteria, they should start antiretroviral therapy as soon as possible for it to be most effective. The therapy should be started soon, even if the woman is in the first trimester of pregnancy. Moreover, antiretroviral resistance testing should be performed in all HIV infected pregnant females before the initiation of antiretroviral therapy. This testing is especially significant if the woman received antiretroviral drugs previously for transmission prophylaxis [22, 23].

In general, HIV infected pregnant women on antiretroviral therapy should use a combination antiretroviral regimen including at least three drugs. A regimen including two Nucleoside Reverse Transcriptase Inhibitors (NRTIs) and either a Non-NRTI (NNRTI) or a Protease Inhibitor (PI) should be used. Evidence exists indicating that a combination of zidovudine with lamivudine is the choice NRTI regimen in pregnancy. In terms of NNRTIs, efavirenz (a preferred NNRTI for non-pregnant women) is recommended for use during the first trimester of pregnancy [22]. Lopinavir/ritonavir is the preferred PI in pregnant women.

For women of unknown HIV sero-status who present during labour, rapid HIV antibody testing should be performed. If the result of the rapid test is positive, intravenous zidovudine should be started without waiting for the results of a confirmatory HIV test. Moreover, some specialists would add a single dose of maternal nevirapine orally to the maternal intravenous zidovudine regimen. Besides, if single dose intrapartum/newborn nevirapine is administered, an antiretroviral tail should be used to lessen the risk of nevirapine resistance. The composition and duration of administration of this tail is not generally accepted, but in the United States the use of maternal postpartum zidovudine/lamivudine for at least seven days is recommended after intrapartum single dose nevirapine. In the United States, infants of HIV infected females should receive six weeks of oral zidovudine, irrespective of maternal use of antiretrovirals through pregnancy and, if antiretrovirals were used during pregnancy, the specific regimen [24].

The timely initiation of prophylaxis with zidovudine is crucial for the infant. Prophylaxis with zidovudine should be started very soon after delivery and within the first 12 hours of life [25]. Besides, the benefits of antiretroviral drugs for HIV infected females and their infants must be weighed against adverse effects associated with these drugs [21, 23 - 25]. Elective caesarean delivery should be considered depleting the risk of perinatal transmission and should be offered at week 38 [26].

4.2. HIV Counseling

Antenatal HIV counseling including testing of pregnant women is an effective medical intervention that contributes to PMTCT of HIV. Counseling and testing are necessary determinants that contribute to the effective treatment and care of HIV positive women and their children.

For sustainable and effective clinical management, HIV infected pregnant women should be counseled on the following issues when possible:

• Using condom to prevent of sexual transmission of HIV and other Sexually

Transmitted Infections (STIs),

- The risk of HIV transmission to the fetus or neonate and how to prevent it,
- The risks and benefits of ARV prophylaxis as part of PMTCT plan,
- The risks of HBV and HCV perinatal transmission and how to decrease them,
- The risks of perinatal syphilis transmission, and the requirement for treatment of syphilis, gonorrhea, chlamydia and other STIs to reduce the risk of HIV transmission,
- The impact of drug use on fetal development, comprising drug withdrawal syndrome and drug interactions,
- Referral to harm reduction and drug-dependence treatment programs, comprising substitution therapy where appropriate [27].

CONCLUSION

PMTCT of HIV is critical to save lives and restrain the impact of the HIV epidemic. Increase of the eligibility of pregnant females with HIV infection to lifelong antiretroviral therapy is recommended. Providing prenatal care and antenatal HIV counselling comprising testing contribute to PMTCT. The extended maternal prophylaxis with HAART for PMTCT among breastfeeding mothers who do not need HAART for their own health should be further gauged and compared with the use of infant postnatal antiretroviral prophylaxis regarding safety and cost-effectiveness [28].

CONFLICT OF INTEREST

The authors confirm that they have no conflict of interest to declare for this publication.

ACKNOWLEDGEMENTS

We gratefully acknowledge the thoughtful comments and advice of Dr. Mehrnaz Rasoulinejad, Professor of Tehran University of Medical Sciences.

REFERENCES

[1]   Oleske J, Minnefor A, Cooper R Jr, *et al.* Immune deficiency syndrome in children. JAMA 1983; 249(17): 2345-9.
       [http://dx.doi.org/10.1001/jama.1983.03330410031024] [PMID: 6834633]

[2]   McKenna MT, Hu X. Recent trends in the incidence and morbidity that are associated with perinatal human immunodeficiency virus infection in the United States. Am J Obstet Gynecol 2007; 197(3) (Suppl.): S10-6.
[http://dx.doi.org/10.1016/j.ajog.2007.02.032] [PMID: 17825639]

[3]   CDC. HIV Among Pregnant Women, Infants, and Children. [Accessed on: Mar 2016]; Available at: http://www.cdc.gov/hiv/risk/gender/pregnantwomen/facts/.

[4]   WHO/UNAIDS. Recommendations on the safe and effective use of short-course ZDV for prevention of mother-to-child transmission of HIV. Wkly Epidemiol Rec 1998; 73(41): 313-20.
[PMID: 9795578]

[5]   CDC. Recommendations for Use of Antiretroviral Drugs in Pregnant HIV-1-Infected Women for Maternal Health and Interventions to Reduce Perinatal HIV Transmission in the United States. [Accessed on: Aug 2012]; Available at: http://aidsinfo.nih.gov/guidelines

[6]   Townsend CL, Cortina-Borja M, Peckham CS, de Ruiter A, Lyall H, Tookey PA. Low rates of mother-to-child transmission of HIV following effective pregnancy interventions in the United Kingdom and Ireland, 2000-2006. AIDS 2008; 22(8): 973-81.
[http://dx.doi.org/10.1097/QAD.0b013e3282f9b67a] [PMID: 18453857]

[7]   Boer K, Nellen JF, Patel D, *et al.* The AmRo study: pregnancy outcome in HIV-1-infected women under effective highly active antiretroviral therapy and a policy of vaginal delivery. BJOG 2007; 114(2): 148-55.
[http://dx.doi.org/10.1111/j.1471-0528.2006.01183.x] [PMID: 17305888]

[8]   Heidari S, Mofenson L, Cotton MF, Marlink R, Cahn P, Katabira E. Antiretroviral drugs for preventing mother-to-child transmission of HIV: a review of potential effects on HIV-exposed but uninfected children. J Acquir Immune Defic Syndr 2011; 57(4): 290-6.
[http://dx.doi.org/10.1097/QAI.0b013e318221c56a] [PMID: 21602695]

[9]   Watts DH. Teratogenicity risk of antiretroviral therapy in pregnancy. Curr HIV/AIDS Rep 2007; 4(3): 135-40.
[http://dx.doi.org/10.1007/s11904-007-0020-y] [PMID: 17883999]

[10]   World Health Organization. Consolidated guidelines on the use of antiretroviral drugs for treating and preventing HIV infection: Recommendations for a public health approach June 2013. Geneva, Switzerland: WHO Press, World Health Organization 2013.

[11]   Recommendations for Use of Antiretroviral Drugs in Pregnant HIV-1-Infected Women for Maternal Health and Interventions to Reduce Perinatal HIV Transmission in the United States NIH. [Accessed on: June 2016]; Available at: https://aidsinfo.nih.gov/guidelines/html/3/perinatal-guidelines/0.

[12]   Nastouli E, Atkins M, Seery P, Hamadache D, Muir D, Lyall H. False-positive HIV antibody results with ultrasensitive serological assays in uninfected infants born to mothers with HIV. AIDS 2007; 21(9): 1222-3.
[http://dx.doi.org/10.1097/QAD.0b013e32810c8cbe] [PMID: 17502739]

[13]   Ou CY, Kwok S, Mitchell SW, *et al.* DNA amplification for direct detection of HIV-1 in DNA of peripheral blood mononuclear cells. Science 1988; 239(4837): 295-7.
[http://dx.doi.org/10.1126/science.3336784] [PMID: 3336784]

[14]   Rogers MF, Ou CY, Rayfield M, *et al.* New York City Collaborative Study of Maternal HIV Transmission and Montefiore Medical Center HIV Perinatal Transmission Study Group. Use of the polymerase chain reaction for early detection of the proviral sequences of human immunodeficiency virus in infants born to seropositive mothers. N Engl J Med 1989; 320(25): 1649-54.
[http://dx.doi.org/10.1056/NEJM198906223202503] [PMID: 2725615]

[15]   Abatemarco DJ, Catov JM, Cross H, Delnevo C, Hausman A. Factors associated with zidovudine receipt and prenatal care among HIV-infected pregnant women in New Jersey. J Health Care Poor Underserved 2008; 19(3): 814-28.
[http://dx.doi.org/10.1353/hpu.0.0039] [PMID: 18677072]

[16]   Sarnquist CC, Cunningham SD, Sullivan B, Maldonado Y. The effectiveness of state and national policy on the implementation of perinatal HIV prevention interventions. Am J Public Health 2007; 97(6): 1041-6.
[http://dx.doi.org/10.2105/AJPH.2005.072371] [PMID: 17463383]

[17]   Kesho Bora Study Group. Eighteen-month follow-up of HIV-1-infected mothers and their children enrolled in the Kesho Bora study observational cohorts. J Acquir Immune Defic Syndr 2010; 54(5): 533-41.
[PMID: 20543706]

[18]   Chibwesha CJ, Giganti MJ, Putta N, *et al.* Optimal time on HAART for prevention of mother-to-child transmission of HIV. J Acquir Immune Defic Syndr 2011; 58(2): 224-8.
[http://dx.doi.org/10.1097/QAI.0b013e318229147e] [PMID: 21709566]

[19]   Guidelines for the Use of Antiretroviral Agents in HIV-1-Infected Adults and Adolescents Aidsinfi. [Accessed on: June 2016]; Available at: http://aidsinfo.nih.gov/ContentFiles/Adultand.

[20]   Guidelines for the Use of Antiretroviral Agents in HIV-1-Infected Adults and Adolescents. [Accessed on: June 2016]; Available at: http://aidsinfo.nih.gov/ContentFiles/Adultand.

[21]   WHO Technical update on treatment optimization. Use of efavirenz during pregnancy: a public health perspective [Accessed on: June 2012]; Available at: http://www.who.int/hiv/pub/treatment2/efavirenz/en/.

[22]   Read JS. Prevention of mother-to-child transmission of HIV: antiretroviral strategies. Clin Perinatol 2010; 37(4): 765-76.
[http://dx.doi.org/10.1016/j.clp.2010.08.007] [PMID: 21078449]

[23]   Nielsen-Saines K, Watts DH, Veloso VG, *et al.* NICHD HPTN 040/PACTG 1043 Protocol Team. Three postpartum antiretroviral regimens to prevent intrapartum HIV infection. N Engl J Med 2012; 366(25): 2368-79.
[http://dx.doi.org/10.1056/NEJMoa1108275] [PMID: 22716975]

[24]   Mirochnick M, Best BM, Clarke DF. Antiretroviral pharmacology: special issues regarding pregnant women and neonates. Clin Perinatol 2010; 37(4): 907-927, xi.
[http://dx.doi.org/10.1016/j.clp.2010.08.006] [PMID: 21078458]

[25]   Fiscus SA, Schoenbach VJ, Wilfert C. Short courses of zidovudine and perinatal transmission of HIV. N Engl J Med 1999; 340(13): 1040-1.
[http://dx.doi.org/10.1056/NEJM199904013401312] [PMID: 10189281]

[26]   Jamieson DJ, Clark J, Kourtis AP, *et al.* Recommendations for human immunodeficiency virus screening, prophylaxis, and treatment for pregnant women in the United States. Am J Obstet Gynecol 2007; 197(3): S26-32.
[http://dx.doi.org/10.1016/j.ajog.2007.03.087] [PMID: 17825647]

[27]   Prevention of HIV Transmission from HIV Infected Mothers to their Infants Clinical Protocol for the WHO European Region [Accessed on: Aug 2015]; Available at: https://aidsinfo.nih.gov/education-materials/fact-sheets/ 20/50/preventing-mother-to-child-transmission-of-hiv.

[28]   Kilewo C, Karlsson K, Ngarina M, *et al.* Mitra Plus Study Team. Prevention of mother-to-child transmission of HIV-1 through breastfeeding by treating mothers with triple antiretroviral therapy in Dar es Salaam, Tanzania: the Mitra Plus study. J Acquir Immune Defic Syndr 2009; 52(3): 406-16.
[http://dx.doi.org/10.1097/QAI.0b013e3181b323ff] [PMID: 19730269]

CHAPTER 5

HIV Infection and Cell Signaling Pathways

Ali Teimoori[1,*], Kazem Baesi[2] and Seyed Younes Hosseini[3]

[1] *Research Center for Infectious Diseases of Digestive System, Ahvaz Jundishapur University of Medical Sciences, Ahvaz, Iran*

[2] *Hepatitis and AIDS Department, Pasteur Institute of Iran, Iran*

[3] *GastroenteroHepatology Research Center, Shiraz University of Medical Sciences, Shiraz, Iran*

Abstract: HIV infects cells of the immune system, particularly T CD4 helper cells. Interaction of viral proteins with the cell, modulate many signaling pathways in the immune system. This interaction facilitate to the HIV replication, trafficking and infection. The starting point in signaling pathways is the attachment of HIV envelope protein gp120 to the CD4 receptor and CCR5 or CXCR4 coreceptor. Such events result in calcium fluctuation and activation of various Protein Kinase C (PKC) isoforms. Moreover, it was reported that gp120 mediates chemotaxis and actin cytoskeleton rearrangement. After the integration of the provirus and gene expression, HIV regulatory and accessory proteins modulate the enzymatic activity of some of the protein kinases. Accessory proteins induction of G2 cell cycle arrest is found to reduce human immune functions through protection against T-cell clonal expansion that would optimize cellular environment for maximal viral replication. Also induced cell cycle arrest *via* a DNA damage-sensitive pathway in HIV infection has been shown. HIV infects and induces apoptosis of circulating CD4 T and CD34 multi-potent hematopoietic progenitor cells.

Keywords: ATM, Caspase, CCR5, CXCR4, gp120, Lymphocyte-specific protein tyrosine kinase, Negative factor, Nuclear factor (NF)-κB, Phospholipase C, Signaling pathways.

* **Correspondence to Ali Teimoori:** Department of Virology, Jundishapur University of Medical Sciences, Ahvaz, Iran; Tel/Fax: +98 (611) 3738313; E-mail: teimoori_ali@yahoo.com

SeyedAhmad SeyedAlinaghi (Ed.)

1. INTRODUCTION

The HIV replication cycle depends on the interactions of viral proteins with a large number of host cell factors. The first interaction between HIV and target cells begins with the linkage of the trimeric viral surface glycoprotein gp120 to the cellular CD4 receptor [1]. This interaction activates conformational changes in gp120, and this enables the recognition of CC -chemokine receptor 5 (CCR5) or CXC-chemokine receptor 4 (CXCR4) co-receptors [2, 3]. Two key biological events will occur, *i.e.* membrane fusion and signaling transduction.

2. SIGNALING PATHWAYS THAT ARE ACTIVATED *VIA* HIV GP120 AND CHEMOKINE CO-RECEPTORS

Chemokine receptor signaling is reported as a moderator for cell migration, transcriptional activation, as well as cell growth and differentiation. Heterotrimeric G-proteins (α, β andγsubunits in a heterotrimeric) are activated through coupling to the G protein-coupled receptor CXCR4. A wide range of classes of Gα are found (Gas, Gai, Gaq, Ga12/13), however, it seems that CXCR4 is specifically linked to Gai and Gaq. The Gaq proteins activate phospholipase C-c (PLC-c), hydrolyzing phosphatidylinositol- 4, 5-biphosphate (PIP2) to inositol triphosphate (IP3) and diacylglyerol (DAG). These events result in calcium fluctuation and activation of different isoforms of Protein Kinase C (PKC) [4]. Gai-coupled Src-family kinases activates the lipid kinase PI3K, also PI3Kc is activated *via* direct coupling of Gβ,γ to the regulatory subunits of PI3Kc [5, 6]. Protein kinase B (PKB/Akt) and mitogen/extracellular signal-regulated kinase (MEK-1) and extracellular signal-regulated kinase (ERK1/2) are downstream of PI3K and function in cell survival and proliferation. Moreover, PI3K stimulates the tyrosine phosphorylation of focal adhesion complex components including proline-rich tyrosine kinase (Pyk2). Pyk2 has an important role for cell migration and cell adhesion [7]. Also, PI3K is upstream of the critical nuclear transcription activator NF-κB, regulating gene expression in the face of inflammation and activating HIV proviral gene expression [8].

Furthermore, coupling of HIV-1 gp120 to CCR5 or CXCR4 causes a faster activation of Pyk2 PI3K, Aktb, Erk-1/2 [9, 10], and CD4/CXCR4-dependent

NFAT (nuclear factor of activated T cells) nuclear translocation [11]. It was reported that gp120 mediates chemotaxis, actin cytoskeleton rearrangement [12, 13] and activation of an actin depolymerization factor cofilin for viral intracellular migration in resting CD4 T cells. Cofilin activation leads to an increase in cortical actin dynamics and actin treadmilling, and thereby promoting the movement of the viral pre-integration complex toward the nucleus [13]. As recently reported, a few HIV particles might be sufficient to activate signaling through CXCR4 [14]. CCR5 signaling has found to foster expression of genes belonging to MAPK signal transduction pathways and genes regulating the cell cycle [11]. Also, HIV infection typically leads to chronic activation of the immune system, with profound changes in quantity and quality in the T cell compartment that the basal level of phosphorylation is found to be increased in CD4 and CD8 T cells, probably due to the elevated levels of immune activation observed in advanced disease [15].

The significance of chemokine co-receptor signaling for viral infection remains controversial. In fact, the inhibition of co-receptor signaling did not inhibit HIV-1 replication [16]. Furthermore, CCR5 mutants without its signaling ability to mobilize calcium show no remarkable impairment in viral entry and replication in Hela-CD4 cells [17]. Besides, many studies have described the modulation of cellular functions by HIV gp120 signaling, from causing neurotoxicity to apoptosis. Also, stimulation of resting CD4 T cells of infected patients with gp120 resulted in induction of viral replication [18]. On the other hand, the gp120-mediated binding of HIV-1 virions to DC-SIGN can greatly stimulate the ability of virus to infect CD4 negative and coreceptor-positive cells that come in contact with the DC-SIGN expressing cell. For viral entry into the dendritic cells, DC-SIGN does not function as a receptor, it rather encourages efficient infection in *trans* of cells that express CD4 and chemokine receptors [19].

3. THE ROLE OF HIV REGULATORY AND ACCESSORY PROTEINS ON CELLULAR SIGNALING PATHWAYS

3.1. The Role of HIV Nef Protein

HIV contains several regulatory and accessory proteins (Tat, Rev, Vif, Nef, Vpr and Vpu) that modulate cell signaling pathways. Nef (Negative factor) protein is as a master regulator affecting the transcription of a series of cellular genes [20]. Membrane coupling, moderated through a covalently attached myristic acid moiety and a cluster of N-terminal basic residues plays a critical role in Nef function [21]. Deletion of the nef gene has a profound effect in the SIV or *Rhesus macaque* animal model system. Monkeys inoculated with nef-deleted mutants develop high-level antibody responses, but produce no detectable circulating virus [22]. The experiments indicate that Nef plays a critical role in initiating and sustaining SIV infection *in vivo*. In tissue cultures, Nef is not required for HIV infection, but enhances viral infectivity. These findings suggest that *nef* viral protein alters a cell signaling pathway(s) [23].

In this line, Nef has been reported to interact with CD4 [24], Lymphocyte-specific protein tyrosine kinase (Lck) [25], p53, Mitogen-activated protein (MAP) Kinase [26], the SH3 domains of Hck and Lyn [27], c-Src [28] and b-COP [29]. Lck, a tyrosine kinase, phosphorylates tyrosine residues of certain proteins related to the intracellular signaling pathways of these lymphocytes. It belongs to the Src family of tyrosine kinases, and is involved in the cytoplasmic tails of the CD4 and CD8 co-receptors on T helper cells and cytotoxic T cells, respectively, to assist signaling from the T Cell Receptor (TCR) complex. When the TCR is engaged by the specific antigen presented by MHC, Lck acts to phosphorylate the intracellular chains of the CD3 and ζ-chains of the TCR complex, allowing another cytoplasmic tyrosine kinase called ZAP-70 to bind to them [30, 31]. Then, Lck phosphorylates and activates ZAP-70 [31], in turn phosphorylating another molecule in the signaling cascade called Linker of Activated T cells (LAT), a trans-membrane protein that serves as a docking site for a number of other proteins, the most important of which are Shc-Grb2-SOS, PI3K, and phospholipase C (PLC) [32].

Numerous studies have investigated the perturbation of cell signaling by Nef in T-cells and the interaction of Nef with the T-cell restricted Lck tyrosine kinase (both *in vitro* and *in vivo*). Analysis of the molecular basis for this interaction confirms the participations of cell-derived Nef in a synergistic manner by the recombinant Src homology 2 (SH2) and SH3 domains from Lck. A functional proline-rich motif and the tyrosine phosphorylation of Nef are regarded as the potential participants in the interaction. The precipitation of Nef by the Lck recombinant proteins was specific, since neither Fyn, Csk, p85 phosphatidylinositol 3-kinase nor phospholipase Cγ SH2 domains co-precipitated Nef from T-cells. Ultimately, depressed Lck kinase activity raised from the existence of Nef, both *in vitro* and in intact cells, and *nef* expression leads to damage in both proximal and distal Lck-mediated signaling events. These findings provide a molecular basis for the Nef-induced T-cell signaling defect and its role in the pathogenesis of AIDS [25].

The mechanism of CD4 down-regulation by Nef is very well understood to date. In this regards, Nef binds to the cytoplasmic tail of CD4 with a KD of about 1 μM. Nef amino acids 57-59, 95, 97, 106, 110, and additional residues in the N terminal flexible arm of Nef form the interface with CD4. This coupling is not found to be sufficient for Nef to down-regulate CD4 from the plasma membrane [33, 34]. In fact, clathrin adaptor complex AP-2 relates with Nef to cause internalization of CD4 [35]. In this system, the interaction of Nef and CD4 was failed in the lack of the co-expression of both AP-2 α and σ2 proteins [36]. Therefore, the internalization of CD4 was induced by this complex p. Moreover, the p21-activated Kinases (PAK) provide critical effectors binding Rho GTPases to cytoskeleton reorganization and nuclear signaling. Complex formation between Nef and PAK2 leads to PAK2 autophosphorylation activation [37]. The HIV-1 Nef protein interaction with PAK2 and its role in T-cell activation, viral replication, apoptosis, and progression to AIDS is however controversial. Nef mutants show dysfunctions due to the involvement of Nef residue F191 in PAK2 coupling [38 - 40]. As reported, the F191H mutation lowers and the F191R mutation damages the interaction of Nef with PAK2 [41]. Above all, HIV-1 Nef mutants replicated efficiently and generated CD4$^+$ T-cell depletion in *ex vivo*-infected human lymphoid tissue. In general, other data indicates no significant role of the interaction of Nef with PAK2 for the activation of in T-cell, viral replication or apoptosis.

The application of a new T cell reporter system show that Nef more than doubles the number of cells expressing the transcription factors NF-κB and NFAT after TCR stimulation. This Nef-induced priming of TCR signaling pathways appeared independently of calcium signaling and related to a very proximal step before activation of protein kinase C. Participation of the TCR by MHC-bound antigen fosters the formation of immunological synapse through using detergent-resistant membrane micro-domains, known as lipid rafts. Approximately, 5-10% of the total cellular pool of Nef is localized within lipid rafts. As found, Nef may be obtained from lipid rafts to the immunological synapse immediately after antibody interaction with the TCR/CD3 and CD28 receptors. This application relied on the N-terminal domain of Nef encompassing its myristoylation moiety. Nef localization resulted in no increase in the number of cell surface lipid rafts or immunological synapses. Research shows a specific interaction of Nef with PAK2 just observed in the lipid rafts. Therefore, the co-recruitment of Nef and key cellular partners (*i.e.* PAK2) into the immunological synapse may encourage the increased frequency of cells expressing transcriptionally active forms of NF-κB and NFAT and the resulting variations in T cell activation [42].

3.2. The Role of NF- κB Transcription Factors and Tat

Transcription of genes associated with the immune and inflammatory response is regulated by the nuclear transcription factors (NF)-κB. The NF-κB family is composed of RelA/p65, c-Rel, RelB, p50 and p52 that share a highly conserved 300-amino acid Rel homology domain (RHD) for homo- or hetero-dimerization and DNA-binding. The transcriptional activity of the NF-κB complex depends on dimer composition since C-terminal unrelated transcriptional activation domains are present exclusively in p65, RelB and c-Rel [43].

Inhibitors of NF-κB (generally IkB proteins) interfere with its coupling to DNA. In the canonical pathway of NF-κB activation, the activated IkB kinase (IKK) phosphorylates IkB at specific serine residues that target the protein for ubiquitination and proteasomal degradation, releasing the functional NF-κB complex in the nucleus [44]. The NF-κB activity is increased by phosphorylation of p65 at Ser276 by Protein Kinase A (PKA) and Mitogen- and Stress-activated protein Kinase-1(MSK1) Ser311 by PKCζ and Ser536 by IKKa [45 - 48]. Stable activation of NF-κB occurs in HIV-1 infected monocytes, macrophages and microglia, that improves NF-κB-responsive gene expression, including pro-inflammatory cytokines, cell adhesion molecules and chemokines [49]. In HIV-1 entry, the linking of the gp120 viral envelope to CD4 encourages the NF-κB activity through activating of IKK and pro-caspase 8 [50, 51].

Another HIV regulatory protein that seems to enhance the efficiency of viral transcription is the Trans-Activator of Transcription (Tat). Tat protein consists of between 86 to 101 amino acids depending on the HIV-1 subtype. The secreted Tat can bind to a variety of cell types by some different receptors. Most of them will allow Tat endocytosis. Upon internalization, low endosomal pH fosters a conformational variation in Tat that results in membrane insertion. Cytosolic Tat can encourage different cell responses [52]. Also, Tat links to RNA stem-loop structures formed by the ′5 end of target transcripts, including the HIV-1 transactivation-responsive element (TAR) [53], tumor necrosis factor β (TNFβ) [54] and interleukin-6 (IL-6) [55] to activate gene transcription. In fact, Tat enhances the onset of transcription and elongation *via* the interaction with transacting factors and cofactors, such as Sp1, TFIID, E2F-4, C/EBPβ, cyclin T1/CDK9 and the histone acetyltransferases p300/CBP and P/CAF [52].

As reported, NF-κB is constitutively active in Jurkat cells that stably expressed the Tat gene [56]. After gene transfection or protein transduction, Tat triggered the IKK activity and proteasomal degradation of IkB-α, and improved the p65 transcriptional activity by inhibiting the SIRT-1-mediated deacetylation of p65 Lys310. Hence, Tat moderates key enzymes associated with NF-κB signaling; however, how Tat can subvert the negative feedback of NF-κB, primarily relied on de novo synthesis of IkB-α, is unclear [57]. It has been found that IkB-α links to Tat and enhances the nuclear export of the viral transactivator. Further, Tat counteracts the post-activation turn off of NF-κB by directly interacting with IkB-α and p65, and thereby improving the DNA coupling and transcriptional activity for the NF-κB complex [58].

3.3. The Role of Vpr

During HIV infection, the Vpr-induced G2 cell cycle arrest is found to decrease human immune functions *via* protection against T-cell clonal expansion, which will optimize cell's environment to maximize viral replication [59]. In this regard, switching from G2 to mitosis relies on cyclin B1-Cdc2 kinase complex activation and its entrance into the nucleus during prophase [60]. The activity of Cdc2 is maintained in an opposing manner by the Cdc25C phosphatase [61] and the Wee1 and Myt-1 kinases [62]. Both variations in their overall phosphorylation, variations in their sub-cellular localization contribute to the regulation of functions of Cdc25C and Wee1. During S phase, Cdc25C predominantly resides in the cytoplasm, reflecting its assembly with a 14-3-3 protein as members of the highly conserved and ubiquitously expressed family of 14-3-3 proteins [63]. Significant shifts were observed in the Vpr-induced changes in intracellular trafficking of Cdc25C and cyclin B1 and localization of Cdc25C and cyclin B1 shifted. It seems that intermittent rupture of the Vpr-induced nuclear envelope herniations resulted in transient missing of the sub-cellular compartmentalization of Cdc25C, cyclin B1, and Wee1 and presumably other soluble cellular components [64].

Biochemical evidences have demonstrated that Vpr mediates G_2 arrest by forming a complex with protein phosphatase 2A (PP2A), an upstream regulator of cdc25. Generally, the active form of cdc25 accumulates in the nucleus and activates cdc2-cyclin B to trigger mitosis. The interaction pf PP2A holoenzyme containing B55 subunits and cdc25 regulates its activity. In HIV-1-infected cells, Vpr associates with PP2A through interacting B regulatory subunits. The Vpr-PP2A interaction improves PP2A catalytic activity and targets the hyperactive holoenzyme to the nucleus where active cdc25 substrate is placed. The lack of cdc25 activation, due to efficient dephosphorylation, remains cdc2-cyclin B in its hyperphosphorylated form, and in turn stop cell entry from mitosis [65].

4. DNA DAMAGE-SIGNALING PATHWAYS AND APOPTOSIS IN HIV INFECTION

DNA damage-signaling pathways compose of a network of interacting and occasionally redundant signals resulting in inactivation of the Cdc2-cyclin B complex and cell cycle arrest in G2 [66]. A key point of regulation of the Cdc2-cyclin B cyclin complex is through inhibitory phosphorylation of Cdc2 on Tyr-15. Furthermore, Phosphorylation of the adjacent residue, Thr-14, associates with the inhibition of Cdc2 activity. Cdc25C, a dual specificity phosphatase, dephosphorylates Cdc2 on both Tyr-15 and Thr-14, resulting in the activation of Cdc2. By inducing the DNA damage checkpoint, several kinases inactivate Cdc25C, such as Chk1 and Chk2, which are under the control of the phosphatidylinositol 3-kinase-like proteins ATR and ATM [67, 68]. ATR and

ATM respond to different abnormal DNA structures and trigger a signaling cascade leading to a DNA damage checkpoint [69]. Their roles are relatively unessential, but with some important distinctions both with regard to substrate preference and the types of the DNA damage to which the kinases respond. In the face to genotoxic stress, ATM perform the phosphorylation of the Chk2 protein kinase, while ATR is responsible for phosphorylation of Chk1. ATR is mainly important for triggering of the cell cycle checkpoint which is activated in the face to intra- S-phase genotoxic stress, as exemplified by stalled replication forks and topoisomerase inhibition [70]. ATM is rather responsible for the ionizing radiation-induced DNA damage checkpoint. Methylxanthines, such as caffeine, can inhibit both proteins. ATR acts in concert with Rad17 and the proliferating cell nuclear antigen-like heterotrimer composed of Rad9, Hus1, and Rad1 to enforce the DNA damage checkpoint [71]. Induction of G2 arrest by Vpr can be overcome by methylxanthines [72]. Accordingly, the above observations suggest that Vpr fosters cell cycle arrest through a DNA damage-sensitive pathway [73], despite the elusive nature of precise signaling pathways . In this regard, a direct binding of Vpr to DNA has been reported [74]. Also, Vpr causes changes in the structure of chromatin, leading to stalled replication. These changes in chromatin structure and replication are sensed by ATR, and thereby activating Chk1. More activation of the ATR/Chk1 cascade can inhibit Cdc2, the key regulator of the G2/M transition [75].

Vpr expression is involved in the down-regulation of genes in the Mitogen-activated Protein Kinase Kinase 2- Extracellular signal-regulated Kinases (MEK2-ERK) pathway and with decreased phosphorylation of the MEK2 effector protein ERK. Exogenous provision of excess MEK2 reverses the cell cycle arrest engaged in Vpr, which supports the impact of the MEK2-ERK pathway in the arrest of Vpr-mediated cell cycle. Therefore, it seems that Vpr arrests the cell cycle at G2/M by two mechanisms, the ATR mechanism and a newly described MEK2 mechanism [76]. This redundancy shows that Vpr-mediated cell cycle arrest contributes to HIV replication and pathogenesis.

In any viral infection, an increase in the destruction of certain cell types may be induced by direct cytotoxicity of infected cells, programmed cell death (either apoptotic or non-apoptotic) enforced in infected cells, or programmed cell death in uninfected, so called 'bystander' cells fostered by soluble or membrane-bound viral or host immune factors [77]. Correspondingly, HIV infects and induces apoptosis of circulating CD4T and CD34 multi-potent hematopoietic progenitor cells. Analysis of viral dynamics *in vivo* shows that a remarkable proportion of CD4 T cell death is stem from viral induced cytotoxicity in the infected cells [77, 78]. Moreover, as indirect evidence confirmed, the induction of G2 arrest and apoptosis are coupled. For example, treatment of cells with either caffeine, an inhibitor of ATR/ATM checkpoint function, or small interfering RNA (siRNA) specific to ATR, relieves both Vpr-induced G2 arrest and apoptosis [79, 80]. Also, it has been found that siRNA knockdown of Wee1, a Cdk1 inhibitor that is activated by DNA damage, abrogated both Vpr-induced G2 arrest and apoptosis [81]. Cell cycle transition into G2 is of importance for the induction of apoptosis by Vpr and blockade of the cell cycle in G1 for 48h effectively prevented apoptosis, and following release of the block enabled apoptosis induction, coinciding with entry into G2. Also, it has been found that efficient removal of Adenine Nucleotide Transporter (ANT) -an essential domain of PTPC- shows no impact on Vpr apoptosis to any degree. The ANT known as the ADP/ATP translocator, extracts ATP from the mitochondrial matrix and distributes ADP into the matrix. ANT is the most plentiful protein in the inner mitochondrial membrane. ANT is a key component of the structure in the mitochondrial permeability transition pore [82], which may open and result in cell mortality through apoptosis.

Unlike the above observations, elimination of Bax -an independent mitochondrial pore-forming protein- cause relatively full decrease in apoptosis. Also, Bax activation relies on the presence of ATR, as induced by apoptosis. Accordingly, this data strongly support a model in which the ATR activation is the apical step toward Vpr-induced apoptosis, followed by the activation of downstream apoptotic mediators such as Bax, Smac, and caspases. As suggested by some other reports, nuclear proteins, such as Rad9 or Histone H1, may shift from the nucleus to the cytoplasm in the face to DNA damage, to interact with mitochondrion-associated Bcl-2 family proteins and encourage cytochrome c release and apoptosis [83].

Two major pathways are introduced for induction of apoptosis, the Fas/Fas ligand pathway and the mitochondrial pathway. In both pathways the activation of caspase 3 as a hallmark and downstream target of these apoptotic pathways. In cells infected with virions that carry Vpr^{wt}, caspase 3 is dramatically elevated and activated [84]. Also, both caspase 8 and caspase 9 are activated with different stimuli. Caspase 8 activity is a downstream indicator of activation of the Fas/Fas ligand apoptotic pathway, whereas caspase 9 is a downstream indicator of the mitochondrial apoptotic pathway. Previous reports found that infection with Vpr^{wt} or Vpr$^-$ viruses failed to induce caspase 8 activity. This suggested that in PBMCs, the HIV-1 Vpr-induced apoptosis is not mediated through the Fas death receptor pathway. Several additional evidences collectively illustrated that Vpr acts independently of the caspase 8 Fas/FADD pathway [85]. The disruption of trans-membrane potential, which indicates the disruption of the membrane integrity, is one of the earliest phenomena in the mitochondrial pathway of apoptosis. HIV-1 Vpr disrupts the mitochondrial membrane potential and may induce apoptosis through mitochondrial disruption [85]. By making the mitochondrial membrane permeable, Vpr would facilitate the release of apoptotic proteins such as cytochrome c, which form a complex with Apaf-1. The complex that activates the mitochondrial apoptosis pathway consists of cytochrome c released from the mitochondria (Apaf-2), the human homolog of Ced-4 (Apaf-1) and proenzyme (Casp9) (Apaf-3). The Apaf-1-cytochrome c complex recruits pro-caspase 9 and induces its auto-activation by aggregation and ultimately affects caspase 9 and later cleaves caspase 3. The Bcl-2 protein family, as an anti-apoptotic protein, regulates mitochondrial potential and early apoptotic changes. These proteins hinder the release of caspases and caspase-activating factors from apoptotic mitochondria [86].

In conclusion, cell fate in HIV infection depends on interaction of virus to signaling pathways. These signaling pathways on T-cell occurred in very well organized and managed manner. After interaction of HIV-1 gp120 to chemokine receptor, T-cell signaling pathways are activated. These events are very important for productive HIV-1 infection as these signaling pathways ultimately regulates several cellular functions such as cytoskeletal rearrangement, cell survival and differentiation, and activation of several cellular transcription factors. The signaling pathways induced by HIV proteins in infected and bystander T cells facilitate disease progression. A better perception of the dynamic interaction between HIV-1 and specific T-cell signaling pathway, may lead to the development of a vaccine and antiviral strategies that can limit HIV-1 pathogenesis.

CONFLICT OF INTEREST

The authors confirm that they have no conflict of interest to declare for this publication.

ACKNOWLEDGEMENTS

Declared none.

REFERENCES

[1]   Dalgleish AG, Beverley PC, Clapham PR, Crawford DH, Greaves MF, Weiss RA. The CD4 (T4) antigen is an essential component of the receptor for the AIDS retrovirus. Nature 1984; 312(5996): 763-7.
        [http://dx.doi.org/10.1038/312763a0] [PMID: 6096719]

[2]   Feng Y, Broder CC, Kennedy PE, Berger EA. HIV-1 entry cofactor: functional cDNA cloning of a seven-transmembrane, G protein-coupled receptor. Science 1996; 272(5263): 872-7.
        [http://dx.doi.org/10.1126/science.272.5263.872] [PMID: 8629022]

[3]   Wu Y, Yoder A. Chemokine coreceptor signaling in HIV-1 infection and pathogenesis. PLoS Pathog 2009; 5(12): e1000520.
        [http://dx.doi.org/10.1371/journal.ppat.1000520] [PMID: 20041213]

[4]   Shahabi NA, McAllen K, Sharp BM. Stromal cell-derived factor 1-alpha (SDF)-induced human T cell chemotaxis becomes phosphoinositide 3-kinase (PI3K)-independent: role of PKC-theta. J Leukoc Biol 2008; 83(3): 663-71.
        [http://dx.doi.org/10.1189/jlb.0607420] [PMID: 18055570]

[5]   Sotsios Y, Whittaker GC, Westwick J, Ward SG. The CXC chemokine stromal cell-derived factor activates a Gi-coupled phosphoinositide 3-kinase in T lymphocytes. J Immunol 1999; 163(11): 5954-63.
        [PMID: 10570282]

[6]   Ganju RK, Brubaker SA, Meyer J, *et al.* The alpha-chemokine, stromal cell-derived factor-1alpha, binds to the transmembrane G-protein-coupled CXCR-4 receptor and activates multiple signal transduction pathways. J Biol Chem 1998; 273(36): 23169-75.
        [http://dx.doi.org/10.1074/jbc.273.36.23169] [PMID: 9722546]

[7]   Lev S, Moreno H, Martinez R, *et al.* Protein tyrosine kinase PYK2 involved in Ca(2+)-induced regulation of ion channel and MAP kinase functions. Nature 1995; 376(6543): 737-45.
        [http://dx.doi.org/10.1038/376737a0] [PMID: 7544443]

[8]   Nabel G, Baltimore D. An inducible transcription factor activates expression of human immunodeficiency virus in T cells. Nature 1987; 326(6114): 711-3.
[http://dx.doi.org/10.1038/326711a0] [PMID: 3031512]

[9]   Davis CB, Dikic I, Unutmaz D, *et al.* Signal transduction due to HIV-1 envelope interactions with chemokine receptors CXCR4 or CCR5. J Exp Med 1997; 186(10): 1793-8.
[http://dx.doi.org/10.1084/jem.186.10.1793] [PMID: 9362541]

[10]   François F, Klotman ME. Phosphatidylinositol 3-kinase regulates human immunodeficiency virus type 1 replication following viral entry in primary CD4+ T lymphocytes and macrophages. J Virol 2003; 77(4): 2539-49.
[http://dx.doi.org/10.1128/JVI.77.4.2539-2549.2003] [PMID: 12551992]

[11]   Cicala C, Arthos J, Martinelli E, *et al.* R5 and X4 HIV envelopes induce distinct gene expression profiles in primary peripheral blood mononuclear cells. Proc Natl Acad Sci USA 2006; 103(10): 3746-51.
[http://dx.doi.org/10.1073/pnas.0511237103] [PMID: 16505369]

[12]   Balabanian K, Harriague J, Décrion C, *et al.* CXCR4-tropic HIV-1 envelope glycoprotein functions as a viral chemokine in unstimulated primary CD4+ T lymphocytes. J Immunol 2004; 173(12): 7150-60.
[http://dx.doi.org/10.4049/jimmunol.173.12.7150] [PMID: 15585836]

[13]   Yoder A, Yu D, Dong L, *et al.* HIV envelope-CXCR4 signaling activates cofilin to overcome cortical actin restriction in resting CD4 T cells. Cell 2008; 134(5): 782-92.
[http://dx.doi.org/10.1016/j.cell.2008.06.036] [PMID: 18775311]

[14]   Melar M, Ott DE, Hope TJ. Physiological levels of virion-associated human immunodeficiency virus type 1 envelope induce coreceptor-dependent calcium flux. J Virol 2007; 81(4): 1773-85.
[http://dx.doi.org/10.1128/JVI.01316-06] [PMID: 17121788]

[15]   Schweneker M, Favre D, Martin JN, Deeks SG, McCune JM. HIV-induced changes in T cell signaling pathways. J Immunol 2008; 180(10): 6490-500.
[http://dx.doi.org/10.4049/jimmunol.180.10.6490] [PMID: 18453567]

[16]   Cocchi F, DeVico AL, Garzino-Demo A, Cara A, Gallo RC, Lusso P. The V3 domain of the HIV-1 gp120 envelope glycoprotein is critical for chemokine-mediated blockade of infection. Nat Med 1996; 2(11): 1244-7.
[http://dx.doi.org/10.1038/nm1196-1244] [PMID: 8898753]

[17]   Farzan M, Choe H, Martin KA, *et al.* HIV-1 entry and macrophage inflammatory protein-1bet--mediated signaling are independent functions of the chemokine receptor CCR5. J Biol Chem 1997; 272(11): 6854-7.
[http://dx.doi.org/10.1074/jbc.272.11.6854] [PMID: 9054370]

[18]   Kinter A, Catanzaro A, Monaco J, *et al.* CC-chemokines enhance the replication of T-tropic strains of HIV-1 in CD4(+) T cells: role of signal transduction. Proc Natl Acad Sci USA 1998; 95(20): 11880-5.
[http://dx.doi.org/10.1073/pnas.95.20.11880] [PMID: 9751759]

[19]   Geijtenbeek TB, Kwon DS, Torensma R, *et al.* DC-SIGN, a dendritic cell-specific HIV-1-binding protein that enhances trans-infection of T cells. Cell 2000; 100(5): 587-97.
[http://dx.doi.org/10.1016/S0092-8674(00)80694-7] [PMID: 10721995]

[20]   Balog K, Minarovits J. Nef: a pleiotropic modulator of primate lentivirus infectivity and pathogenesis. Acta Microbiol Immunol Hung 2006; 53(1): 51-75.
[http://dx.doi.org/10.1556/AMicr.53.2006.1.4] [PMID: 16696550]

[21]   Welker R, Harris M, Cardel B, Kräusslich HG. Virion incorporation of human immunodeficiency virus type 1 Nef is mediated by a bipartite membrane-targeting signal: analysis of its role in enhancement of viral infectivity. J Virol 1998; 72(11): 8833-40.
[PMID: 9765428]

[22]   Kestler HW III, Ringler DJ, Mori K, *et al.* Importance of the nef gene for maintenance of high virus loads and for development of AIDS. Cell 1991; 65(4): 651-62.
[http://dx.doi.org/10.1016/0092-8674(91)90097-I] [PMID: 2032289]

[23]   Skowronski J, Parks D, Mariani R. Altered T cell activation and development in transgenic mice expressing the HIV-1 nef gene. EMBO J 1993; 12(2): 703-13.
[PMID: 8095017]

[24]   Harris MP, Neil JC. Myristoylation-dependent binding of HIV-1 Nef to CD4. J Mol Biol 1994; 241(2): 136-42.
[http://dx.doi.org/10.1006/jmbi.1994.1483] [PMID: 8057354]

[25]   Collette Y, Dutartre H, Benziane A, *et al.* Physical and functional interaction of Nef with Lck. HIV-1 Nef-induced T-cell signaling defects. J Biol Chem 1996; 271(11): 6333-41.
[http://dx.doi.org/10.1074/jbc.271.11.6333] [PMID: 8626429]

[26]   Greenway A, Azad A, McPhee D. Human immunodeficiency virus type 1 Nef protein inhibits activation pathways in peripheral blood mononuclear cells and T-cell lines. J Virol 1995; 69(3): 1842-50.
[PMID: 7853525]

[27]   Lee CH, Leung B, Lemmon MA, *et al.* A single amino acid in the SH3 domain of Hck determines its high affinity and specificity in binding to HIV-1 Nef protein. EMBO J 1995; 14(20): 5006-15.
[PMID: 7588629]

[28]   Du Z, Lang SM, Sasseville VG, *et al.* Identification of a nef allele that causes lymphocyte activation and acute disease in macaque monkeys. Cell 1995; 82(4): 665-74.
[http://dx.doi.org/10.1016/0092-8674(95)90038-1] [PMID: 7664345]

[29]   Benichou S, Bomsel M, Bodéus M, *et al.* Physical interaction of the HIV-1 Nef protein with beta-COP, a component of non-clathrin-coated vesicles essential for membrane traffic. J Biol Chem 1994; 269(48): 30073-6.
[PMID: 7982906]

[30]   Zamoyska R, Basson A, Filby A, Legname G, Lovatt M, Seddon B. The influence of the src-family kinases, Lck and Fyn, on T cell differentiation, survival and activation. Immunol Rev 2003; 191: 107-18.
[http://dx.doi.org/10.1034/j.1600-065X.2003.00015.x] [PMID: 12614355]

[31]   Wang H, Kadlecek TA, Au-Yeung BB, *et al.* ZAP-70: an essential kinase in T-cell signaling. Cold Spring Harb Perspect Biol 2010; 2(5): a002279.
[http://dx.doi.org/10.1101/cshperspect.a002279] [PMID: 20452964]

[32]   Mustelin T, Taskén K. Positive and negative regulation of T-cell activation through kinases and phosphatases. Biochem J 2003; 371(Pt 1): 15-27.
[http://dx.doi.org/10.1042/bj20021637] [PMID: 12485116]

[33]   Grzesiek S, Stahl SJ, Wingfield PT, Bax A. The CD4 determinant for downregulation by HIV-1 Nef directly binds to Nef. Mapping of the Nef binding surface by NMR. Biochemistry 1996; 35(32): 10256-61.
[http://dx.doi.org/10.1021/bi9611164] [PMID: 8756680]

[34]   Preusser A, Briese L, Baur AS, Willbold D. Direct *in vitro* binding of full-length human immunodeficiency virus type 1 Nef protein to CD4 cytoplasmic domain. J Virol 2001; 75(8): 3960-4.
[http://dx.doi.org/10.1128/JVI.75.8.3960-3964.2001] [PMID: 11264384]

[35]   Lindwasser OW, Smith WJ, Chaudhuri R, Yang P, Hurley JH, Bonifacino JS. A diacidic motif in human immunodeficiency virus type 1 Nef is a novel determinant of binding to AP-2. J Virol 2008; 82(3): 1166-74.
[http://dx.doi.org/10.1128/JVI.01874-07] [PMID: 18032517]

[36]   Chaudhuri R, Mattera R, Lindwasser OW, Robinson MS, Bonifacino JS. A basic patch on alpha-adaptin is required for binding of human immunodeficiency virus type 1 Nef and cooperative assembly of a CD4-Nef-AP-2 complex. J Virol 2009; 83(6): 2518-30.
[http://dx.doi.org/10.1128/JVI.02227-08] [PMID: 19129443]

[37]   Arora VK, Molina RP, Foster JL, *et al.* Lentivirus Nef specifically activates Pak2. J Virol 2000; 74(23): 11081-7.
[http://dx.doi.org/10.1128/JVI.74.23.11081-11087.2000] [PMID: 11070003]

[38]   Agopian K, Wei BL, Garcia JV, Gabuzda D. A hydrophobic binding surface on the human immunodeficiency virus type 1 Nef core is critical for association with p21-activated kinase 2. J Virol 2006; 80(6): 3050-61.
[http://dx.doi.org/10.1128/JVI.80.6.3050-3061.2006] [PMID: 16501114]

[39]   Foster JL, Molina RP, Luo T, *et al.* Genetic and functional diversity of human immunodeficiency virus type 1 subtype B Nef primary isolates. J Virol 2001; 75(4): 1672-80.
[http://dx.doi.org/10.1128/JVI.75.4.1672-1680.2001] [PMID: 11160665]

[40]   O'Neill E, Kuo LS, Krisko JF, Tomchick DR, Garcia JV, Foster JL. Dynamic evolution of the human immunodeficiency virus type 1 pathogenic factor, Nef. J Virol 2006; 80(3): 1311-20.
[http://dx.doi.org/10.1128/JVI.80.3.1311-1320.2006] [PMID: 16415008]

[41]   Schindler M, Rajan D, Specht A, *et al.* Association of Nef with p21-activated kinase 2 is dispensable for efficient human immunodeficiency virus type 1 replication and cytopathicity in *ex vivo*-infected human lymphoid tissue. J Virol 2007; 81(23): 13005-14.
[http://dx.doi.org/10.1128/JVI.01436-07] [PMID: 17881449]

[42]   Fenard D, Yonemoto W, de Noronha C, Cavrois M, Williams SA, Greene WC. Nef is physically recruited into the immunological synapse and potentiates T cell activation early after TCR engagement. J Immunol 2005; 175(9): 6050-7.
[http://dx.doi.org/10.4049/jimmunol.175.9.6050] [PMID: 16237100]

[43]   Vallabhapurapu S, Karin M. Regulation and function of NF-kappaB transcription factors in the

immune system. Annu Rev Immunol 2009; 27: 693-733.
[http://dx.doi.org/10.1146/annurev.immunol.021908.132641] [PMID: 19302050]

[44]   Li Q, Verma IM. NF-kappaB regulation in the immune system. Nat Rev Immunol 2002; 2(10): 725-34.
[http://dx.doi.org/10.1038/nri910] [PMID: 12360211]

[45]   Zhong H, Voll RE, Ghosh S. Phosphorylation of NF-kappa B p65 by PKA stimulates transcriptional activity by promoting a novel bivalent interaction with the coactivator CBP/p300. Mol Cell 1998; 1(5): 661-71.
[http://dx.doi.org/10.1016/S1097-2765(00)80066-0] [PMID: 9660950]

[46]   Vermeulen L, De Wilde G, Van Damme P, Vanden Berghe W, Haegeman G. Transcriptional activation of the NF-kappaB p65 subunit by mitogen- and stress-activated protein kinase-1 (MSK1). EMBO J 2003; 22(6): 1313-24.
[http://dx.doi.org/10.1093/emboj/cdg139] [PMID: 12628924]

[47]   Duran A, Diaz-Meco MT, Moscat J. Essential role of RelA Ser311 phosphorylation by zetaPKC in NF-kappaB transcriptional activation. EMBO J 2003; 22(15): 3910-8.
[http://dx.doi.org/10.1093/emboj/cdg370] [PMID: 12881425]

[48]   Sakurai H, Chiba H, Miyoshi H, Sugita T, Toriumi W. IkappaB kinases phosphorylate NF-kappaB p65 subunit on serine 536 in the transactivation domain. J Biol Chem 1999; 274(43): 30353-6.
[http://dx.doi.org/10.1074/jbc.274.43.30353] [PMID: 10521409]

[49]   DeLuca C, Roulston A, Koromilas A, Wainberg MA, Hiscott J. Chronic human immunodeficiency virus type 1 infection of myeloid cells disrupts the autoregulatory control of the NF-kappaB/Rel pathway *via* enhanced IkappaBalpha degradation. J Virol 1996; 70(8): 5183-93.
[PMID: 8764027]

[50]   Bossis G, Salinas S, Cartier C, Devaux C, Briant L. NF-kappaB activation upon interaction of HIV-1 envelope glycoproteins with cell surface CD4 involves IkappaB kinases. FEBS Lett 2002; 516(1-3): 257-64.
[http://dx.doi.org/10.1016/S0014-5793(02)02566-8] [PMID: 11959143]

[51]   Bren GD, Trushin SA, Whitman J, Shepard B, Badley AD. HIV gp120 induces, NF-kappaB dependent, HIV replication that requires procaspase 8. PLoS One 2009; 4(3): e4875.
[http://dx.doi.org/10.1371/journal.pone.0004875] [PMID: 19287489]

[52]   Debaisieux S, Rayne F, Yezid H, Beaumelle B. The ins and outs of HIV-1 Tat. Traffic 2012; 13(3): 355-63.
[http://dx.doi.org/10.1111/j.1600-0854.2011.01286.x] [PMID: 21951552]

[53]   Berkhout B, Silverman RH, Jeang KT. Tat trans-activates the human immunodeficiency virus through a nascent RNA target. Cell 1989; 59(2): 273-82.
[http://dx.doi.org/10.1016/0092-8674(89)90289-4] [PMID: 2478293]

[54]   Buonaguro L, Buonaguro FM, Giraldo G, Ensoli B. The human immunodeficiency virus type 1 Tat protein transactivates tumor necrosis factor beta gene expression through a TAR-like structure. J Virol 1994; 68(4): 2677-82.
[PMID: 8139045]

[55] Ambrosino C, Ruocco MR, Chen X, *et al.* HIV-1 Tat induces the expression of the interleukin-6 (IL6) gene by binding to the IL6 leader RNA and by interacting with CAAT enhancer-binding protein beta (NF-IL6) transcription factors. J Biol Chem 1997; 272(23): 14883-92.
[http://dx.doi.org/10.1074/jbc.272.23.14883] [PMID: 9169458]

[56] Scala G, Ruocco MR, Ambrosino C, *et al.* The expression of the interleukin 6 gene is induced by the human immunodeficiency virus 1 TAT protein. J Exp Med 1994; 179(3): 961-71.
[http://dx.doi.org/10.1084/jem.179.3.961] [PMID: 8113688]

[57] Sun SC, Ganchi PA, Ballard DW, Greene WC. NF-kappa B controls expression of inhibitor I kappa B alpha: evidence for an inducible autoregulatory pathway. Science 1993; 259(5103): 1912-5.
[http://dx.doi.org/10.1126/science.8096091] [PMID: 8096091]

[58] Fiume G, Vecchio E, De Laurentiis A, *et al.* Human immunodeficiency virus-1 Tat activates NF-κB via physical interaction with IκB-α and p65. Nucleic Acids Res 2012; 40(8): 3548-62.
[http://dx.doi.org/10.1093/nar/gkr1224] [PMID: 22187158]

[59] Goh WC, Rogel ME, Kinsey CM, *et al.* HIV-1 Vpr increases viral expression by manipulation of the cell cycle: a mechanism for selection of Vpr *in vivo.* Nat Med 1998; 4(1): 65-71.
[http://dx.doi.org/10.1038/nm0198-065] [PMID: 9427608]

[60] Pines J, Hunter T. Human cyclins A and B1 are differentially located in the cell and undergo cell cycle-dependent nuclear transport. J Cell Biol 1991; 115(1): 1-17.
[http://dx.doi.org/10.1083/jcb.115.1.1] [PMID: 1717476]

[61] Russell P, Nurse P. cdc25+ functions as an inducer in the mitotic control of fission yeast. Cell 1986; 45(1): 145-53.
[http://dx.doi.org/10.1016/0092-8674(86)90546-5] [PMID: 3955656]

[62] Lew DJ, Kornbluth S. Regulatory roles of cyclin dependent kinase phosphorylation in cell cycle control. Curr Opin Cell Biol 1996; 8(6): 795-804.
[http://dx.doi.org/10.1016/S0955-0674(96)80080-9] [PMID: 8939679]

[63] Peng CY, Graves PR, Thoma RS, Wu Z, Shaw AS, Piwnica-Worms H. Mitotic and G2 checkpoint control: regulation of 14-3-3 protein binding by phosphorylation of Cdc25C on serine-216. Science 1997; 277(5331): 1501-5.
[http://dx.doi.org/10.1126/science.277.5331.1501] [PMID: 9278512]

[64] de Noronha CM, Sherman MP, Lin HW, *et al.* Dynamic disruptions in nuclear envelope architecture and integrity induced by HIV-1 Vpr. Science 2001; 294(5544): 1105-8.
[http://dx.doi.org/10.1126/science.1063957] [PMID: 11691994]

[65] Hrimech M, Yao XJ, Branton PE, Cohen EA. Human immunodeficiency virus type 1 Vpr-mediated G(2) cell cycle arrest: Vpr interferes with cell cycle signaling cascades by interacting with the B subunit of serine/threonine protein phosphatase 2A. EMBO J 2002; 21(14): 3918.
[PMID: 12110603]

[66] Zhou BB, Elledge SJ. The DNA damage response: putting checkpoints in perspective. Nature 2000; 408(6811): 433-9.
[http://dx.doi.org/10.1038/35044005] [PMID: 11100718]

[67] Sanchez Y, Wong C, Thoma RS, *et al.* Conservation of the Chk1 checkpoint pathway in mammals:

linkage of DNA damage to Cdk regulation through Cdc25. Science 1997; 277(5331): 1497-501. [http://dx.doi.org/10.1126/science.277.5331.1497] [PMID: 9278511]

[68] Baber-Furnari BA, Rhind N, Boddy MN, Shanahan P, Lopez-Girona A, Russell P. Regulation of mitotic inhibitor Mik1 helps to enforce the DNA damage checkpoint. Mol Biol Cell 2000; 11(1): 1-11. [http://dx.doi.org/10.1091/mbc.11.1.1] [PMID: 10637286]

[69] Westphal CH. Cell-cycle signaling: Atm displays its many talents. Curr Biol 1997; 7(12): R789-92. [http://dx.doi.org/10.1016/S0960-9822(06)00406-4] [PMID: 9382823]

[70] Cliby WA, Lewis KA, Lilly KK, Kaufmann SH. S phase and G2 arrests induced by topoisomerase I poisons are dependent on ATR kinase function. J Biol Chem 2002; 277(2): 1599-606. [http://dx.doi.org/10.1074/jbc.M106287200] [PMID: 11700302]

[71] Zou L, Cortez D, Elledge SJ. Regulation of ATR substrate selection by Rad17-dependent loading of Rad9 complexes onto chromatin. Genes Dev 2002; 16(2): 198-208. [http://dx.doi.org/10.1101/gad.950302] [PMID: 11799063]

[72] Zhu Y, Gelbard HA, Roshal M, Pursell S, Jamieson BD, Planelles V. Comparison of cell cycle arrest, transactivation, and apoptosis induced by the simian immunodeficiency virus SIVagm and human immunodeficiency virus type 1 vpr genes. J Virol 2001; 75(8): 3791-801. [http://dx.doi.org/10.1128/JVI.75.8.3791-3801.2001] [PMID: 11264368]

[73] Poon B, Jowett JB, Stewart SA, Armstrong RW, Rishton GM, Chen IS. Human immunodeficiency virus type 1 vpr gene induces phenotypic effects similar to those of the DNA alkylating agent, nitrogen mustard. J Virol 1997; 71(5): 3961-71. [PMID: 9094673]

[74] Zhang S, Pointer D, Singer G, Feng Y, Park K, Zhao LJ. Direct binding to nucleic acids by Vpr of human immunodeficiency virus type 1. Gene 1998; 212(2): 157-66. [http://dx.doi.org/10.1016/S0378-1119(98)00178-4] [PMID: 9611258]

[75] Roshal M, Kim B, Zhu Y, Nghiem P, Planelles V. Activation of the ATR-mediated DNA damage response by the HIV-1 viral protein R. J Biol Chem 2003; 278(28): 25879-86. [http://dx.doi.org/10.1074/jbc.M303948200] [PMID: 12738771]

[76] Yoshizuka N, Yoshizuka-Chadani Y, Krishnan V, Zeichner SL. Human immunodeficiency virus type 1 Vpr-dependent cell cycle arrest through a mitogen-activated protein kinase signal transduction pathway. J Virol 2005; 79(17): 11366-81. [http://dx.doi.org/10.1128/JVI.79.17.11366-11381.2005] [PMID: 16103188]

[77] Cummins NW, Badley AD. Mechanisms of HIV-associated lymphocyte apoptosis: 2010. Cell Death Dis 2010; 1: e99. [http://dx.doi.org/10.1038/cddis.2010.77] [PMID: 21368875]

[78] Perelson AS, Neumann AU, Markowitz M, Leonard JM, Ho DD. HIV-1 dynamics *in vivo*: virion clearance rate, infected cell life-span, and viral generation time. Science 1996; 271(5255): 1582-6. [http://dx.doi.org/10.1126/science.271.5255.1582] [PMID: 8599114]

[79] Andersen JL, Zimmerman ES, DeHart JL, *et al.* ATR and GADD45alpha mediate HIV-1 Vpr-induced apoptosis. Cell Death Differ 2005; 12(4): 326-34. [http://dx.doi.org/10.1038/sj.cdd.4401565] [PMID: 15650754]

[80]   Andersen JL, DeHart JL, Zimmerman ES, *et al*. HIV-1 Vpr-induced apoptosis is cell cycle dependent and requires Bax but not ANT. PLoS Pathog 2006; 2(12): e127.
[http://dx.doi.org/10.1371/journal.ppat.0020127] [PMID: 17140287]

[81]   Yuan H, Kamata M, Xie YM, Chen IS. Increased levels of Wee-1 kinase in G(2) are necessary for Vpr- and gamma irradiation-induced G(2) arrest. J Virol 2004; 78(15): 8183-90.
[http://dx.doi.org/10.1128/JVI.78.15.8183-8190.2004] [PMID: 15254189]

[82]   Kaukonen J, Juselius JK, Tiranti V, *et al*. Role of adenine nucleotide translocator 1 in mtDNA maintenance. Science 2000; 289(5480): 782-5.
[http://dx.doi.org/10.1126/science.289.5480.782] [PMID: 10926541]

[83]   Konishi A, Shimizu S, Hirota J, *et al*. Involvement of histone H1.2 in apoptosis induced by DNA double-strand breaks. Cell 2003; 114(6): 673-88.
[http://dx.doi.org/10.1016/S0092-8674(03)00719-0] [PMID: 14505568]

[84]   Stewart SA, Poon B, Song JY, Chen IS. Human immunodeficiency virus type 1 vpr induces apoptosis through caspase activation. J Virol 2000; 74(7): 3105-11.
[http://dx.doi.org/10.1128/JVI.74.7.3105-3111.2000] [PMID: 10708425]

[85]   Muthumani K, Hwang DS, Desai BM, *et al*. HIV-1 Vpr induces apoptosis through caspase 9 in T cells and peripheral blood mononuclear cells. J Biol Chem 2002; 277(40): 37820-31.
[http://dx.doi.org/10.1074/jbc.M205313200] [PMID: 12095993]

[86]   Gross A, McDonnell JM, Korsmeyer SJ. BCL-2 family members and the mitochondria in apoptosis. Genes Dev 1999; 13(15): 1899-911.
[http://dx.doi.org/10.1101/gad.13.15.1899] [PMID: 10444588]

CHAPTER 6

Determinants of HIV Pathogenesis Related to Disease Progression

Zahra Goodarzi[1], Seyed Hadi Razavi[2,*] and Asghar Abdoli[3]

[1] *Applied Virology Research Center, Baqyatallah University of Medical Sciences, Tehran, Iran*

[2] *Department of Microbiology, Faculty of Medicine, Golestan University of Medical Sciences, Gorgan, Iran*

[3] *Department of Hepatitis and AIDS, Pasteur Institute of Iran, Tehran, Iran*

Abstract: HIV infection is regarded as one of the most important causes of mortality disease worldwide. The pathogenesis of HIV infection is complex and a multi-factorial process that is influenced by both viral and host factors. These factors play an important role in disease progression in HIV infected people. The HIV infected individuals eventually develop AIDS in a different progressive rate. The biological correlates to progression rate toward AIDS remain to be elusive. A variety of factors including host genetic susceptibility, immune function, viral genetic variability and co-infections with several microbial agents may affect the rate of progression of infection. This chapter provides information on most important factors that regulate the rate of progression of HIV infection toward AIDS.

Keywords: AIDS, CCR5, CXCR4, Cytokines, Dendritic cells, HIV, HLA-B27 antigen, HLA-B 57 antigen, Interferon gamma, Pathogenesis.

1. INTRODUCTION

In 1981, a new syndrome was observed in the United States that was determined by a profound unexplained immune deficiency [1]. Patients presented with abnormal infections and cancers such as *Pneumocystis jiroveci* (carinii)

---

* **Correspondence to Seyed Hadi Razavi:** Faculty of Medical Sciences, Tarbiat Modares University, Tehran, Iran; Tel/Fax: +98(21)82883581; E-mail: hadi_razavi@yahoo.com.

SeyedAhmad SeyedAlinaghi (Ed.)

pneumonia and Kaposi's sarcoma. This Acquired Immune Deficiency Syndrome (AIDS) consisted of a marked reduction in CD4 T cell numbers and enhanced B-cell proliferation and hyper-gammaglobulinemia. This latter finding most likely reflects immune activation, which has recently been reappreciated as a major cause of the pathogenic pathway. In this regard, chronic inflammation has received better attention as a cause of cancer, cardiovascular diseases, and other co-morbidities appearing in long-term HIV infected people [2 - 4]. HIV-1 infection has increasingly developed around the world and become a dominant cause of death in infectious diseases in some areas. Following infection with HIV-1, the clinical course and the rate of progression toward AIDS seem to be highly variable among patients.

In fact, the rate of progression toward AIDS includes three basic types: (i) classical progression course (the most common clinical course), when AIDS becomes apparent after an interval of three to 10 years after seroconversion; (ii) long-term non-progression (LTNP) when seropositive patients remain AIDS-free for more than 10 years. In this group there are two subgroups: 1, virologic controllers who maintain the viral load below 2,000 RNA copies/mL and 2, elite controllers who have undetectable viral load or below 50 RNA copies/mL; and (iii) rapid progression (RP), where AIDS spreads within two to three years of infection [5 - 7]. Such clinical courses of progression toward AIDS depend on possible combinations of viral, host and environmental factors. In this chapter, we outline the most important factors that seem to regulate the HIV-1 infection rate of progress to AIDS.

2. DETERMINANTS OF HIV PATHOGENESIS

2.1. Host Genetic

Generally speaking, the host genetic variability contributes to determine whether an individual is susceptible or resistant to potentially pathogenic infections. Host genetic factors have a great role in the consequences of complicated or multi-factorial diseases such as AIDS which are also regarded as important to regulate disease progression rates. With regard to AIDS, several reports have shown the strong and/or weak associations between certain host genes and the variable rates of progression toward AIDS. The selective host genes and factors which are suspected to contribute to the progression rate from HIV infection to AIDS can be divided into two categories:

A. Genes which encode cell-surface receptors or their ligands
B. Genes within human leukocyte antigens (HLA) and Killer cell Immunoglobulin-like Receptors (KIRs) regulating host immune responses to infection.

A. Genes Encoding Cell-surface Receptors or their Ligands

The entrance of HIV into cells occurs through an interaction with both CD4 and chemokine receptors of seven trans-membrane family, CCR5 and CXCR4. CCR5 exhibits different variants in its coding region, the deletion of a 32-bp segment named CCR5-Δ32 (CCR5 delta 32) results in a nonfunctional receptor, and multiple studies suggest that the existence of a single copy of this mutation causes the progression toward AIDS to dealy by about two years as it prevents HIV infection; rather, two copies of the gene establish a strong protection against HIV entry, albeit it is not a complete protection. This allele is observed in about 10% of Europeans, although rare in Africans and Asians. Beyond the genetic determinants of CCR5 expression, it is suggested that an increased number of CCL3L1 gene copy (encoding the natural ligand of CCR5, MIP-1α) may decrease the risk of HIV infection and cause a delay in clinical progression in HIV-infected subjects [5, 8 - 10].

B. Genes within Human Leukocyte Antigens (HLA) that Regulate Host Immune Responses to Infection

Host defenses have a great role in the course of HIV acquisition. The importance of diversity of T-cell recognition in disease control was suggested after realizing that homozygosity for class I HLA molecules is associated with an accelerated disease course [11]. On the other hand, certain class I HLA types are associated with a more benign disease course. It has been reported that HLA-B*27, HLA-B*57and HLA-Bw*4 exert a preventive impact with regard to progressive AIDS in patients with HIV-1 infection [12]. An immunological description for the defective role HLA B27 plays in HIV disease is that B27[+] patients show certain and robust CTL responses against a p24 epitope and p24 protein is highly conserved among HIV isolates [13].

The significance of the HLA-B*57 restricted epitopes is relatively resulted from the fitness cost of evade from mutations taking place in regions of Gag. It seems that the frequency of Gag specific CD8$^+$ T cells is associated with the capability of primary CD8$^+$ T cells to prevent viral replication [7]. Further, the importance of HLA-B*27, HLA-B*57 and HLA-Bw*4 is accompanied by the NK cell responses. Inhibiting NK lysis of autologous targets, these HLA alleles function as certain ligands for NK cell inhibitory receptors or KIRs [14 - 16]. On the contrary to the above reports, a large number of studies have also highlighted the significance of certain HLA alleles in accelerated progression of HIV-1 infection to AIDS. It appears that the strongest susceptibility is conferred by HLA-B*3- -Px, Cw*04 allele which contiibutes to virus escape from the defective immunity through lowering the NK cell activity against HIV-1 [17, 18].

A very small proportion of infected persons seem to maintain HIV replication under the lack of antiretroviral treatment. Elite Suppressors (ES) refer untreated HIV-1-infected subjects who control viremia to levels below the limit of detection for currently available assays [11, 19]. A growing body of evidence supports the idea that T-cell-mediated responses against HIV are important determinants of elite control [20]. Approximately, half of these elite controllers express HLA-B57, HLA-B5801 or HLA-B27. Thus, certain HLA class I alleles are more prevalent in HIV controllers and are associated with strong HIV-specific T cells responses [21].

2.2. Cytokines and Immune Cell Responses

It was identified that the progression of HIV infection to AIDS may be maintained by establishing an equilibrium between type 1 cytokines (primarily enhancing cell-mediated immunity) and type 2 cytokines (primarily augmenting antibody production). Therefore, HIV progression was observed with a decrease in *in vitro* production of interleukin-2 (IL-2), IL-12 and interferon gamma (IFN-γ) (type 1 cytokines) and an increase in the production of IL-4, IL-5, IL-6 and IL-10 (type 2 cytokines) by peripheral blood mononuclear cells of HIV-seropositive subjects.

Thus, the type 1 to type 2 shifts may be determinants for these events: (i) decline in the number of CD4; (ii) accelerated progression to AIDS; (iii) poor prognosis and mortality. In fact, high concentrations of type 2 cytokines correlate with lower counts of CD4 cells in HIV infection [22]. A decrease in IFN-γ production rate was accompanied with an increase in the risk of CD4 counts below 100 cells/mm3 and mortality. Thus, alterations in the production of IFN-γ seem to be associated with the risk of disease progression in HIV infection. IL-1β and TNFα are considered as pro-inflammatory cytokines, they play a critical role in the pathogenesis and progression of HIV-1 infection. TNF-α and IL-1β can improve the permeability of blood brain barrier for HIV-1 infected mononuclear-macrophages to enter the brain, and meanwhile they can enhance the virus replication, and stimulate inflammatory reaction working together with chemotatic factors . In addition, TNF-α can boost the injury sensitivity of glial cells, and cause neurons apoptosis through the glutamic acid, calcium disorders and oxidative stress mechanism. IL-1β can affect cell migration, stimulate nerve cell proliferation, and mediate the virus neurotoxic action and neurodegeneration [23].

2.3. The Role of NK Cell and Dendritic Cells

Decreased counts of NK cells in the blood is associated with a quick disease progression, it means that defective non-MHC restricted cytotoxicity is involved in acceleration of HIV infection progression [24]. Furthermore, the findings suggest that loss of Plasmacytoid Dendritic Cells (pDC) in HIV infection may contribute to disease progression [25]. Historically, the pDCs have been regarded as natural interferon-producing cells, responding to stimulation of Toll-like Receptor (TLR)-7 and -9 in humans, which is responsible for the response to a wide range of enveloped viruses such as HIV [26]. The production of type I IFN in to the face of HIV acquisition *in vitro* and *in vivo* demonstrates the role pDCs play in anti-HIV immunity. If type I IFN production is low then the disease progression is accelerated. This could be explained because pDCs express CD4 and the chemokine receptors CCR5 and CXCR4, they show multinuclear cell syncytia formation and death following infection. The decreased number of pDCs and type I IFN is inversely correlated with viral load and progression to AIDS [27, 28].

2.4. Chronic Immune Activation

High-level immune activation and T cell apoptosis indicate a progressive HIV infection. Chronic immune activation predicts disease outcome. As recent studies reported, *nef* alleles from primate lentiviruses, such as HIV-2, down-regulate TCR-CD3 of infected T cells, leading to blocked responsiveness to the activation. On the other hand, *nef* alleles from HIV-1 fail to down-regulate TCR-CD3 and to inhibit cell death [27, 29]. Therefore, Nef-mediated suppression of T cell activation represents a critical characteristic of primate lentiviruses potentially associated with maintaining viral persistence in intact host immune systems. Furthermore, opportunistic infection or their circulating products which are propagated from the gastrointestinal tract, cause systemic chronic immune activation [30]. Opportunistic pathogens and their components intruding across disrupted intestinal mucosa stimulate innate immunity and create a milieu having markedly elevated pro-inflammatory cytokines and chemokines. Broad innate immune activation results in acceleration of thymic T cell regeneration and naïve T cell delivery to mucosa sites. This compensatory renewal fuels targets for HIV infection, further increasing the level of specific or non-specific immune activation and gradually exacerbating the problem [31].

2.5. Intrinsic Intracellular Factors

The important role of intrinsic intracellular anti-HIV resistance factors has recently been determined. APOBEC3G and 3F, a cytosine deaminase, alters single stranded DNA synthesis during reverse transcription and causes the production of an inactive DNA product that is degraded by the cell [32]. APOBEC3G prevents viral cDNA synthesis via deaminating deoxycytidines (dC) in the minus-strand retroviral cDNA replication intermediate. As a result, it creates stop codons or G-A transitions in the newly synthesized viral cDNA which is then subject to elimination by host DNA repair machinery. APOBEC3G confers its antiviral effect by encapsidating into the virus particles through interaction with viral Gag protein and thus, APOBEC3G represents an innate host defense mechanism against HIV infection. However, the virus has also developed an offensive strategy to suppress the antiviral effect of APOBEC3G through Vif. Recent studies suggested that a higher expression of APOBEC3G within the cell is associated with lower viral replication during acute infection [33].

2.6. Other Factors Related to Host

Many observational studies have found that low blood levels of vitamins, in particular vitamin A and D are associated with rapid HIV disease progression and death. Vitamin A is important for immunity, growth and development, and the production of red blood cells. It is a major factor in the development and differentiation of white blood cells, such as lymphocytes, necessary for immunity responses. The first line of body protection against infection is exhibited by the skin and mucosa, the integrity of which is maintained by vitamin A. The antimicrobial impacts of vitamin D have been well documented and related research report that lower levels of 25D3 and/or 1,25D3 influences innate immunity in response to HIV acquisition and its deficiency is related with inflammation and quick progression of HIV infection. Therefore, multivitamin supplements seem to delay the spread of HIV, especially in poorer populations [34 - 40]. In addition to nuritional components, age plays a great role to determine the survival and disease progression rates. In fact, patients over 40 years of age at sero-conversion exhibit a more rapid progression toward AIDS [41, 42].

3. VIRUS DETERMINANTS

3.1. HIV-1 Evolution

At least 10 different genetic HIV-1 subtypes (A-J) have a role in the AIDS pandemic. The HIV-1 subtype contributes to the progression rate to AIDS. Subjects with subtypes C, D and G infections are eight times more likely to progress AIDS compared to those infected with subtype A [43]. In addition, occasional variability in disease course may be owing to variations in HIV itself. Certain deletions in the nef gene and mutations in the vpr gene have been associated with a slower disease course [44 - 46]. These data show that survival after HIV infection is also correlated with the HIV genome.

HIV changes in the use of coreceptors have been previously shown during the infection, and such adaptation is involved in the progression to AIDS. Primary isolates of HIV-1 exhibit distinguished variations in their biological properties *in vitro*, such as differences in replication kinetics, tropism, and syncytium- inducing capacity. Macrophage-tropic, nonsyncytium- inducing (NSI) viruses are most commonly transmitted and predominate in early infection [47]. Syncytium-inducing (SI) isolates are usually detectable in the late stage of infection and may acquire a wide tropism *in vitro*, such as the ability to replicate in CD4 T cell lines [48]. HIV-1 tropism is heavily dependent on the env gene, which encodes the surface (gp120) and transmembrane (gp41) envelope glycoproteins [12, 49]. The T cell Line Adapted (TCLA) SI strains of HIV-1 infect CD4 T cells throught the CXCR-4 coreceptor. Another molecule-CCR5- has been defined as a co-receptor for macrophage-tropic, NSI strains of HIV-1. Disease progression in many HIV-1 infected individuals is accompanied with a shift in the viral phenotype from NSI to SI [32, 50, 51].

3.2. CD4$^+$ T cell Depletion

The Mucosal-associated Lymphoid Tissue (MALT) houses the majority of CD4$^+$ T cells in the body. More than half of the total T lymphocytes reside in GALT and a considerable part of these cells has an activated or memory phenotype. This abundance of substrate provides a histological basis for massive CD4$^+$ T cell depletion during acute infection because HIV preferentially targets activated CD4$^+$ T cells [31]. Destruction of CD4$^+$ T cells is a primary reason for the opportunistic infections and cancers associated with HIV infection. Many factors can be involved in this CD4$^+$ cell loss (Table **1**).

Table 1. Potential factors involved in HIV-induced loss of CD4$^+$ lymphocyte number and function.

Direct cytopathic effects of HIV and its proteins on CD4$^+$ cells and progenitor cells
Effect of HIV on cell membrane permeability; enhanced fragility of CD4$^+$ cells
Induction of apoptosis *via* immune activation
Destruction of bone marrow (*e.g.*, stem cells, stromal cells)
Cytokine cytotoxicity
Destruction of lymphoid tissue (*e.g.*, thymus) and reduced Production of new cells
Anti- CD4$^+$ cell cytotoxic activity (CD8$^+$ and CD4$^+$ cells; NK cells)
Anti- CD4$^+$ cell autoantibodies

For example certain cytokines (*i.e.* TNF-a) and HIV proteins (*i.e.* Tat, Nef, Vpr,

Vpu) can influence the extent of HIV replication and CD4$^+$ cell death. Other processes involved in this CD4$^+$ cell loss can include the conventional disruption in metabolic processes and cell membrane integrity by HIV causing necrosis. In many cases, apoptosis results from direct viral infection or an indirect effect of immune activation. More recently, autophagy has been noted as a possible cause of bystander CD4$^+$ cell death with HIV infection [52]. Another reason can be CD8$^+$ Cytotoxic T cell (CTL) activity against normal CD4$^+$ cells [53]. The reduction in the peripheral blood CD4$^+$ cell count over time also results from a block in T cell restoration processes in the thymus [54].

4. THE EFFECT OF CO-INFECTIONS ON PROGRESSION RATES

Co-infection and the subsequent immune activation may enhance viral replication, the immunopathogenesis, transmission and faster progression to AIDS. This activation results in facilitating the three key stages of the viral life cycle: entrance into cells, reverse transcription and pro-viral transcription [55]. Chemokine receptors have a critical role in the entry of HIV into cells. Their expression is the product of immune activation, which would augment the number of cells potentially infected by HIV-1. For example, the expression of CXCR4 and CCR5 were elevated on CD4 T cells in blood samples from patients with tuberculosis. As suggested, the up-regulation of CXCR4 and CCR5 on CD4 T cells cause an increase in HIV viremia related to tuberculosis, and hence leading to accelerated progression of HIV infection [55 - 57]. Thus, the influence of co-infections by micro-organisms including Mycobacterium tuberculosis is of great importance in disease progression, especially for those with a high prevalence of chronic and recurrent acute infections and poor access to medical care.

In an infected cell, both reverse transcription of the HIV-1 genome and the rate of transcription of proviral DNA rely upon the activation of the cell. This observation is explained by an increase in the cytoplasmic concentrations of mediators required for reverse transcription of the HIV genome in activated cells [58, 59]. Activated cells also release IFN-alpha which up-regulates the rates of physiologically active NF-kappa B that in turn activates both host cell genes and HIV-1 LTR [47, 60 - 62]. Co-infection with some DNA viruses such type 1 herpes simplex virus, varicella zoster virus, Epstein-Barr virus (EBV), JC virus,

BK virus, papilloma virus, and cytomegalovirus can stimulate the expression of HIV and therefore increase viral loads as they may encode proteins capable to trans-activate the expression of the HIV-1 pro-viral DNA [63, 64].

CONCLUDING REMARKS AND FUTURE PERSPECTIVES

As this chapter illustrated, an enormous amount of information has been obtained over the past two decades regarding the molecular and biological aspects of the HIV-1 pathogenesis. The pathogenesis of HIV infection is a multi-factorial process that is influenced by both viral and host factors and is reflected by the highly variable rates of disease progressions that are observed in individuals infected with HIV. The importance of viral and host factors in modulating rates of disease progression is further underscored by the observation that even individuals who were apparently infected from a common source may experience widely variant clinical outcomes. Recent insights into the pathogenesis of HIV infection highlight several new and promising areas of investigation.

CONFLICT OF INTEREST

The authors confirm that they have no conflict of interest to declare for this publication.

ACKNOWLEDGEMENTS

Declared none.

REFERENCES

[1]   Centers for Disease Control (CDC). Pneumocystis pneumonia--Los Angeles. MMWR Morb Mortal Wkly Rep 1981; 30(21): 250-2.
        [PMID: 6265753]

[2]   Barre-Sinoussi F, Chermann JC, Rey F, *et al.* Isolation of a T-lymphotropic retrovirus from a patient at risk for acquired immune deficiency syndrome (AIDS). 1983 Revista de investigacion clinica; organo del Hospital de Enfermedades de la Nutricion 2004; 56(5): 9-126.

[3]   Gallo RC, Salahuddin SZ, Popovic M, *et al.* Frequent detection and isolation of cytopathic retroviruses (HTLV-III) from patients with AIDS and at risk for AIDS. Science 1984; 224(4648): 500-3.
        [http://dx.doi.org/10.1126/science.6200936] [PMID: 6200936]

[4]   Levy JA, Hoffman AD, Kramer SM, Landis JA, Shimabukuro JM, Oshiro LS. Isolation of lymphocytopathic retroviruses from San Francisco patients with AIDS. Science 1984; 225(4664): 840-

2.
[http://dx.doi.org/10.1126/science.6206563] [PMID: 6206563]

[5]   Hunt PW, Carrington M. Host genetic determinants of HIV pathogenesis: an immunologic perspective. Curr Opin HIV AIDS 2008; 3(3): 342-8.
[http://dx.doi.org/10.1097/COH.0b013e3282fbaa92] [PMID: 19372988]

[6]   Morgan D, Mahe C, Mayanja B, Okongo JM, Lubega R, Whitworth JA. HIV-1 infection in rural Africa: is there a difference in median time to AIDS and survival compared with that in industrialized countries? AIDS 2002; 16(4): 597-603.
[http://dx.doi.org/10.1097/00002030-200203080-00011] [PMID: 11873003]

[7]   O'Connell KA, Bailey JR, Blankson JN. Elucidating the elite: mechanisms of control in HIV-1 infection. Trends Pharmacol Sci 2009; 30(12): 631-7.
[http://dx.doi.org/10.1016/j.tips.2009.09.005] [PMID: 19837464]

[8]   Liu R PW, Choe S, Ceradini D, *et al.* Homozygous defect in HIV-1 coreceptor accounts for resistance of some multiply-exposed individuals to HIV-1 infection cell 1996; 86(3): 367-77.

[9]   Wasik TJ, Smoleń J, Kruszyński P, Bratosiewicz-Wasik J, Beniowski M. Effects of CCR5-delta32, CCR2-64I and SDF-1-3'A polymorphic alleles on human immunodeficiency virus 1 (HIV-1) infection in the Polish population. Wiad Lek 2005; 58(9-10): 500-7.
[PMID: 16529059]

[10]   Reiche EM, Bonametti AM, Voltarelli JC, Morimoto HK, Watanabe MA. Genetic polymorphisms in the chemokine and chemokine receptors: impact on clinical course and therapy of the human immunodeficiency virus type 1 infection (HIV-1). Curr Med Chem 2007; 14(12): 1325-34.
[http://dx.doi.org/10.2174/092986707780597934] [PMID: 17504215]

[11]   Lackner AA LM, Rodriguez B. HIV pathogenesis: the host. Cold Spring Harb Perspect Med 2012; 2(9): a007005.
[http://dx.doi.org/10.1101/cshperspect.a007005]

[12]   Gao X, Bashirova A, Iversen AK, *et al.* AIDS restriction HLA allotypes target distinct intervals of HIV-1 pathogenesis. Nat Med 2005; 11(12): 1290-2.
[http://dx.doi.org/10.1038/nm1333] [PMID: 16288280]

[13]   den Uyl D, van der Horst-Bruinsma IE, van Agtmael M. Progression of HIV to AIDS: a protective role for HLA-B27? AIDS Rev 2004; 6(2): 89-96.
[PMID: 15332431]

[14]   Martin MP, Qi Y, Gao X, *et al.* Innate partnership of HLA-B and KIR3DL1 subtypes against HIV-1. Nat Genet 2007; 39(6): 733-40.
[http://dx.doi.org/10.1038/ng2035] [PMID: 17496894]

[15]   D'Andrea A CC, Franz-Bacon K, McClanahan T, Phillips JH, Lanier LL. A natural killer cell receptor for HLA-B allotypes J Immunol 1995; 1155(5): 2306-10.

[16]   Martin MP, Gao X, Lee JH, *et al.* Epistatic interaction between KIR3DS1 and HLA-B delays the progression to AIDS. Nat Genet 2002; 31(4): 429-34.
[PMID: 12134147]

[17]   Gao X, Nelson GW, Karacki P, *et al.* Effect of a single amino acid change in MHC class I molecules

on the rate of progression to AIDS. N Engl J Med 2001; 344(22): 1668-75.
[http://dx.doi.org/10.1056/NEJM200105313442203] [PMID: 11386265]

[18]   K. C. Host genetic factors in susceptibility to HIV-1 infection and progression to AIDS. J Genet 2010;
20(2): 26-9.

[19]   Blankson JN, Bailey JR, Thayil S, *et al*. Isolation and characterization of replication-competent human
immunodeficiency virus type 1 from a subset of elite suppressors. J Virol 2007; 81(5): 2508-18.
[http://dx.doi.org/10.1128/JVI.02165-06] [PMID: 17151109]

[20]   Blankson JN. Control of HIV-1 replication in elite suppressors. Discov Med 2010; 9(46): 261-6.
[PMID: 20350494]

[21]   Emu B, Sinclair E, Hatano H, *et al*. HLA class I-restricted T-cell responses may contribute to the
control of human immunodeficiency virus infection, but such responses are not always necessary for
long-term virus control. J Virol 2008; 82(11): 5398-407.
[http://dx.doi.org/10.1128/JVI.02176-07] [PMID: 18353945]

[22]   Clerici M, Fusi ML, Ruzzante S, *et al*. Type 1 and type 2 cytokines in HIV infection -- a possible role
in apoptosis and disease progression. Ann Med 1997; 29(3): 185-8.
[http://dx.doi.org/10.3109/07853899708999334] [PMID: 9240622]

[23]   Zhao L, Pu SS, Gao WH, *et al*. Effects of HIV-1 tat on secretion of TNF-α and IL-1β by U87 cells in
AIDS patients with or without AIDS dementia complex. Biomed Environ Sci 2014; 27(2): 111-7.
[PMID: 24625401]

[24]   Bruunsgaard H, Pedersen C, Skinhøj P, Pedersen BK. Clinical progression of HIV infection: role of
NK cells. Scand J Immunol 1997; 46(1): 91-5.
[http://dx.doi.org/10.1046/j.1365-3083.1997.d01-98.x] [PMID: 9246213]

[25]   Donaghy H, Pozniak A, Gazzard B, *et al*. Loss of blood CD11c(+) myeloid and CD11c(-)
plasmacytoid dendritic cells in patients with HIV-1 infection correlates with HIV-1 RNA virus load.
Blood 2001; 98(8): 2574-6.
[http://dx.doi.org/10.1182/blood.V98.8.2574] [PMID: 11588058]

[26]   Steinman RM, Granelli-Piperno A, Pope M, *et al*. The interaction of immunodeficiency viruses with
dendritic cells. Curr Top Microbiol Immunol 2003; 276: 1-30.
[http://dx.doi.org/10.1007/978-3-662-06508-2_1] [PMID: 12797441]

[27]   Schmidt B, Scott I, Whitmore RG, *et al*. Low-level HIV infection of plasmacytoid dendritic cells:
onset of cytopathic effects and cell death after PDC maturation. Virology 2004; 329(2): 280-8.
[http://dx.doi.org/10.1016/j.virol.2004.08.016] [PMID: 15518808]

[28]   Müller-Trutwin M, Hosmalin A. Role for plasmacytoid dendritic cells in anti-HIV innate immunity.
Immunol Cell Biol 2005; 83(5): 578-83.
[http://dx.doi.org/10.1111/j.1440-1711.2005.01394.x] [PMID: 16174110]

[29]   Schindler M, Münch J, Kutsch O, *et al*. Nef-mediated suppression of T cell activation was lost in a
lentiviral lineage that gave rise to HIV-1. Cell 2006; 125(6): 1055-67.
[http://dx.doi.org/10.1016/j.cell.2006.04.033] [PMID: 16777597]

[30]   Brenchley JM, Price DA, Schacker TW, *et al*. Microbial translocation is a cause of systemic immune
activation in chronic HIV infection. Nat Med 2006; 12(12): 1365-71.

[http://dx.doi.org/10.1038/nm1511] [PMID: 17115046]

[31]   Li C, Hu Q-X. Driving forces of AIDS pathogenesis: Massive CD4⁺ T lymphocyte depletion and abnormal immune activation. Virol Sin 2009; 24(6): 501-8.
[http://dx.doi.org/10.1007/s12250-009-3063-y]

[32]   Berger EA, Murphy PM, Farber JM. Chemokine receptors as HIV-1 coreceptors: roles in viral entry, tropism, and disease. Annu Rev Immunol 1999; 17: 657-700.
[http://dx.doi.org/10.1146/annurev.immunol.17.1.657] [PMID: 10358771]

[33]   Bergner A, Huber RM. Regulation of the endoplasmic reticulum Ca(2⁺)-store in cancer. Anticancer Agents Med Chem 2008; 8(7): 705-9.
[http://dx.doi.org/10.2174/187152008785914734] [PMID: 18855571]

[34]   Annan RA. Vitamin A supplementation and disease progression in HIV-infected adults. World Health Organization 2011.

[35]   Fawzi WW MG, Spiegelman D, Wei R, *et al.* A randomized trial of multivitamin supplements and HIV disease progression and mortality N Engl J Med 2004; 1135(4): 23-32.

[36]   Fawzi W, Msamanga G, Spiegelman D, Hunter DJ. Studies of vitamins and minerals and HIV transmission and disease progression. J Nutr 2005; 135(4): 938-44.
[PMID: 15795466]

[37]   Mehta S FW. Effects of vitamins, including vitamin A, on HIV/AIDS patients J Nutr 2007; 75: 355-83.

[38]   Viard JP SJ, Kirk O, Reekie J, *et al.* EuroSIDA Study Group. Vitamin D and clinical disease progression in HIV infection results from the EuroSIDA study. AIDS 2011; 1925(10): 1305-15.

[39]   Ansemant T, Mahy S, Piroth C, *et al.* Severe hypovitaminosis D correlates with increased inflammatory markers in HIV infected patients. BMC Infect Dis 2013; 13(10): 7.
[http://dx.doi.org/10.1186/1471-2334-13-7] [PMID: 23295013]

[40]   Campbell GR, Spector SA. Toll-like receptor 8 ligands activate a vitamin D mediated autophagic response that inhibits human immunodeficiency virus type 1. PLoS Pathog 2012; 8(11): e1003017.
[http://dx.doi.org/10.1371/journal.ppat.1003017] [PMID: 23166493]

[41]   Time from HIV-1 seroconversion to AIDS and death before widespread use of highly-active antiretroviral therapy: a collaborative re-analysis. Collaborative Group on AIDS Incubation and HIV Survival including the CASCADE EU Concerted Action. Concerted Action on SeroConversion to AIDS and Death in Europe Lancet 2000; 355(9210): 1131-7.

[42]   Pezzotti P GN, Vlahov D, Rezza G, Lyles CM, Astemborski J. Direct comparison of time to AIDS and infectious disease death between HIV seroconverter injection drug users in Italy and the United States: results from the ALIVE and ISS studies. AIDS Link to Intravenous Experiences. Italian Seroconversion Study J Acquir Immune Defic Syndr Hum Retrovirol 1999; 20(3): 275-82.
[http://dx.doi.org/10.1097/00042560-199903010-00010]

[43]   Kanki PJ, Hamel DJ, Sankalé JL, *et al.* Human immunodeficiency virus type 1 subtypes differ in disease progression. J Infect Dis 1999; 179(1): 68-73.
[http://dx.doi.org/10.1086/314557] [PMID: 9841824]

[44] Deacon NJ TA, Solomon A, Smith K, *et al.* Genomic structure of an attenuated quasi species of HIV-1 from a blood transfusion donor and recipients Science 1995; 270(5238): 988-91.

[45] Kirchhoff F, Greenough TC, Brettler DB, Sullivan JL, Desrosiers RC. Brief report: absence of intact nef sequences in a long-term survivor with nonprogressive HIV-1 infection. N Engl J Med 1995; 332(4): 228-32.
[http://dx.doi.org/10.1056/NEJM199501263320405] [PMID: 7808489]

[46] Lum JJ, Cohen OJ, Nie Z, *et al.* Vpr R77Q is associated with long-term nonprogressive HIV infection and impaired induction of apoptosis. J Clin Invest 2003; 111(10): 1547-54.
[http://dx.doi.org/10.1172/JCI16233] [PMID: 12750404]

[47] Groenink M, Fouchier RA, de Goede RE, *et al.* Phenotypic heterogeneity in a panel of infectious molecular human immunodeficiency virus type 1 clones derived from a single individual. J Virol 1991; 65(4): 1968-75.
[PMID: 2002552]

[48] Cornelissen M, Mulder-Kampinga G, Veenstra J, *et al.* Syncytium-inducing (SI) phenotype suppression at seroconversion after intramuscular inoculation of a non-syncytium-inducing/SI phenotypically mixed human immunodeficiency virus population. J Virol 1995; 69(3): 1810-8.
[PMID: 7853521]

[49] Zhuang K FA, Toma J, Frantzell A, Huang W, Sodroski J, Cheng-Mayer C. Identification of interdependent variables that influence coreceptor switch in R5 SHIV(SF162P3N)-infected macaques. Retrovirology 2012; 09(106): 9-4690. 106
[http://dx.doi.org/10.1186/1742-4690-9-106]

[50] Connor RI SK, Ceradini D, Choe S, Landau NR. Change in coreceptor use correlates with disease progression in HIV-1--infected individuals. J Exp Med 1997; 185(4): 621-8.

[51] Xiao L RD, Owen SM, Spira TJ, Lal RB. Adaptation to promiscuous usage of CC and CXC-chemokine coreceptors *in vivo* correlates with HIV-1 disease progression. J Exp Med 1998; 12(13): 137-43.

[52] Espert L, Denizot M, Grimaldi M, *et al.* Autophagy is involved in T cell death after binding of HIV-1 envelope proteins to CXCR4. J Clin Invest 2006; 116(8): 2161-72.
[http://dx.doi.org/10.1172/JCI26185] [PMID: 16886061]

[53] Zinkernagel RM, Hengartner H. T-cell-mediated immunopathology *versus* direct cytolysis by virus: implications for HIV and AIDS. Immunol Today 1994; 15(6): 262-8.
[http://dx.doi.org/10.1016/0167-5699(94)90005-1] [PMID: 7915115]

[54] McCune JM. The dynamics of CD4$^+$ T-cell depletion in HIV disease. Nature 2001; 410(6831): 974-9.
[http://dx.doi.org/10.1038/35073648] [PMID: 11309627]

[55] Lawn SD, Butera ST, Folks TM. Contribution of immune activation to the pathogenesis and transmission of human immunodeficiency virus type 1 infection. Clin Microbiol Rev 2001; 14(4): 753-77.
[http://dx.doi.org/10.1128/CMR.14.4.753-777.2001] [PMID: 11585784]

[56] Juffermans NP, Speelman P, Verbon A, *et al.* Patients with active tuberculosis have increased expression of HIV coreceptors CXCR4 and CCR5 on CD4($^-$) T cells. Clin Infect Dis 2001; 32(4): 650-

2.
[http://dx.doi.org/10.1086/318701] [PMID: 11181132]

[57]   Wolday D TB, Kassu A, Messele T, Coutinho R, van Baarle D, Miedema F. Expression of chemokine receptors CCR5 and CXCR4 on CD4$^+$ T cells and plasma chemokine levels during treatment of active tuberculosis in HIV-1-coinfected patients J Acquir Immune Defic Syndr Hum Retrovirol 2005; 39(3): 265-71.

[58]   Arlen PA BD, Gao LY, Vatakis D, Brown HJ, Zack JA. Rapid expression of human immunodeficiency virus following activation of latently infected cells. J Virol 2006; 80(3): 603-1599.
[http://dx.doi.org/10.1128/JVI.80.3.1599-1603.2006]

[59]   Kinoshita S, Chen BK, Kaneshima H, Nolan GP. Host control of HIV-1 parasitism in T cells by the nuclear factor of activated T cells. Cell 1998; 95(5): 595-604.
[http://dx.doi.org/10.1016/S0092-8674(00)81630-X] [PMID: 9845362]

[60]   He G, Ylisastigui L, Margolis DM. The regulation of HIV-1 gene expression: the emerging role of chromatin. DNA Cell Biol 2002; 21(10): 697-705.
[http://dx.doi.org/10.1089/104454902760599672] [PMID: 12443539]

[61]   Greene WC. Regulation of HIV-1 gene expression. Annu Rev Immunol 1990; 8: 453-75.
[http://dx.doi.org/10.1146/annurev.iy.08.040190.002321] [PMID: 2188670]

[62]   Dahl V, Josefsson L, Palmer S. HIV reservoirs, latency, and reactivation: prospects for eradication. Antiviral Res 2010; 85(1): 286-94.
[http://dx.doi.org/10.1016/j.antiviral.2009.09.016] [PMID: 19808057]

[63]   Gendelman HE, Phelps W, Feigenbaum L, *et al.* Trans-activation of the human immunodeficiency virus long terminal repeat sequence by DNA viruses. Proc Natl Acad Sci USA 1986; 83(24): 9759-63.
[http://dx.doi.org/10.1073/pnas.83.24.9759] [PMID: 2432602]

[64]   Scala G, Quinto I, Ruocco MR, *et al.* Epstein-Barr virus nuclear antigen 2 transactivates the long terminal repeat of human immunodeficiency virus type 1. J Virol 1993; 67(5): 2853-61.
[PMID: 8386279]

CHAPTER 7

HIV Systems Biology

Asghar Abdoli[1,*], Zahra Goodarz[2], Mohammad Reza Aghasadeghi[1], Amin Farzanegan[3] and **Seyed Hadi Razavi[3]**

[1] *Department of Hepatitis and AIDS, Pasteur Institute of Iran, Tehran, Iran*

[2] *Applied Virology Research Center, Baqyatallah University of Medical Sciences, Tehran, Iran*

[3] *Faculty of Medical Sciences, Tarbiat Modares University, Tehran, Iran*

Abstract: The human immunodeficiency virus (HIV) belongs to the lentivirus a subgroup of Retroviruses belongs to the Retroviridae family that attacks the immune system. The last stage of HIV infection is AIDS. HIV is absurdly simple, albeit surprisingly complex. The virus is composed of nine genes encoding 15 different proteins. The literature has reported a large number of protein interactions of HIV and human proteins. Accordingly, many human host factors have been described to be important for HIV infection and replication. Systems biology (also known as Systeomics) is an approach to study systematically complex interactions within biological systems, and to integrate and analyze complex data sets from multiple experimental sources. Long-term non progressors are patients who remain AIDS-free for more than 10 years. In this group there are two subgroups: 1. virologic controllers who maintain the viral load below 2,000 RNA copies/mL and 2. elite controllers who have undetectable viral load or below 50 RNA copies/mL. Systems biology study of elite controllers provides an opportunity to analyze the immune system response which is uniquely endowed with the capacity to retain a long-term control of HIV replication.

Keywords: AIDS, Antiretroviral therapy, Elite controllers, HIV, Host cell, Immune system, Interactions, Long-term non progressors, Replication, Retroviridae, Retroviridae, Systems biology.

---

* **Correspondence to Asghar Abdoli:** Department of Hepatitis and AIDS, Pasteur Institute of Iran, Iran; Tel/Fax: +98 (21) 66969291; E-mail: asghar.abdoli7@gmail.com.

SeyedAhmad SeyedAlinaghi (Ed.)

1. INTRODUCTION

Systems biology refers to an interdisciplinary approach whose focuses is to systematically describe complex interactions between all parts of biological systems, as to elucidate novel biological rules appropriate to estimate the behavior of biological systems [1]. The approaches of systems biology represent the integration of different data types and it is the most challenging field to discover interactions between genes, transcripts, proteins, metabolites, and epigenetic regulators [2]. A hypothesis-driven analysis understands relationships intuitively and then tests them; in this regard, systems biology discloses relationships between independent sets of observations to model complex networks [3, 4]. Major advances in high throughput technologies may generate large amounts of data and a wide variety of multi-dimensional assays are available for an accurate characterization of many of the elements essential to biological systems such as: A) genomics including Single Nucleotide Polymorphisms (SNPs), recombination and Chromosomal Copy Number Variation (CNV); B) epigenomics and DNA post-translational modifications such as methylation and acetylation, C) transcriptomics including mRNA expression, microRNA expression, differential transcript detection, RNA interference screening, D) Proteomics including protein expression and localization, protein-protein interaction and E) Bioinformatics. This list can be extended with newly emerging trends, such as lipidomics, metabolomics, interactomics, localizomics, phosphoproteomics, and poly-chromatic flow cytometry made possible by newly available, high-throughput, multi-dimensional technologies [5, 6].

Complex interactions take place between HIV-1 and host target cells, where all stages of the virus infection cycle rely on the strengthen of cellular proteins and basic machineries by viral proteins [7, 8]. Once host cells infected by HIV-1, active interactions between the host and pathogen occur. The efficiency of viral infection and following progression are determined by the ultimate equilibrium among the interactions. To respond viral invasion, HIV infected cells develop different antiviral tactics including antiviral mechanisms in innate, cellular and humoral immune defenses. In contrast, the virus uses strategies against such host cellular responses [9, 10]. The pathogenesis mechanism of HIV disease is multifactorial and multiphasic and it changes in different stages of the infection

[11]. Many factors, including host genetics and epigenetics, HIV strain variation, reservoirs of pro-viral DNA integrated into the human genome and co-infection with hepatitis C virus (HCV) affect the pathogenesis of AIDS [12]. Comprehensive network analysis by system biology approach establishes a promising source to assess the interactions between the host and HIV infection and the role their functions play in the pathogenesis of AIDS. Research efforts focus on a system biology approach designed for identifying multi-parametric signatures of the efficacy of protection, prevention, and treatment through classifying wide range of observations and describing mutual relations in what formerly regarded as distinct [13, 14].

2. HIV-1-HUMAN PROTEIN INTERACTION NETWORK

HIV is absurdly simple, but surprisingly complex. The virus contains a mere 9000 bases of RNA - one millionth the amount of human cell's genetic material-and a small place of nine genes coding a few 15 proteins [10]. Nevertheless, Ptak and *et al.*, identified 1448 human proteins interacting with HIV-1 composed of 2589 unique interactions between HIV-1 to human protein. Data analysis determined direct physical interactions (binding) and indirect interactions (up-regulation through signaling pathway activation) by 32% and 68%, respectively. Surprisingly, it was found that 37% of human proteins in the database interacted with more than one HIV-1 protein. The mitogen-activated protein kinase 1, for example, shows significantly different interactions with 10 various HIV-1 proteins. Furthermore, many interactions have been reported for the HIV-1 regulatory protein Tat and envelope proteins: 30% and 33% of total interactions were identified, respectively. The database is readily accessible at http://www.ncbi.nlm.nih.gov/RefSeq/HIVInteractions/ and it is cross-linked to other National Center for Biotechnology Information databases and softwares *via* Entrez Gene. The study aims to define main factors to improve therapeutic interventions and to develop an effective vaccine [15 - 18].

3. MICRORNAS AND HIV-1: COMPLEX INTERACTIONS

Cellular miRNAs maintain the replication of HIV in two ways: target of HIV RNA or targeting the mRNAs which encode host cell factors involved in HIV replication (Table **1**) [19].

Table 1. miRNAs associated with the HIV-1 regulatory expression [adapted from Ref. 20].

Targeting	miRNAs	Target	Function
DIRECT	miR-29a	nef	Lowering HIV infectivity rate
	miR-28 miR-125b* miR-150 miR223 miR382	3'LTR	Latency in primary resting CD4$^+$ T cells Limiting HIV-1 replication in monocytes
	miR-133b miR-138 miR-149 miR-326	3'LTR**	Lowering HIV replication rate
INDIRECT	miR-17-5p miR-20a	PCAF	Lowering HIV infection rate
	miR-198	Cyclin T1	Limiting HIV-1 replication in monocytes
	miR-27b	Cyclin T1	Limiting HIV-1 replication in resting CD4$^+$ T cells
	miR-29b miR-150 miR-223	Cyclin T1***	
	miR-15a miR-15b miR-16 miR-20a miR-93 miR-106b	Pur-α	Limiting HIV-1 replication in monocytes
	miR-217	SIRT-1	Improving HIV-1 expression in MAGI cells

*miR-125b was involved in HIV-1 restriction in resting T cells only.
**This study specifically examined only the miR-326 target site.
*** Indirect regulation of cyclin T1 by miR-29b, miR-150, and miR-223.

Thus, cellular miRNAs can affect viral replication; and conversely, HIV-1 infection changes cellular miRNA profiles. For HIV-1, the viral Tat protein has been suggested to have RNAi-suppressing activity. The treatment of a neuronal cell line with soluble Vpr protein up-regulated 30 and down-regulated 15 miRNA [21 - 23].

Taken together, the findings suggest that, in divergent cells and in varying contexts, different miRNAs may selectively regulate HIV-1 replication through direct targeting of viral sequences and conversely, infection by HIV-1 could alter the cell's miRNA expression.

4. EPIGENETIC REGULATION OF HIV-1 LATENCY

Epigenetic modifications refers to reversible modifications on DNA or histones which impact the gene expression, although the DNA sequence do not suffer changes [24]. DNA methylation and histone modification are examples of two of the most well-known epigenetic modifications. In HIV-infected individuals, HIV-1 plasma titers are remarkably reduced by Highly Active Anti-retroviral Therapy (HAART), leading to decreased morbidity and mortality. But, the persistence of a reservoir of latent virus within resting CD4 T cells contributes to the reappearance of viremia upon quitting HAART [25 - 27]. In resting CD4 T cells, different factors maintain HIV-1 in a latent state, inhibiting the expression of virus gene after integrated in cell's DNA. This reservoir must be cleared for the removal of infection [28]. The HIV-1 is epigenetically regulated in its promoter located at the 5′ long terminal repeat region *via* histone protein modifications and the presence of inhibitory nucleosomes and DNA methylation in CpG islands flanking the transcription start site. This contributes to the establishment, maintenance, and reactivation of HIV latency [29, 30].

The induction of DNA methylation inhibitors might improve the removal of HIV-1 from infected individuals, such as 5-aza-29′deoxycytidine (aza-CdR) and Valproic acid both drugs belong to a class called Histone Deacetylase (HDAC) inhibitors [31, 32]. Unfortunately, it is already known that long-term valproic acid therapy is insufficient to decrease the size of the viral reservoir [33].

5. SYSTEMATIC PROFILING OF IMMUNE SYSTEM IN HIV INFECTION

HIV can harshly nibble at immune cells until the collapse of whole system, this paves the ground for a vast array of illnesses and finally death [10]. Retroviruses have evolved effective strategies to evade the host immune response, such as high variability and latent infection. In addition, primate lentiviruses, such as HIV-1, have acquired several ''accessory'' genes that antagonize antiviral host restriction factors and facilitate viral immune evasion (Table **2**), thereby allowing continuous and efficient viral replication despite apparently strong innate and acquired immune responses [34 - 36]. Moreover, Glycosylation of the envelop protein of HIV-1 can avoid immune recognition through taking benefits from the host glycosylation machinery for protection against potential protein antigenic epitopes. Furthermore, enveloped viruses exploit host secretory pathways to fold and assemble their heavily glycosylated coat proteins. The application of glycosylation inhibitors to prevent the folding of viral envelope proteins might show a potential antiviral effect for the hepatitis B virus (HBV) and the HIV [37 - 39].

Table 2. Host defenses and mechanisms of primate lentiviral evasion or antagonism [adapted from Ref. 34].

Immune Response	Host Defense	Antiviral Effect	Viral Evasion or Antagonist Mechanism	Viral Factor(s) or Properties
Innate	NK cells	lysis of infected cells	selective downmodulation of HLA-A and -B, but not HLA-C and -E	Nef
Intrinsic	ABOBEC 3G	lethal hypermutations	Polyubiquitination and degradation	Vif
	TRIM5α	Untimely uncoating	variation in capsid	High variability
	tetherin	Bocks virion release	Sequestration from the site of virion budding	Vpu,Nef,Env
Acquired	Cytotoxic CD8+ T cells	lysis of infected cells, inhibitory cytokines	MHC-I downmodulation, escape mutations, latent infection	Nef, High variability
	CD4+ helper T cells	helper function to promote antibody and CTL responses	destruction by infection or bystander apoptosis; downmodulation of CD4, CD3, CD28, and CXCR4	Nef,Vpu,viral cytopathicity
	B cells, antibodies	neutralization	antigenic variation, glycosylation, shielding of functional epitopes, inhibition of IgG2, and IgA switching	High variability, N-lined glycosylation sites, Env structure, Nef
	Antigen-presenting cells	viral antigen presentation, helper T cell activation	Upmodulation of li surface expression	Nef

The practice of systems biology requires capturing and integrating global sets of biological data from as many hierarchical levels as possible for the visualization of 'emergent properties' not exhibited by their individual parts and unpredicted from the parts alone [40].

6. THE BEST APPROACH TO STUDY HIV INFECTION BY SYSTEM BIOLOGY

The identification and dissection of the immune mechanisms which are responsible for protecting against the progression of HIV disease requires to focus on rare individuals being able to naturally control HIV infection (with no therapy). About viral evolution and immune control, our knowledge has been primarily obtained from the investigations on groups of elite controllers (ECs) maintaining the viral loads at undetectable levels for a long time after seroconversion; long-term non-progressors (LTNPs) and viremic non-progressors (VNPs), who succeed in retaining a functional CD4 T cell compartment and persist asymptomatic over time with no antiretroviral treatment, despite detectable viral loads [41]. These subjects offer research opportunities to analyze an immune system richly preserved with the capacity to develop a tradeoff between viral replication control in the long term as ECs and a functional immune system in response to continued viral replication as VNPs [3].

Hyrcza and co-worker in 2007 used a systems biology approach [42] to understand dissimilar transcriptional profiles in purified CD4+ and CD8+ T cells from subjects with various clinical and progression data. The study included five early infected individuals, five chronically infected and progressing individuals, five LTNPs, and five HIV-negative controls, all patients naïve to antiretroviral treatment. A microarray analysis was performed for the identification of differential gene expression with pair-wise comparisons. Four genes were just surprisingly identified with differential regulation among the groups in the early and chronic stages, while no genes were differentially regulated between the LTNP and HIV-negative groups. Next, the researchers merged the groups to enhance statistical significance values and they obtained two distinctive gene-expression signatures; one characterized LTNP and HIV-negative T cells, and the second linked with the early HIV and chronic HIV. The comparative results revealed a higher number of differential gene expressions for CD8+ than CD4+ T cells. Also, down-regulation in the expressions was only obvious in the CD8+ subset. Interferon-stimulated genes (ISGs) were unregulated in early and chronic HIV-infected subjects, in comparison to two LTNP and HIV-negative samples. The result led us to assess whether the application of an ISG gene signature alone achieves an un superintended clustering of the CD4+ and CD8+ subjects. In fact, the selective application of ISG signatures provided an access to a hierarchical cluster analysis of the early and chronic subjects from those of LTNP and HIV-negative samples. The results gain an insight into the regulatory function and major role of the CD8 T-cell compartment in the pathogenesis of HIV. By using gene categories to distinguish the expression of genes of thymocytes *versus* peripheral T cells, the authors investigated the gene expression profiles associated with T-cell differentiation [43]. The database of gene-expression data obtained from the early and chronic subjects was over-represented in a gene cluster which was up-regulated at single-positive thymocytes. In contrast, LTNP subjects obtained a similar gene-expression profile as circulating peripheral T cells. This is consistent with the higher T-cell turnover in progressive HIV infection and it may be relatively resulted from augmentation of recent thymic emigrants which is considered as a compensatory mechanism for the loss of peripheral and mucosal CD4 T-cells [44]. Importantly, the gene families clustered in different clinical categories were observed in pathways involved in apoptotic, cell cycling, and DNA replication. The current research revealed numerous major mechanisms which provide natural protection against HIV transmission. At first, the study found a differential gene-expression profiles of the populations of CD4+ and CD8+ T-cells had the capability to discriminate progressors from non-progressors. Furthermore, a similar gene expression profile was observed among LTNPs in their peripheral blood and HIV-negative subjects. Third, as suggested, ISG signatures in the peripheral blood are unique to subjects with early and chronic infection as compared to LTNPs, and type I IFN chronic exposure signature are identified in both patients. Through an analysis on the global profiles of gene-expression for CD4+ and CD8+ T cells sorted from LTNPs and HIV-negative donors, Wu *et al.*, [45] compared the profiles to both viremic and ART treated subjects. As the profiles of gene expression from purified cells normalized, they were presented to pair wise comparisons of the fold changes with an aim to describe differential gene expressions. Unlike Hyrcza *et al.*, Wu *et al.*, detected a smaller number of genes differentially regulated among LTNPs and HIV-negative subjects. An investigation on the enriched gene ontology categories from the viremic groups compared to LTNP samples showed that the C1qA/B/C complex induction and complement activation were observed in CD4+ T cells, and that its catalytic activity and response to stimuli such as the proteasome core complex were enhanced in CD8+ T cells. Gene Set Enrichment Analysis (GSEA) represented a wide range of metabolic pathways associated with disease progression like the OXPHOS pathway in cellular energy production and the tricarboxylic acid (TCA) cycle. The research suggested that the up-regulation of metabolic pathways on HIV progression can be considered as a compensatory mechanism in the face of mitochondrial dysfunction resulted from HIV infection and/or ART. Furthermore, GSEA showed that pathways associated with immunity were significantly correlated with progression; including cell cycle, apoptosis, cytotoxicity, complement activation, interleukin and interferon response, and cell adhesion. Compared to LTNP samples, CD4+ T cells revealed the up-regulation of apoptotic genes such as TNFR1, BCL2, and BID in the viremic subjects. Despite the little number of enriched pathways in the T cell compartments of LTNPs, the study found that genes in the MAPK pathways related to the ERK, JNK, and p38 branches were significantly up-regulated in the LNTPs. The WNT-β-catenin pathway which plays a role in promoting self-renewal is selectively enriched in T cells extracted from LTNPs and regulated by the MAPK pathway. As the study proposed, activation of T cell signaling pathways enhances the efficacy of the antiviral response and also promotes effector T cell survival.

As a major consequence of HIV-1 infection is CD4 T cell depletion early after infection, the profiles of gene expression in LTNPs in the intestinal mucosal tissue was assessed by the first analyses on systems biology about natural protection against HIV infection [46]. A comparative microarray gene-expression study was conducted by Sankaran *et al.*, using jejunal biopsy samples from four antiretroviral therapy-naïve HIV-1 seropositive patients, four HIV-1 seronegative subjects and three LTNPs. In general, the profiles of mucosal gene expression obtained from the High Viral Load (HVL) individuals revealed the up-regulation of 369 genes in comparison to HIV-negative donors, while the LTNP group showed the up-regulation of 150 genes. Compared to HIV-negative controls, in contrast, 411 genes down-regulated in LTNPs were shown and 196 genes down-regulated in HVLs. Next, a hierarchical clustering study was carried out to examine the up-regulation of genes associated with homeostasis, digestion, and innate immune responses in both LTNP and HVL patients. A variety of features were appeared in the gene-expression profiles of the two groups. The induction of multiple array of immune response gene expression was found in the gut mucosa of both patients, including the interferon pathway (IFITM2 and OAS2), cell surface receptor expression (PD-1, leukocyte immunoglobulin receptor, B2), and chemotaxis (Eotaxin, MCP-1). Rather, down-regulation of numerous genes related to lymphocyte activation and inflammation was observed within LTNP, whereas it was up-regulated in HVL patients compared to HIV- negative controls. An example of this case is RANTES, the major ligand for CCR5, which was down-regulated in two out of three LTNPs, but up-regulated in three out of four HVLs. In summary, the high levels of viral replication in the Gut-associated Lymphoid Tissue (GALT) resulted in inflammatory gene expression profiles in HVL patients. For both LTNP and HVL subjects, regular expressions exhibited down-regulated genes involve in nutrient absorption and lipid metabolism in the GALT, while the down regulation in those related to amino acid metabolism were observed in tissues extracted from HVLs, rather than LTNPs. As suggested, HIV infection sequelae contributed to the pathology of gastrointestinal diseases and the deregulation of metabolic gene expressions in both groups, even with the lack of viral replication. Furthermore, the authors found an increased gene expression in HVL subjects for cell cycling (CCNA2 and MCM4), growth, and cell adhesion, but no evidence for this in the LTNP subjects. Despite attractive trends outlined for differential gene regulation involved in metabolism, growth, cell cycle and trafficking, the down-regulation of immune response genes in the LTNP group exhibited the most profound differences between the profiles of LTNP and HVL tissues *versus* both HVLs and HIV-negative controls.

7. AN ANIMAL MODEL FOR STUDYING HIV INFECTION BY SYSTEM BIOLOGY: NON-HUMAN PRIMATE MODELS OF SIV INFECTION

Comparisons of gene expression profiles in pathogenic *versus* non-pathogenic SIV infection in natural host species provides a powerful approach to assess HIV infection and to describe potential correlates of natural protection [47]. Despite of significant viral loads and robust viral replication, SIV infection in sooty mangabeys monkeys and African green monkeys (AGMs) is non-pathogenic, while infection of *rhesus macaques* usually results in chronic progressive disease. To characterize the pathogenic *rhesus macaques* model consists of T lymphocytes apoptosis and increased T cell activation and proliferation. On the other hand, the apoptotic loss of CD4+ T cells does not appear with SIV-infected sooty mangabeys and AGMs and a lack of chronic immune activation was exhibited in response to persistently high rate of virus replication [48]. In recent years, two studies with an comparative longitudinal whole-genome expression analysis were conducted on non-pathogenic (AGM and sooty mangabey) and pathogenic (*rhesus macaque*) SIV infection. As both suggested, non-pathogenic infection was characterized by the complete down-regulation of immune activation following early infection [49, 50]. An analysis of SIV transcription in whole blood, lymph nodes, and/or purified CD4+ T cells from the susceptible subjects compared with non-susceptible species showed a robust profile of the antiviral immune response in both groups early after infection. Although same profiles were obtained in acute infection, significant variation was observed for gene expressions during the transition from the acute to the chronic phase. Surprisingly, Jacquelin *et al.*, found a normalization in the expression of ISG in AGMs to baseline levels in some animals over 28 days after infection. Remarkably, the up-regulation of multiple immune regulatory genes in sooty mangabeys showed a potential mechanism to attenuate immune responses. Moreover, for AGMs and sooty mangabeys with non-pathogenic infection, Bosinger *et al.*, suggested the induction of a variety of immune-regulatory molecules, including ADAR (negative regulator of ISGs), IDO (immunoregulatory molecule induced in myeloid cells by IFN-γ), and TIM3 (immune inhibitory molecule). In summary, the researches mentioned above gained an insight into mechanisms limiting susceptibility to virus infection in the host, as well as required an effectively regulation of inflammatory responses in order to prevent against HIV/SIV disease progression [3].

CONCLUSION

In conclusion, analyses of systems biology shed new light on the monitoring of pathogenesis and interaction of HIV with host cell at various clinical stages and disease progression rates. In addition, appropriate analysis and modeling of host and HIV interaction network by systems biology will be applied to generate novel vaccines and drugs or re-generate vaccination and drugs, transferring treatment from the "empirical" to the "knowledge-based".

CONFLICT OF INTEREST

The authors confirm that they have no conflict of interest to declare for this publication.

ACKNOWLEDGEMENTS

Declared none.

REFERENCES

[1] Pulendran B, Li S, Nakaya HI. Systems vaccinology. Immunity 2010; 33(4): 516-29.
     [http://dx.doi.org/10.1016/j.immuni.2010.10.006] [PMID: 21029962]

[2] Buonaguro L, Wang E, Tornesello ML, Buonaguro FM, Marincola FM. Systems biology applied to vaccine and immunotherapy development. BMC Syst Biol 2011; 5(1): 146.
     [http://dx.doi.org/10.1186/1752-0509-5-146] [PMID: 21933421]

[3] Peretz Y, Cameron C, Sékaly R-P. Dissecting the HIV-specific immune response: a systems biology approach. Curr Opin HIV AIDS 2012; 7(1): 17-23.
     [http://dx.doi.org/10.1097/COH.0b013e32834ddb0e] [PMID: 22134339]

[4] Nakaya HI, Pulendran B. Systems vaccinology: its promise and challenge for HIV vaccine development. Curr Opin HIV AIDS 2012; 7(1): 24-31.
     [http://dx.doi.org/10.1097/COH.0b013e32834dc37b] [PMID: 22156839]

[5] Oberg AL, Kennedy RB, Li P, Ovsyannikova IG, Poland GA. Systems biology approaches to new vaccine development. Curr Opin Immunol 2011; 23(3): 436-43.
     [http://dx.doi.org/10.1016/j.coi.2011.04.005] [PMID: 21570272]

[6] Querec TD, Akondy RS, Lee EK, *et al.* Systems biology approach predicts immunogenicity of the yellow fever vaccine in humans. Nat Immunol 2009; 10(1): 116-25.
     [http://dx.doi.org/10.1038/ni.1688] [PMID: 19029902]

[7] Goff SP. Host factors exploited by retroviruses. Nat Rev Microbiol 2007; 5(4): 253-63.
     [http://dx.doi.org/10.1038/nrmicro1541] [PMID: 17325726]

[8] Zhang L, Zhang X, Ma Q, Zhou H. Host proteome research in HIV infection. Genomics Proteomics Bioinformatics 2010; 8(1): 1-9.
     [http://dx.doi.org/10.1016/S1672-0229(10)60001-0] [PMID: 20451157]

[9] Zhao RY, Bukrinsky M, Elder RT. HIV-1 viral protein R (Vpr) & host cellular responses. Indian J Med Res 2005; 121(4): 270-86.
     [PMID: 15817944]

[10]   Cohen J. Virology. HIV gets by with a lot of help from human host. Science 2008; 319(5860): 143-4.
[http://dx.doi.org/10.1126/science.319.5860.143] [PMID: 18187626]

[11]   Appay V, Sauce D. Immune activation and inflammation in HIV-1 infection: causes and consequences. J Pathol 2008; 214(2): 231-41.
[http://dx.doi.org/10.1002/path.2276] [PMID: 18161758]

[12]   Shapshak P, Chiappelli F, Commins D, *et al.* Molecular epigenetics, chromatin, and NeuroAIDS/HIV: translational implications. Bioinformation 2008; 3(1): 53-7.
[http://dx.doi.org/10.6026/97320630003053] [PMID: 19052667]

[13]   Arrell DK, Terzic A. Network systems biology for drug discovery. Clin Pharmacol Ther 2010; 88(1): 120-5.
[http://dx.doi.org/10.1038/clpt.2010.91] [PMID: 20520604]

[14]   Qian X, Yoon B-J. Comparative analysis of protein interaction networks reveals that conserved pathways are susceptible to HIV-1 interception. BMC Bioinformatics 2011; 12 (Suppl. 1): S19.
[http://dx.doi.org/10.1186/1471-2105-12-S1-S19] [PMID: 21342548]

[15]   Ptak RG, Fu W, Sanders-Beer BE, *et al.* Cataloguing the HIV type 1 human protein interaction network. AIDS Res Hum Retroviruses 2008; 24(12): 1497-502.
[http://dx.doi.org/10.1089/aid.2008.0113] [PMID: 19025396]

[16]   Fu W, Sanders-Beer BE, Katz KS, Maglott DR, Pruitt KD, Ptak RG. Human immunodeficiency virus type 1, human protein interaction database at NCBI. Nucleic Acids Res 2009; 37(Database issue) (Suppl. 1): D417-22.
[http://dx.doi.org/10.1093/nar/gkn708] [PMID: 18927109]

[17]   Pinney JW, Dickerson JE, Fu W, Sanders-Beer BE, Ptak RG, Robertson DL. HIV-host interactions: a map of viral perturbation of the host system. AIDS 2009; 23(5): 549-54.
[http://dx.doi.org/10.1097/QAD.0b013e328325a495] [PMID: 19262354]

[18]   Liang WS, Maddukuri A, Teslovich TM, *et al.* Therapeutic targets for HIV-1 infection in the host proteome. Retrovirology 2005; 2(1): 20.
[http://dx.doi.org/10.1186/1742-4690-2-20] [PMID: 15780141]

[19]   Hariharan M, Scaria V, Pillai B, Brahmachari SK. Targets for human encoded microRNAs in HIV genes. Biochem Biophys Res Commun 2005; 337(4): 1214-8.
[http://dx.doi.org/10.1016/j.bbrc.2005.09.183] [PMID: 16236258]

[20]   Klase Z, Houzet L, Jeang K-T. MicroRNAs and HIV-1: complex interactions. J Biol Chem 2012; 287(49): 40884-90.
[http://dx.doi.org/10.1074/jbc.R112.415448] [PMID: 23043098]

[21]   Yeung ML, Bennasser Y, Myers TG, Jiang G, Benkirane M, Jeang K-T. Changes in microRNA expression profiles in HIV-1-transfected human cells. Retrovirology 2005; 2(1): 81.
[http://dx.doi.org/10.1186/1742-4690-2-81] [PMID: 16381609]

[22]   Yeung ML, Bennasser Y, Le SY, Jeang KT. siRNA, miRNA and HIV: promises and challenges. Cell Res 2005; 15(11-12): 935-46.
[http://dx.doi.org/10.1038/sj.cr.7290371] [PMID: 16354572]

[23]   Mukerjee R, Chang JR, Del Valle L, *et al.* Deregulation of microRNAs by HIV-1 Vpr protein leads to the development of neurocognitive disorders. J Biol Chem 2011; 286(40): 34976-85.
[http://dx.doi.org/10.1074/jbc.M111.241547] [PMID: 21816823]

[24]   Vaissière T, Sawan C, Herceg Z. Epigenetic interplay between histone modifications and DNA methylation in gene silencing. Mutat Res 2008; 659(1-2): 40-8.
[http://dx.doi.org/10.1016/j.mrrev.2008.02.004] [PMID: 18407786]

[25]   Huang J, Wang F, Argyris E, *et al.* Cellular microRNAs contribute to HIV-1 latency in resting primary CD4+ T lymphocytes. Nat Med 2007; 13(10): 1241-7.
[http://dx.doi.org/10.1038/nm1639] [PMID: 17906637]

[26]   Zhang L, Ramratnam B, Tenner-Racz K, *et al.* Quantifying residual HIV-1 replication in patients receiving combination antiretroviral therapy. N Engl J Med 1999; 340(21): 1605-13.
[http://dx.doi.org/10.1056/NEJM199905273402101] [PMID: 10341272]

[27]   Furtado MR, Callaway DS, Phair JP, *et al.* Persistence of HIV-1 transcription in peripheral-blood mononuclear cells in patients receiving potent antiretroviral therapy. N Engl J Med 1999; 340(21): 1614-22.
[http://dx.doi.org/10.1056/NEJM199905273402102] [PMID: 10341273]

[28]   Marcello A. Latency: the hidden HIV-1 challenge. Retrovirology 2006; 3(1): 7.
[http://dx.doi.org/10.1186/1742-4690-3-7] [PMID: 16412247]

[29]   Kauder SE, Bosque A, Lindqvist A, Planelles V, Verdin E. Epigenetic regulation of HIV-1 latency by cytosine methylation. PLoS Pathog 2009; 5(6): e1000495.
[http://dx.doi.org/10.1371/journal.ppat.1000495] [PMID: 19557157]

[30]   Hakre S, Chavez L, Shirakawa K, Verdin E. Epigenetic regulation of HIV latency. Curr Opin HIV AIDS 2011; 6(1): 19-24.
[http://dx.doi.org/10.1097/COH.0b013e3283412384] [PMID: 21242889]

[31]   Archin NM, Eron JJ, Palmer S, *et al.* Valproic acid without intensified antiviral therapy has limited impact on persistent HIV infection of resting CD4+ T cells. AIDS 2008; 22(10): 1131-5.
[http://dx.doi.org/10.1097/QAD.0b013e3282fd6df4] [PMID: 18525258]

[32]   Fernandez G, Zeichner SL. Cell line-dependent variability in HIV activation employing DNMT inhibitors. Virol J 2010; 7(1): 266.
[http://dx.doi.org/10.1186/1743-422X-7-266] [PMID: 20942961]

[33]   Sagot-Lerolle N, Lamine A, Chaix ML, *et al.* Prolonged valproic acid treatment does not reduce the size of latent HIV reservoir. AIDS 2008; 22(10): 1125-9.
[http://dx.doi.org/10.1097/QAD.0b013e3282fd6ddc] [PMID: 18525257]

[34]   Kirchhoff F. Immune evasion and counteraction of restriction factors by HIV-1 and other primate lentiviruses. Cell Host Microbe 2010; 8(1): 55-67.
[http://dx.doi.org/10.1016/j.chom.2010.06.004] [PMID: 20638642]

[35]   Malim MH, Bieniasz PD. HIV restriction factors and mechanisms of evasion. Cold Spring Harb Perspect Med 2012; 2(5): a006940.
[http://dx.doi.org/10.1101/cshperspect.a006940] [PMID: 22553496]

[36]   Martin N, Sattentau Q. Cell-to-cell HIV-1 spread and its implications for immune evasion. Curr Opin HIV AIDS 2009; 4(2): 143-9.
[http://dx.doi.org/10.1097/COH.0b013e328322f94a] [PMID: 19339954]

[37]   Vigerust DJ, Shepherd VL. Virus glycosylation: role in virulence and immune interactions. Trends Microbiol 2007; 15(5): 211-8.
[http://dx.doi.org/10.1016/j.tim.2007.03.003] [PMID: 17398101]

[38]   Reitter JN, Means RE, Desrosiers RC. A role for carbohydrates in immune evasion in AIDS. Nat Med 1998; 4(6): 679-84.
[http://dx.doi.org/10.1038/nm0698-679] [PMID: 9623976]

[39]   Rudd PM, Elliott T, Cresswell P, Wilson IA, Dwek RA. Glycosylation and the immune system. Science 2001; 291(5512): 2370-6.
[http://dx.doi.org/10.1126/science.291.5512.2370] [PMID: 11269318]

[40]   Zak DE, Aderem A. Systems biology of innate immunity. Immunol Rev 2009; 227(1): 264-82.
[http://dx.doi.org/10.1111/j.1600-065X.2008.00721.x] [PMID: 19120490]

[41]   Deeks SG, Walker BD. Human immunodeficiency virus controllers: mechanisms of durable virus control in the absence of antiretroviral therapy. Immunity 2007; 27(3): 406-16.
[http://dx.doi.org/10.1016/j.immuni.2007.08.010] [PMID: 17892849]

[42]   Hyrcza MD, Kovacs C, Loutfy M, *et al.* Distinct transcriptional profiles in *ex vivo* CD4+ and CD8+ T cells are established early in human immunodeficiency virus type 1 infection and are characterized by a chronic interferon response as well as extensive transcriptional changes in CD8+ T cells. J Virol 2007; 81(7): 3477-86.
[http://dx.doi.org/10.1128/JVI.01552-06] [PMID: 17251300]

[43]   Lee MS, Hanspers K, Barker CS, Korn AP, McCune JM. Gene expression profiles during human CD4+ T cell differentiation. Int Immunol 2004; 16(8): 1109-24.
[http://dx.doi.org/10.1093/intimm/dxh112] [PMID: 15210650]

[44]   Dion M-L, Poulin J-F, Bordi R, *et al.* HIV infection rapidly induces and maintains a substantial suppression of thymocyte proliferation. Immunity 2004; 21(6): 757-68.
[http://dx.doi.org/10.1016/j.immuni.2004.10.013] [PMID: 15589165]

[45]   Wu JQ, Dwyer DE, Dyer WB, Yang YH, Wang B, Saksena NK. Genome-wide analysis of primary CD4+ and CD8+ T cell transcriptomes shows evidence for a network of enriched pathways associated with HIV disease. Retrovirology 2011; 8(1): 18.
[http://dx.doi.org/10.1186/1742-4690-8-18] [PMID: 21410942]

[46]   Sankaran S, Guadalupe M, Reay E, *et al.* Gut mucosal T cell responses and gene expression correlate with protection against disease in long-term HIV-1-infected nonprogressors. Proc Natl Acad Sci USA 2005; 102(28): 9860-5.
[http://dx.doi.org/10.1073/pnas.0503463102] [PMID: 15980151]

[47]   Pendyala G, Trauger SA, Kalisiak E, Ellis RJ, Siuzdak G, Fox HS. Cerebrospinal fluid proteomics reveals potential pathogenic changes in the brains of SIV-infected monkeys. J Proteome Res 2009; 8(5): 2253-60.
[http://dx.doi.org/10.1021/pr800854t] [PMID: 19281240]

[48]   Sodora DL, Allan JS, Apetrei C, *et al.* Toward an AIDS vaccine: lessons from natural simian immunodeficiency virus infections of African nonhuman primate hosts. Nat Med 2009; 15(8): 861-5.
[http://dx.doi.org/10.1038/nm.2013] [PMID: 19661993]

[49]   Bosinger SE, Li Q, Gordon SN, *et al.* Global genomic analysis reveals rapid control of a robust innate response in SIV-infected sooty mangabeys. J Clin Invest 2009; 119(12): 3556-72.
[http://dx.doi.org/10.1172/JCI40115] [PMID: 19959874]

[50]   Jacquelin B, Mayau V, Targat B, *et al.* Nonpathogenic SIV infection of African green monkeys induces a strong but rapidly controlled type I IFN response. J Clin Invest 2009; 119(12): 3544-55.
[http://dx.doi.org/10.1172/JCI40093] [PMID: 19959873]

CHAPTER 8

HIV/TB Co-Infection

Katayoun Tayeri[*]

Iranian Research Center for HIV/AIDS, Iranian Institute for Reduction of High Risk Behaviors, Tehran University of Medical Sciences, Tehran, Iran

Abstract: In HIV infected patients, tuberculosis is the leading cause of death through the world. According to some World Health Organization (WHO) reports, the risk of tuberculosis disease in People Living with HIV (PLHIV) is about 10-20 times greater than people without HIV. The risk of developing tuberculosis disease in PPD positive HIV infected is about 10% annually but in HIV un-infected people is about 10% throughout their life. HIV accelerates the progression of tuberculosis infection toward disease both in recent and latent infection of TB. Pulmonary tuberculosis is the most common type of TB and its symptoms are related to the immune status of the patients and the level of progression to AIDS. Usually, signs and symptoms of tuberculosis are mild and it is difficult to diagnose. In smear negative pulmonary TB which is mostly observed in advanced HIV infection, mortality and morbidity would be higher due to the delay in establishing the diagnosis. Considering that reactivation of Latent TB (LTB) to active tuberculosis is more prevalent in PLHIV compared to HIV negative people, the diagnosis of LTB infection would be an important priority and screenings for TB should be done periodically among PLHIV as a priority. Any PLHIV with suspected LTB is eligible for isoniazid (INH) prophylaxis. All PLHIV with tuberculosis disease should be under Antiretroviral Therapy (ART) irrespective of CD4 cell count.

Keywords: AFB, AIDS, ART, CD4 cell, LTB, PLHIV, Prophylaxis, PPD, Tuberculosis, XDR-TB.

1. INTRODUCTION

In HIV infected patients, tuberculosis is the leading cause of death through the

---

[*] **Correspondence to to Katayoun Tayeri:** Iranian Research Center for HIV/AIDS (IRCHA), Imam Khomeini Hospital, Keshavarz Blvd., Tehran, Iran; Tel/Fax: +98 (21) 66947984; E-mail: katayon_tayeri@yahoo.com.

SeyedAhmad SeyedAlinaghi (Ed.)

world. Overall, at least one third of 34 million people who are living with HIV are infected with tuberculosis. According to the WHO report, during 2012 about 8.6 million new cases of tuberculosis were diagnosed globally, and 13% of them (1.1 million) were co-infected with HIV. On the other hand, among 1.1 million deaths due to tuberculosis, 24% (350000 cases) were co-infected with HIV. Also, about 1.8 million people died from HIV infection in 2010 among whom 35000 cases were due to tuberculosis [1 - 4].

In susceptible people, *Mycobacterium tuberculosis* is transmitted through cough, sneezing, crying, shouting and singing. After entering the body, in 2-12 weeks the immune system identifies the microorganism and initiates a response. In people with normal immune status, the immune response controls the infection and thus the signs and symptoms of the disease are not manifest. But, viable bacilli may remain in several tissues of the hosts' body without producing any symptoms for several decades [5]. This situation is known as Latent TB infection (LTB), and the people with latent TB infection do not transmit the infection [6]. After several years, if the immune system is defective for some reason such as malnutrition, malignancies, chemotherapy and HIV infection, LTB can turn into tuberculosis disease [7, 8]. With regard to HIV infection, tuberculosis may be seen in any stage of HIV infection with any CD4 count, although the symptoms of the patients can be related to the CD4 cell count. It is noteworthy that poverty and crowding are the two major predisposing factors for tuberculosis [8].

2. INTERACTION OF TB AND HIV

2.1. The Effect of HIV Infection on Active Tuberculosis

HIV accelerates the progression of tuberculosis infection toward disease both in recent and latent infection of TB. In fact, HIV infection is the most important risk factor of tuberculosis reactivation. In co-infected TB/HIV patients, the risk of reactivation of tuberculosis is about 8-10% annually, but in HIV negative people, it would be about 5-10% throughout their life.

2.2. The Effect of HIV Infection on Tuberculosis Transmission

Tuberculosis is one of the most common opportunistic infections in People Living with HIV (PLHIV), especially in areas with high prevalence of TB. By increasing the number of tuberculosis disease, the chance of TB transmission would increase throughout community and of course the rate of multi-drug resistance TB would also increase due to inappropriate treatment [9].

2.3. The Effect of HIV Infection on Tuberculosis Symptoms

Pulmonary tuberculosis is the most common type of TB and its symptoms are related to the immune status of the patients. The pulmonary TB in PLHIV with CD4>350, is similar to HIV negative patients; but in people with CD4<200 the manifestations are different. In lower CD4 cells count, patients would usually have negative sputum smears without cavitation, with middle or lower lobe infiltration in addition to lymphadenopathy. In advanced HIV infection, the rates of extra-pulmonary TB increase [10].

2.4. The Effect of Tuberculosis on HIV Infection

In HIV/TB co-infection, HIV related immunodeficiency is exacerbated and tends to manifest more opportunistic infections such as candida esophagitis, cryptoccocal meningitis and *pneumocystis jiroveci* infection [11 - 13].

3. CLINICAL SIGNS AND SYMPTOMS

In LTB, the patient has inactive microorganism in some parts of body without any sign and symptom while in active tuberculosis, the signs and symptoms are related to the CD4 cell count. When CD4>350, the clinical manifestations are similar to HIV negative patients, hence upper lobe infiltration with or without cavitation is seen [14]. The symptoms of extra-pulmonary TB are mostly relate to the site of infection.

The important types of HIV/TB co-infection are pulmonary TB, smear negative pulmonary TB and extra-pulmonary TB. In pulmonary TB, typical signs include productive cough, fever, night sweat, chest pain and hemoptysis may be seen and are related to the stage of HIV infection. However, the patient may sometimes be asymptomatic, and in 22% of the co-infected patients with pulmonary TB, chest X-ray can be normal [14]. In smear negative pulmonary TB which is mostly observed in advanced HIV infection, mortality and morbidity would be higher due to the delay in establishing the diagnosis [15]. The extrapulmonary tuberculosis is more common in PLHIV and may be concomitantly present with pulmonary TB. In total, 40-80% of TB infection is extra-pulmonary in PLHIV, while this figure is 10-20% among HIV negative people. Irrespective to the CD4 count, the prevalence of extra-pulmonary TB is more among PLHIV, and the most common type is lymphadenitis.

4. DIAGNOSIS

4.1. Diagnosis of LTB

Considering that reactivation of LTB to active tuberculosis is more prevalent in PLHIV compared to HIV negative people, the diagnosis of LTB infection would be an important priority and should be done periodically among PLHIV. Diagnostic criteria for the possibility of LTB in the absence of clinical signs and symptoms include:

- *PPD Test:* An induration of 5mm or more after 48-72 hour is considered positive. If PPD is negative and CD4>200, PPD test should be done annually. In CD4<200, PPD test should be repeated after antiretroviral therapy (ART) and achieving higher CD4 levels (*i.e.* CD4>200) [16 - 18].
- *Recent Exposure to Smear Positive Pulmonary TB Patient:* At first, active tuberculosis should be ruled out in any HIV positive exposed patient and then patient eligible for INH prophylaxis regardless of PPD result.
- *Interferon Gamma Assay (IGRA):* several studies showed IGRA is a valuable test in diagnosis of LTB due to its excellent specificity for *Mycobacterium tuberculosis,* but this test is very expensive and cannot be used in many developing countries [19].

4.2. Diagnosis of Active Tuberculosis

All PLHIV should be regularly evaluated about active tuberculosis. In this regard, the best tools include the history of patient's signs and symptoms, and intensified case finding. In each visit, patient should be evaluated about certain symptoms such as fever, weight loss, cough and night sweat. Such history taking would have 79% sensitivity and 50% specificity for active TB case finding. In countries where the prevalence of TB in PLHIV in about 5%, the negative predictive value of this method would be 97.7%, which means that the PLHIV who do not report to have any of this symptoms, do not have active TB and isoniazid (INH) prophylaxis can be started. Adding abnormal chest x-ray finding to the above symptoms increases the sensitivity of case finding to 91%, but decreases specificity to 39%. Using chest x-ray finding besides clinical finding in high TB prevalence areas is thereby recommended. Of course normal chest x-ray cannot alone rule out the active TB [20, 21]. For each patient with above findings and/or pulmonary symptoms, sputum smear and culture for Acid-Fast Bacilli (AFB) should be done. By improving the quality of sputum smear exam method and also LED microscopy, sensitivity of diagnosing the active TB is increased.

Gen Xpert MTB/RIF

This is the newer method for diagnosis of *Mycobacterium tuberculosis,* that in addition to rapid diagnosis of the organism (about 100 hours in comparison to culture that takes at least two months), determines the resistance to rifampin. According to the WHO recommendation, Gen Xpert MTB/RIF is the preferred method of TB diagnosis in PLHIV with suspected TB and the first step for diagnosis of Multi-Drug Resistance TB (MDR-TB) [21 - 23].

TB-LAM Assay

In this method, certain particles of the *Mycobacterium tuberculosis* cell wall can be detected in a sample of patient's urine. It is easily done with a dip stick method. This methods is especially helpful in PLHIVs with CD4<50. Combination of TB-LAM assay with direct sputum smear are equal to Gen Xpert MTB/RIF in PLHIV with CD4<100. Also, it is a reliable method for ruling out active TB and initiation of INH prophylaxis in PLHIV with CD4>200, besides the other methods [21, 22, 24].

5. TREATMENTS

5.1. Treatment of LTB

Any PLHIV with suspected LTB is eligible for INH prophylaxis. According to

WHO guidelines, having a positive PPD test is not necessary to initiation of INH prophylaxis and when active tuberculosis is ruled out, INH prophylaxis can be initiated. But still PPD test is the main determining factor in deciding for INH prophylaxis.

The drug of choice for latent TB prophylaxis is INH 5mg/kg/day for nine months. INH should be prescribed with caution and is contraindicated in:

• Active hepatitis
• Continuous consumption of alcohol
• When symptoms of peripheral neuropathy are present [20].

Every patient with INH prophylaxis should receive pyridoxine (vitamin B6) through the course of prophylaxis. For LTB, some researchers have recommended other regimens including INH+RIM for three months, especially in specific situations such as prisons [25].

5.2. Treatment of Active Tuberculosis

In addition to higher prevalence of MDR-TB in PLHIV, incomplete or incorrect treatments, lower adherence to therapies and absence of treatment are more common in PLHIV; accordingly performing the DOTS program through the whole course of the treatment is of great value in this group of patients [20]. In order to provide a more effective therapeutic setting, treatment supporters may be assigned to aid the patients in receiving their regular treatments. The treatment supporter may be selected as a social worker, health interface or from patients' relatives.

The treatment regimen of tuberculosis in adults co-infected with HIV is similar to that of HIV negative patients. Treatment course last six months; the first two months with INH, rifampin (RIF), pyrazinamide (PZA) and ethambutol (EMB) followed by four months of INH and RIF. The course of therapy should be extended to nine months in cases of cavitary disease and delayed response to therapy (positive smear culture at the end of second month after initiating the therapy). Moreover, in extra-pulmonary tuberculosis such as miliary TB and skeletal TB the duration of the treatment is extended to 9-12 months [20].

5.3. Simultaneous Treatment of HIV and TB

In PLHIV with TB, the priority is to treat TB. In fact, although ART is very important in improving the quality of life of PLHIV, but initiating the anti-tuberculosis regimen, if indicated, should be regarded as the first priority. Scenarios of tuberculosis treatment in PLHIV include:

Patient has already received the ART:

ART should be continued and when indicated, anti-TB drugs should be started; but some cautions need to be considered:

○ If patients' ART regimen does not include a Protease Inhibitor (PI), there are no changes required in usual ART and anti-TB drug regimen.

○ If patients' ART regimen contains a PI, rifampin must be replaced with rifabutin. If needed (when rifabutin is not available), the PI should be replaced with efavirenz. In this situation, in patients with weight > 60kg, efavirenz dosage should be increased to 800 mg/day [26].

Patient has not already received ART:

Usually after starting anti-TB regimen, ART should be initiated as soon as possible:

○ In patients with CD4<50/cc, ART should be started within the first two weeks of anti-tuberculosis therapy.

○ In patients with CD4>50/cc with severe symptoms like severe inability, anemia, hypo-albuminemia and organ failure, ART should be started during the first 2-4 weeks of anti-tuberculosis therapy.

○ In patients with CD4>50/cc without symptoms, ART can be postponed after 2-4 weeks of anti-tuberculosis therapy, but not to more than 8-12 weeks.

○ In patient with MDR-TB or extensive-drug resistance TB (XDR-TB), ART should be started during the first 2-4 weeks [21, 26, 27].

Co-trimoxazole

Co-trimoxazole prophylaxis should be considered for all PLHIV throughout the whole course of anti-tuberculosis therapy [26].

5.4. Tuberculosis Immune Reconstitution Syndrome (IRIS)

Usual signs and symptoms of tuberculosis IRIS are high fever, new lymphadenitis or worsening of previous lymphadenopathy, increasing pulmonary infiltration and pleural effusion. IRIS in under treatment patients usually occurs during the first three months of anti-tuberculosis therapy, especially when CD4<50. In all cases anti-tuberculosis should be continued. For severe symptoms, Non-steroidal anti-inflammatory Drugs (NSAIDs) and/or prednisone 1mg/kg/day are prescribed for two weeks.

The underlying factors that increase the risk of TB IRIS include:

- CD4<50
- CD4 percent <7%
- Hb<10
- Clinical stage 3 or 4 of HIV infection
- Body Mass Index<18 kg/m^2
- Higher viral load

5.5. Prophylaxis from Exposure to *Mycobacterium Tuberculosis*

All confirmed or suspected cases of tuberculosis should be isolated from all PLHIV. For returning the tuberculosis cases to public places, especially HIV communities, treatment must be continued for at least two weeks with concomitant improvement of clinical symptoms. If the TB infected patient has to refer to places like prison, he/she must have three consecutive negative sputum smears (taken within eight hours interval).

5.6. BCG Vaccination

BCG vaccination is contraindicated in all PLHIV and those who are suspected to have HIV infection [28].

A Few Tips

Co-infection of HIV/TB/HCV or HBV

Before starting therapies such as interferon, especially when CD4<200, patient should be evaluated for tuberculosis and other opportunistic diseases. In HBV/HCV/TB co-infection, there is a 14-fold increase in the rate of hepatic toxicity.

Diabetes Mellitus with HIV/TB Co-infection:

In this situation, a poor response to anti-tuberculosis therapy is anticipated; so, the risk of MDR-TB increases. This group of patients needs to be more closely monitored during treatment.

HIV/TB with Alcoholism:

The presence of alcoholism and active tuberculosis should always be considered; hence alcohol can worsen the course of TB and also HIV infection. In this situation the risk of rifampin hepatic toxicity is increased.

CONFLICT OF INTEREST

The author confirms that author has no conflict of interest to declare for this publication.

ACKNOWLEDGEMENTS

Declared none.

REFERENCES

[1]   WHO. TB/HIV fact sheet Available at:www.who.int/tb/challenges/hiv/factsheets/en/.

[2]   World Health Organization. Global tuberculosis control 2012. [Accessed on: Jan 2012]; Available at: http://www.who. int/tb/publications/global_report/2010/en/index.html.

[3]   UNAIDS. Chapter 2: epidemic update. UNAIDS report on the global AIDS epidemic 2010. [Accessed on: Jan   2012];   Available   at: http://www.unaids.org/documents/20101123_GlobalReport_Chap2_em.pdf.

[4]   Aaron L, Saadoun D, Calatroni I, *et al.* Tuberculosis in HIV-infected patients: a comprehensive review. Clin Microbiol Infect 2004; 10(5): 388-98.
       [http://dx.doi.org/10.1111/j.1469-0691.2004.00758.x] [PMID: 15113314]

[5]   Marchal G. [Pathophysiology and immunology of tuberculosis]. Rev Mal Respir 1997; 14 (Suppl. 5): S19-26.
       [PMID: 9496588]

[6]   Dye C, Scheele S, Dolin P, Pathania V, Raviglione MC. Consensus statement. Global burden of tuberculosis: estimated incidence, prevalence, and mortality by country. WHO Global Surveillance and Monitoring Project. JAMA 1999; 282(7): 677-86.
[http://dx.doi.org/10.1001/jama.282.7.677] [PMID: 10517722]

[7]   Roberts T, Beyers N, Aguirre A, Walzl G. Immunosuppression during active tuberculosis is characterized by decreased interferon- gamma production and CD25 expression with elevated forkhead box P3, transforming growth factor- beta, and interleukin-4 mRNA levels. J Infect Dis 2007; 195(6): 870-8.
[http://dx.doi.org/10.1086/511277] [PMID: 17299718]

[8]   Whalen CC, Zalwango S, Chiunda A, et al. Secondary attack rate of tuberculosis in urban households in Kampala, Uganda. PLoS One 2011; 6(2): e16137.
[http://dx.doi.org/10.1371/journal.pone.0016137] [PMID: 21339819]

[9]   Sonnenberg P, Glynn JR, Fielding K, Murray J, Godfrey-Faussett P, Shearer S. How soon after infection with HIV does the risk of tuberculosis start to increase? A retrospective cohort study in South African gold miners. J Infect Dis 2005; 191(2): 150-8.
[http://dx.doi.org/10.1086/426827] [PMID: 15609223]

[10]   Jones BE, Young SM, Antoniskis D, Davidson PT, Kramer F, Barnes PF. Relationship of the manifestations of tuberculosis to CD4 cell counts in patients with human immunodeficiency virus infection. Am Rev Respir Dis 1993; 148(5): 1292-7.
[http://dx.doi.org/10.1164/ajrccm/148.5.1292] [PMID: 7902049]

[11]   Badri M, Ehrlich R, Wood R, Pulerwitz T, Maartens G. Association between tuberculosis and HIV disease progression in a high tuberculosis prevalence area. Int J Tuberc Lung Dis 2001; 5(3): 225-32.
[PMID: 11326821]

[12]   López-Gatell H, Cole SR, Hessol NA, et al. Effect of tuberculosis on the survival of women infected with human immunodeficiency virus. Am J Epidemiol 2007; 165(10): 1134-42.
[http://dx.doi.org/10.1093/aje/kwk116] [PMID: 17339383]

[13]   Vanham G, Edmonds K, Qing L, et al. Generalized immune activation in pulmonary tuberculosis: co-activation with HIV infection. Clin Exp Immunol 1996; 103(1): 30-4.
[http://dx.doi.org/10.1046/j.1365-2249.1996.907600.x] [PMID: 8565282]

[14]   Getahun H, Kittikraisak W, Heilig CM, et al. Development of a standardized screening rule for tuberculosis in people living with HIV in resource-constrained settings: individual participant data meta-analysis of observational studies. PLoS Med 2011; 8(1): e1000391.
[http://dx.doi.org/10.1371/journal.pmed.1000391] [PMID: 21267059]

[15]   Mtei L, Matee M, Herfort O, et al. High rates of clinical and subclinical tuberculosis among HIV-infected ambulatory subjects in Tanzania. Clin Infect Dis 2005; 40(10): 1500-7.
[http://dx.doi.org/10.1086/429825] [PMID: 15844073]

[16]   Pai M, Kalantri S, Dheda K. New tools and emerging technologies for the diagnosis of tuberculosis: part I. Latent tuberculosis. Expert Rev Mol Diagn 2006; 6(3): 413-22.
[http://dx.doi.org/10.1586/14737159.6.3.413] [PMID: 16706743]

[17]   Moline JM, Markowitz SB. Medical surveillance for workers exposed to tuberculosis. Occup Med

1994; 9(4): 695-721.
[PMID: 7878496]

[18]   Markowitz N, Hansen NI, Wilcosky TC, *et al.* Pulmonary Complications of HIV Infection Study Group. Tuberculin and anergy testing in HIV-seropositive and HIV-seronegative persons. Ann Intern Med 1993; 119(3): 185-93.
[http://dx.doi.org/10.7326/0003-4819-119-3-199308010-00002] [PMID: 8100692]

[19]   Dheda K, van Zyl Smit R, Badri M, Pai M. T-cell interferon-gamma release assays for the rapid immunodiagnosis of tuberculosis: clinical utility in high-burden *vs.* low-burden settings. Curr Opin Pulm Med 2009; 15(3): 188-200.
[http://dx.doi.org/10.1097/MCP.0b013e32832a0adc] [PMID: 19387262]

[20]   WHO. Guidelines for intensified tuberculosis case finding and isoniazid preventive therapy for people living with HIV in resource- constrained settings 2011. Available at: http://whqlibdoc. who.int/publications/2011/9789241500708_eng.pdf

[21]   WHO. Early detection of tuberculosis: an overview of approaches, guideline and tools 2011. Available at: http://whqlibdoc.who.int/hq/2011/WHO_HTM_STB_PSI_2011.21_eng.pdf.

[22]   HIV & AIDS treatment in practice. Xpert MTB/RIF diagnostic test for TB: a global updateIssue 193, May, 2012. Available at: http://www.aidsmap.com/Xpert-MTBRIF-diagnostic-test-for-TB-a-global-update/page/2685513/

[23]   Tuberculosis diagnostics automated DNA test WHO endorsement and recommendations, 2010. Available at: http://www.who.int/tb/features_archive/xpert_factsheet.pdf

[24]   Lawn SD. Point-of-care detection of lipoarabinomannan (LAM) in urine for diagnosis of HIV-associated tuberculosis: a state of the art review. BMC Infect Dis 2012; 12: 103.
[http://dx.doi.org/10.1186/1471-2334-12-103] [PMID: 22536883]

[25]   Sterling TR, Villarino ME, Borisov AS, *et al.* TB Trials Consortium PREVENT TB Study Team. Three months of rifapentine and isoniazid for latent tuberculosis infection. N Engl J Med 2011; 365(23): 2155-66.
[http://dx.doi.org/10.1056/NEJMoa1104875] [PMID: 22150035]

[26]   WHO policy on collaborative TB/HIV activities. guidelines for national programmes and other stakeholders 2012. Available at: http://www.who.int/tb/publications/2012/tb_hiv_policy_9789241503006/en/

[27]   Panel on Antiretroviral Guidelines for Adults and Adolescents. Guidelines for the use of antiretroviral agents in HIV-1-infected adults and adolescents Department of Health and Human Services , 2014 [10/12/2014]; Available at:http://aidsinfo.nih.gov/ContentFiles/Adultand AdolescentGL.pdf

[28]   Panel on Opportunistic Infections in HIV-Exposed and HIV-Infected Children. Guidelines for the Prevention and Treatment of Opportunistic Infections in HIV-Exposed and HIV-Infected Children. Department of Health and Human Services , 2014 [10/12/2014]; Available at :http://aidsinfo.nih.gov/contentfiles/ lvguidelines/oi_guidelines_pediatrics.pdf

HIV and Hepatitis Viruses Co-infection: A Closer View of Their Interactions and Clinical Consequences

Seyed Younes Hosseini[1,2], **Katayoun Tayeri**[3,*], **Ali Teimoori**[4] and **Kazem Baesi**[5]

[1] *GastroenteroHepatology Research Center, Shiraz University of Medical Sciences,Shiraz, Iran*

[2] *Department of Bacteriology & Virology, Shiraz University of Medical Sciences, Shiraz, Iran*

[3] *Iranian Research Center for HIV/AIDS, Iranian Institute for Reduction of High Risk Behaviors, Tehran University of Medical Sciences, Tehran, Iran*

[4] *Department of Virology, Jundishapur University of Medical sciences, Ahvaz, Iran*

[5] *Hepatitis and AIDS Department, Pasteur Institute of Iran*

Abstract: Due to sharing common routes for transmission, a significant portion of HIV infected patients are co-infected with hepatitis related viruses. It is well documented that the prognosis, pathological pathways, immunological aspects and finally drug responsiveness are different between mono versus co-infected patients. Although the detailed mechanisms regarding disease exacerbation during HIV and hepatitis virus co-infection remain uncovered, recent findings are promising in the better understanding of the interactions that, in turn maybe valuable in drug discovery.

Close interaction of viruses at common site of replication, synergic actions of proteins, changing the immune response and remodeling the cell milieu through miRNA profile are among possible manners of cooperation/counteraction between HIV and hepatitis viruses that are taken into consideration here.

As HIV infection tends to accelerate the progression of HCV and HBV infections, clinical management of this patient group must be considered more seriously. All HIV cases should be tested for HCV and HBV serological/molecular markers for further

---

[*] **Correspondence to Katayoun Tayeri:** Iranian Research Center for HIV/AIDS (IRCHA), Imam Khomeini Hospital, Keshavarz Blvd., Tehran, Iran; Tel/Fax: +98 (21) 66947984; E-mail: katayon_tayeri@yahoo.com.

SeyedAhmad SeyedAlinaghi (Ed.)

management in clinical setting and special therapeutic trend for virus control also should be employed as well.

Keywords: Anti-retroviral therapy, Apoptosis, Co-infection, HBV, HCV, Hepatitis, Hepatocyte, HIV, Immune modulation, Stellate cell.

1. INTRODUCTION

With more than 30 million infected patients worldwide, the Human immunodeficiency virus (HIV) remains as a major human pathogen in the 21st century. Among the clinically important pathogens that may affect HIV infection, hepatitis-related viruses are of considerable importance. In fact, many previous studies have provided evidence that the prognosis, pathological pathways, immunological aspects, and finally, drug responsiveness are different between HIV infected and HIV/hepatitis co-infected patients [1 - 3]. Despite the significant adverse clinical consequences of HIV/HBV and HIV/HCV co-infections, the details of underlying molecular mechanisms of pathogenesis during viral co-infections remain unidentified [2, 4]. In special groups such as IV drug users (IDUs), HCV co-infection is higher and several studies showed that almost 50-90% of HIV infected people with positive history of needle sharing are also co-infected with HCV [2, 3].

In this chapter, we discuss the main molecular interactions between HIV and hepatitis-related viruses, as well as its consequences on the course of pathogenesis and clinical significance.

2. THE CLINICAL SIGNIFICANCE OF CO-INFECTION WITH HIV AND HEPATITIS-RELATED VIRUSES

Due to sharing common routes for transmission, approximately 30% of patients infected with HIV are also co-infected with HCV in some western nations [5]. Also, among the HIV-infected populations, HBV co-infection ranges from 6% to 14% in low prevalence areas [1]. Nonetheless, both HCV and HBV co-infections accelerate the progression of HIV infection toward AIDS and AIDS-related diseases [1, 2]. On the other hand, the complications of chronic hepatitis such as liver fibrosis, steatosis and Hepatocelluar Carcinoma (HCC) tend to develop faster in co-infected patients [1, 2, 4, 6].

The molecular mechanisms related to pathogenesis and clinical manifestation of HIV and HCV-related diseases seem to be completely different among mono-infected and dually infected patients, indicating the clinical importance of their interactions [4, 6]. In co-infected HIV/HCV patients, the desirable control of viral replication seems to be less achievable, both theoretically and in experimental settings. To date, epidemiological studies have supported an association between lower CD4 counts, higher HCV persistence and faster progression of liver disease, suggesting an important role for HIV co-infection in the pathogenesis of chronic liver disease [7]. On the other hand, HCV chronic infection may lead to over activation of CD4 cells which results in consequent depletion that would finally accelerate the progression of AIDS [6, 8, 9]. HIV infection tends to accelerate the progression of HCV infection. Higher HCV viral loads in serum and liver cells, exacerbation of progression toward fibrosis (at least three times more than mono-infected HCV patients) and rapid progression to cirrhosis are seen in co-infection with HIV/HCV [10 - 12].

Similar to HCV, HIV infection may exacerbate HBV infection which is always associated with an accelerated fibrosis, liver malfunction and development of HCC, albeit the mechanisms remain largely unidentified [3, 13]. The anticipated immunodeficiency following HIV infection, highly affects of natural course the HBV infection including longitudinal viral persistence, viral reactivation, less seroconversion and therapy unresponsiveness. High viral DNA load and low HBeAg clearance rate have been reported in association with lower CD4 count in untreated HIV/HBV patients [3]. Overall HIV tends to accelerate the progression of chronic HBV infection and liver failure. Also, HIV tends to increase HBV viral load in serum, while an increased risk for cirrhosis and earlier liver failure are anticipated. Additionally, the rate of reactivation of HBV in chronic carriers is increased. But several studies did not support the direct impact of HBV on HIV progression. Overall in HIV patients co-infected with HCV or HBV, the progression to end stage liver disease seems to be faster than mono infection [3].

GB Virus C (GBV-C) is a human flavivirus, recently separated from other flaviviruses and categorized in the *Pegivirus* genus. The GBV-C is a lymphotropic agent replicating in CD4+ and CD8+ T cells and in B cells with the capability of establishment a persistent infection. The GBV-C infection is a prevalent condition with a range of 20–40% among HIV-positive patients [14]. It was first introduced as a hepatitis inducer agent, but soon afterward, no association was found between liver and GBV-C infection. Surprisingly, pioneer investigators suggested that GBV-C viremia is associated with improved markers of HIV infection, including higher CD4 counts, lower HIV viral load, and delayed progression toward AIDS, as later concluded in plenty of publications [15].

Although the detailed mechanisms regarding disease exacerbation during HIV and hepatitis virus co-infection remain uncovered, recent findings are promising in further understanding the molecular interactions that maybe useful for novel drug development.

3. COMMON SITE OF REPLICATION: A BACKYARD FOR CLOSE INTERACTIONS?

Considering that in first instance HIV and hepatitis-related viruses target different cells, it is unlikely direct interactions between these viruses in the same cells; however, recently published studies have confirmed the presence and replication of HIV inside hepatocytes, which are the major site for hepatitis-related viruses replication as well as the stellate cells, the key player in development of liver fibrosis [16]. In depth analysis also showed that even though HIV does not establish a productive infection inside hepatocytes, it may propagate itself slowly in association with other hepatitis viruses [17, 18]. Such reports also demonstrated that activated Hematopoetic Stem Cells (HSCs) should be considered as a susceptible and permissive target for HIV infection [16]. In fact, other HIV-1 invaded cells residing in the liver tissue such as Kupffer and sinusoidal cells may further affect the liver matrix. Accordingly, HIV infection of the cells in the liver tissue is considered to play an important role in the accelerated pathogenesis of liver that results in fibrosis among co-infected patients.

Neurologic disorders of the HIV/HCV co-infected patients have also been of immense interest, especially after realizing that both HIV and HCV may replicate in the Central Nervous System (CNS), and detailed assays have indicated the presence of viral genomes and proteins in human microglia and astrocytes [19]. Although several experiments confirmed the presence of HCV core and NS3 proteins in human microglia and astrocytes, the immune-histochemical methods were unable to demonstrate the expression of receptors required for HCV entry into both cells [19, 20]. Furthermore, *in vitro* screening of neural cells for their ability to support HCV infection have indeed supported the idea of possible replication site for HCV in the CNS. It was demonstrated that two independent neuroepithelioma cell lines provided HCV candidate receptors like CD81, scavenger receptor B-I and occludin rather than other necessary replication apparatus [21]. This finding indeed supports the idea of a possible extrahepatic replication site for HCV in the Brain. Brain microvascular endothelial cells in Blood Brain Barrier (BBB) support HCV and HIV infection *in vitro* [22]. Stepwise replication, assembly of infectious particles and final cell lysis after HCV infection suggested the possible contribution of HCV in neuropathogenesis *via* direct viral infection or leakiness of the BBB.

It has been previously shown that specialized cells such as monocytes, liver Kupffer cells and even dendritic cells may be a site of replication for HIV, HCV, HBV or GBV-C; accordingly their close interactions and passive viral movement would be possible [23 - 25]. These Extra hepatic viral reservoirs are particularly important for the recurrence of viral infection especially after liver transplantation [25]. However, it should be noted that Antigen Presenting Cells (APCs) may not always support the replication of hepatitis-related virus, and because of that their residual multiplication is avoidable. In this regard, several publications have reported the presence of HBV genome and minus sense RNA of HCV in PBMCs; therefore they may come in direct contact with HIV at the same time, which would eventually affect the dynamics of their replication [26, 27].

Various studies provided evidence that HIV and hepatitis-related viruses may accelerate their replication. However, HIV/hepatitis-related viruses' interactions are less likely to result in the alleviation of HIV pathogenesis, a situation which is evident in the case of HIV/GBV-C infection of T cells. The T cells may support the replication cycle of GBV-C, although they are not susceptible to other hepatitis-related viruses due to lack of surface receptors. Accordingly, it may be concluded that direct viral interactions occur particularly in the case of

HIV/GBV-C co-infection. The fact that GBV-C replicates in CD4+ cells has encouraged investigators to seek further potentially effective anti-HIV therapeutic options [25].

It has been shown that HIV infection of the HBV harboring hepatic cell lines significantly increases the intracellular HBsAg, but does not result in accelerated HBV DNA synthesis. Cells harboring replicating HBV may be infected and efficiently support the productive infection of HIV, suggesting the absence of direct viral interference at least *in vitro* [28]. An *in vitro* study showed that HBX antigen from HBV, might contribute to the faster HIV replication *via* activating long terminal repeat (LTR) *via* the aid of some viral and host factors (*i.e.* Tat and cell mitogenic factor) [3]. Among the HCV proteins, association of NS3/4A enzyme with Vpu may stimulate transcription from LTR that may influence replication of HIV [29]. On the contrary, the GBV-C infection of PBMCs inhibits the replication of HIV in a co-infection culture model. Further reports revealed that inhibition of HIV does not result from direct GBV-C replication, but maybe explained by the alteration of HIV entry receptors following GBV-C infection. In fact, reduced expression of the two HIV entry co-receptors (CCR5 and CXCR4) and high plasma level of their ligands (RANTES, SDF-1, CCL3 and CCL4) are associated with GBV-C infection, which would in turn abrogate the HIV replication indirectly [15, 30]. These findings have changed our insights for discovering common pathways for targeting viral replications regarding the pathogenesis of HIV/hepatitis viruses' co-infections.

4. NEUROTOXIC EFFECTS ASSOCIATED WITH HIV/HEPATITIS-RELATED VIRUSES CO-INFECTION

Productive HIV replication has been detected in different stages of the neurological disorders among various CNS-residing cells types [31, 32]. Resident brain macrophages and microglia particularly support HIV-1 infection, which plays a major role in the spread of viral infection [32]. Even though the HIV transcripts and proteins have been detected in astrocytes, neuronal permission for HIV replication remains unclear.

It is well-known that HIV-1 usually exerts its direct neurotoxic effects through several viral proteins including gp120, Tat, Nef and Vpr. The HIV-1 Vpr, Tat and gp120 trigger neuronal cell apoptosis that leads to neurobehavioral defects in animal models [32]. Different pathways of Tat dependent cell death [32] that consequently augment the neuronal death have been identified. Among such pathways, the over-expression of TRAIL, activation of NF-κB signaling pathway, dys-regulation of neuronal calcium homeostasis, mitochondrial hyper-polarization as well as the up-regulation of p53 have been reported. Tat also causes indirect neuronal injury through boosting the secretion of the specific matrix metalloproteinases MMP-2 and MMP-9. Astrocytes stimulated by HIV serve as main sources of these enzyme, and their increased secretion may lead to either neurotoxic effects or tissue remodeling of the brain [33]. Moreover, Tat has been found to increase the levels of miR-34a in a transgenic mice model. This miRNA was demonstrated to be involved in neurological disorders, as the suppression of the expression of the target genes may lead to serious neuronal dys-regulation and eventually the development of HIV-associated neurologic diseases [34].

The HIV-infected astrocytes and microglia may exert their direct and indirect effects that lead to neuronal injury through releasing soluble toxic viral proteins (*i.e.* Tat and gp120) [35] and pro-inflammatory molecules (*i.e.* cytokines and chemokines), respectively. HIV-activated microglia are capable of producing a wide range of potential neurotoxins including eicosanoids, platelet-activating factor (PAF), pro-inflammatory cytokines, quinolinic acid, free radicals (*e.g.* nitric oxide and superoxide anion), glutamate-like agonist l-cysteine (an endogenous neurotoxin) and neurotoxic amines [32]. In the case of HIV/HCV co-infection, the HIV/HCV interaction would lead to HIV-related neuropathy exacerbation and promotion of disease progression [36]. The HCV/HIV co-infected individuals scored lower in neuro-cognitive tests and revealed considerable cognitive and motor impairment compared to mono-infected patients, which further highlights the syngenic effect of HCV proteins on HIV neuro-pathogenic deterioration [19].

Most recently, the HCV RNA genome and proteins were detected in the brains of HIV/HCV co-infected patients. Detailed molecular assays have indicated that NS3 and NS5A proteins are expressed in human microglia and astrocytes, which are also considered as important sites of HIV replication, but not in neurons or oligodendrocytes [20]. It has also been shown that direct HCV infection of the

BBB endothelial cells occurs frequently and results in apoptosis and barrier dis-integrity that would permit entry of HIV viral particles, inflammatory cytokines and other neurotoxic substances [22].

The persistently higher serum levels of pro-inflammatory cytokines among HIV/HCV co-infected patients compared to the HIV patients has been associated with worse neuro-cognitive diseases, which suggests that synergistic viral interactions may be fulfilled through inducing inflammatory responses [37, 38]. The HCV core protein plays an important role in the activation of human glial cells and induces the expression of pro-inflammatory cytokines in microglia, which may further contribute to HIV-associated neuropathy [20, 37]. Also, core protein overwhelms neuronal membrane currents in addition to decreasing the expression of tubulin and autophagy proteins which finally cause neuronal cell death [20, 36]. Surprisingly, core neurotoxicity and inflammatory properties were increased by HIV Vpr protein. It is likely that Vpr and core act through different mechanisms to result in cumulative neurotoxic effects [20]. Further *in vitro* analysis demonstrated that core protein neurotoxicity may be mediated by activation of TLR2-IRAK1 signaling pathway [36]. Detailed description of this pathway will provide an opportunity for identification of novel molecular targets with regard to halting the HCV neuro-pathogenesis in the CNS [36].

The presence of lipopolysaccharides (LPS) in plasma indicates microbial translocation that arises after gut mucosal leakage during HIV infection and induces monocyte activation and movement. This phenomenon is frequently higher in HCV co-infection suggested a special role of HCV in the movement of activated monocytes toward the brain which possibly cause more progressive HIV-associated dementia [39]. On the contrary to the existing evidence suggesting the mutual role of HIV and HCV in neuronal pathogenesis, there are no data concerning the replication of HBV in the CNS. A recently published study outlined the possible role of CNS as either a source of HBV replication or reservoir, particularly for drug-resistant mutants [40].

5. HIV INFECTION AND HEPATIC PATHOGENESIS

HCV and HBV-associated liver disease is accelerated in HIV co-infected individuals; whereas hepatic steatosis -a common complication of HCV infection- is not necessarily more common in co-infected cases [6]. Although detailed mechanisms of accelerated liver disease in co-infected patients are not well understood, it may include direct viral protein effects, indirect immune alterations, chronic inflammation, enhanced cell apoptosis and diminished specific T-cell responses [1, 6, 11, 41].

In spite of T cell tropism, *in vivo* studies support the presence of HIV pro-viral DNA in liver tissue cells, particularly Kupffer cells and isolated hepatocytes. In addition, HIV proteins have been detected in parenchymal and non-parenchymal liver cells by immunohistochemistry [17]. Increasing evidence suggests that HIV replicates in hepatocytes and Hepatic Stellate Cells (HSC), two major liver cells that play significant roles in hepatic pathogenesis [1, 17]. Also, HIV expresses proteins that may induce apoptosis of hepatocytes and the release of inflammatory cytokines which would eventually promote fibrosis [17, 18]. Furthermore, HIV/HCV co-infection may increase hepatocyte apoptosis by TRAIL and Fas/FasL signaling that accounts for the accelerated liver damage [42]. With regard to HIV/HBV co-infection, the *in vitro* investigations on liver biopsy samples have discovered no more HSCs, Kupffer cells and intra-hepatic T cells activation, but hepatocyte apoptosis accelerated in HIV/HBV co-infected patients [1]. Beside the direct pathogenic role of HIV proteins, immune modulation through alteration of cytokine levels (*i.e.* IL-4, IL-5, IL-13 and TGF-β) would change the liver milieu, resulting in further immune activation [6, 41]. The TGF-β -a key mediator in liver fibrosis- is profoundly increased in the liver matrix following HIV infection. Also, the elevated plasma LPS level during HIV infection could promote HCV and HBV-related liver pathogenesis through direct cytotoxic effects of LPS on hepatocytes or enhancing immune activation [39].

6. STELLATE CELLS CO-INFECTION: UNDERSTANDING THE HIV-INDUCED LIVER FIBROSIS

The Hepatic Stellate Cell (HSC) is a key player in liver fibrosis. Following liver injury, the HSCs are activated and secrete extraordinarily high amounts of extracellular matrix containing remodeling proteins such as MMPs and TIMP, further promoting the process of cirrhosis [16]. The HIV-1 infects HSCs and induces the expression of collagen I and other markers of activation [16]. While some reports suggested that activated HSCs express both CCR5 and CXCR4 HIV coreceptors, quiescent HSCs are not sensitive to HIV infection based on *in vitro* experiments because HIV entry into HSCs is mainly independent on CD4/chemokine coreceptor. Both X4 and R5 tropic HIV have been demonstrated to enter activated HSC LX2 cells so they may contribute to the exacerbation of fibrosis [16].

The effects of HIV proteins on the activity of HSC have been investigated previously. The HIV gp120 has been shown to induce HSCs activity in a receptor-dependent manner and promote their fibrogenetic propensity. Furthermore, the HSCs permissiveness for HIV replication turns them into a prominent intra-hepatic source of HIV proteins (such as gp120) that have been shown to transmit fibrosis inducing stimuli to the neighboring cells. In fact, HIV infection induces a significant increase in TGF-β1 production, a central mediator of fibrogenesis that enhances both the fibrosis and HCV replication [43]. Moreover, HIV/HCV co-infection further increases fibrosis through increased production of reactive oxygen species by HSCs *via* a NFκB-dependent pathway [44].

7. DIRECT INTERACTIONS BETWEEN VIRAL REPLICATION CYCLES

It has been previously shown that the Long Terminal Repeat (LTR) of HIV genome are tightly controlled by the binding of several viral and cellular transcription factors such as USF, c-Myb, NF-AT, and AP-1. The HCV NS3/4A protein can indirectly activate HIV-1 transcription from its LTR region, while the serine protease domain is essential for this purpose. This activation effect of NS3/4A can be explained by its ability to enhance DNA binding of some transcription factors such as AP-1 [29]. On the other hand, the HIV Rev protein activates HCV gene expression by binding to the internal loop of the HCV 5'-untranslated region (5'-UTR). In depth analysis revealed that Rev may increase the HCV IRES-mediated translation [45]. The IRES regulatory sequence provides non-canonical scan independent translation, which provides HCV a big advantage over the cell traditional translation system. Also, the HIV/HCV co-infection is associated with increased expression of IP-10 mRNA and enhanced replication of HCV in liver cells. Among the HIV-1 protein candidates, Tat confirmed to be an activator of HCV replication indirectly through up-regulating the IP-10 production [46].

Among the HBV proteins, HBX protein enhances HIV transcription and might contribute to the rapid HIV progression *via* transcriptional activation of the LTR [47]. The HBX protein may accomplish this function synergistically with other factors such as HIV Tat and protein members of the C/EBP and ATF/CREB families. Additionally, the HBV Covalently Closed Circular DNA (cccDNA) persists in PBMCs for a long period, which in turn accommodates HBX for further trans-activation of the LTR [48]. Moreover, while HBV X protein acts synergistically with Tat in promoting HIV replication, the effect of this synergy on HBV life cycle remains obscure.

It was soon identified that the HIV infection of HBV-infected hepatic cell lines significantly increases intracellular HBsAg titer but does not increase the HBV DNA viral load in supernatant [28]. The increased intra-hepatic HBsAg production may accelerate liver damage in HIV/HBV co-infected patients. The mechanism by which HIV infection alters transcription of the HBsAg is unknown. It is possible that HIV directly influences the transcription of the HBsAg mRNA by improving the binding of the cell trans-activating proteins to its promoter.

During HBV replication in HIV infected patients more mutant strains of HBV may also be enriched in virus population [49]. Recently, HBX and HBS mutations has also been reported in coinfection with undetermined clinical significance but suggesting the impact of coinfection on increasing the virus population heterogenesity [3].

The majority of publications acclaimed that GBV-C proteins inhibit HIV replication due to common site of replication independent of the GBV-C effect on surface CD4 receptor. Also, the E1 and E2, attachment proteins of GBV-C directly inhibit HIV pseudo virus entry. Subsequently, specific peptides derived from both proteins could interfere with HIV cellular binding and fusion [50].

By contrast, GBV-C NS5A regulatory protein expression down regulates CXCR4 surface expression and induces the secretion of SDF-1 and CXCR4 ligand from blood mononuclear cells which ultimately expand the population of cells with HIV resistant phenotype through co-receptor occupation and/or diminution [51]. Surprisingly, expression of a 16 amino acid domain within NS5A is sufficient to prevent HIV replication in a dose-dependent manner, suggesting therapeutic potential of this small molecule to postpone HIV progression. Recently the GBV-C NS3 serine protease has shown inhibition of HIV replication without decreasing HIV receptor expression [52]. Cumulatively in spite of synergistic effect of HBV and HCV proteins in HIV replication, GBV-C protein derivatives has potentiality to be exploited in HIV molecular targeting in future.

8. ON THE IMPORTANCE OF APOPTOSIS

Programmed cell death is an inevitable outcome of viral infection that highly affects the tissue matrix and the surrounding cells. Previous studies suggested that hepatitis viruses need to prevent host apoptosis, in order to ensure lifelong virus spread in the liver; accordingly, they have evolved as non-cytolytic viruses. The induction of apoptosis by HCV and HBV has been evaluated in plenty of experiments and it was revealed that even similar proteins may play dual function both as inducer and inhibitor of apoptosis, depending on the viral and cell cycle stages.

Several HIV-1 proteins, including gp120, protease and the accessory proteins such as Tat, Nef and Vpr have been demonstrated to directly induce neuronal, hepatocyte and lymphocyte cell death [32, 35, 53]. Several mechanisms have been proposed for their pro-apoptotic properties including up-regulation of Fas, increased expression of TRAIL, molecular mimicry of gp 120 with Fas, cell cycle arrest at the G2 phase (gp120), decreased Bcl-2 family expression (protease, Nef, gp120, Vpr), mitochondrial membrane rupture following lysosomal perme-abilization (Nef), generation of reactive oxygen intermediates (gp120), phosphorylation of mTOR and p53 (gp120, Tat), increased expression of the pro-apoptotic proteins like PUMA (gp120) and activation of p38 [32, 53]. Tat protein also causes neuronal cell death through induction of MMPs [33].

Various signaling pathways may be important in inducing the programmed cell death in different target cells. Different HIV proteins can activate the mitochondrial-dependent apoptosis by involvement of TRAIL R2 signaling pathway that requires JNK kinase [32, 42]. In the liver tissue, programmed death is accelerated *via* different pathways, especially a Fas/FasL- dependent pathway that seems to account for the exacerbation of liver damage in co-infected patients. Also, in co-infected intra-hepatic milieu, HIV causes a G-protein independent cell death *via* p38 protein following the binding of gp120 to CXCR4 [42]. Surprisingly, the HIV/GBV-C co-infection is negatively correlated to Fas expression and Fas-mediated apoptosis in PBMCs [54].

The direct effects of HCV and HIV envelope proteins on hepatocytes apoptosis have been studied using an *in vitro* developed model of co-infection [17]. Following simultaneous treatment of cells with E2 and gp120 proteins, an enhanced level of apoptosis was noticed, indicating the synergistic effect of these proteins when compared to the control group. Another study showed that these proteins induce extraordinary expression of FasL on different cells surface and DISC complex formation when applied together which promotes extrinsic pathway of apoptosis [55]. Furthermore, HCV E2 and HIV gp120 proteins are able to up-regulate the expression of Bax, Bid and Bak pre-apoptotic proteins, leading to mitochondrial membrane permeabilization and apoptosis [4]. With regard to HCV, different proteins such as E2, core, NS5A and NS3 have been reported to trigger apoptosis *via* multiple pathways. The NS4A has been shown to induce cytochrom C release from mitochondrial membrane and trigger apoptosome complex formation by an unknown mechanism [4], while core and NS3 accelerate apoptosis in different cell types by different mechanisms [4].

It is noteworthy that the process of apoptosis depends largely on the outer environment of target cells. A new study in HIV/HBV co-infected individuals was performed to assess T-cell, NK cells and HSCs activation on liver biopsy samples and revealed no evidence of intrahepatic activation, but detected a significant increase in apoptosis especially among hepatocytes [56]. It is unlikely that apoptosis of hepatocytes was caused by the HBV itself, as HBV is generally considered a non-cytopathic agent. However, previous studies showed that HBV sensitizes hepatocytes to TRAIL-mediated apoptosis through up-regulating of Bax by HBX protein [57, 58]. Furthermore, intra-hepatic accumulation of HBV proteins such as HBsAg-as recently demonstrated *in vitro* may potentially facilitate hepatocyte apoptosis *via* stressing the endoplasmic reticulum during HIV/HBV co-infection.

9. THE ROLE OF MIRNAS IN HIV/HEPATITIS RELATED VIRUSES CO-INFECTION

Alike other human viruses, HIV, HCV and HBV may influence and exploit total miRNA transcription inside the host cells for optimal reproduction. Although different viral strains induce the up or down regulation of a wide spectrum of miRNAs, investigations have revealed a partial overlap among them [59]. A recent report demonstrated a significant overlap between up-regulated micro RNAs in HCV infected hepatoma lines and blood PBMCs from HIV-1 infected patients that indicates a similar route of control over host by these viruses [60]. It has been recently accepted that miRNA-122 plays a critical role in promoting the HCV life cycle [61, 62]. It is proposed that maybe miRNA-122 boosts HCV polycistronic transcripts translation or protects them from early RNA degradation, but the exact mechanisms have not been established so far [62]. Interestingly, HIV-1 infection of T cells significantly up-regulated the expression of miR-122 that implies a possible role of miR-122 in HIV replication cycle. On the contrary to miR-122, the miR-29 over-expression reduces the HCV replication in hepatocytes and targets the 3'UTR HIV transcripts for degradation [61, 63]. Thus, as a novel therapeutic strategy, the over-expression of miR-29 may be considered as a valuable option among the co-infected patients [61].

The role of exosomes and exosomal pathways in cell-to-cell communication has been well characterized. The exosomal pathways may also be exploited by viruses to transmit miRNA messages to the neighboring cells [64, 65]. Thus, depending on the tropism of HIV-1 and HCV viruses, it is possible that circulating miRNAs in exosomes are secreted by non-hepatocyte HIV-1 sources and are taken by HCV-infected hepatocytes or *vice versa* [61]. This phenomenon may eventually affect the neighboring hepatocyte or PBMCs, which may ultimately exacerbate disease outcome. In addition, the levels of miR-34a -a miRNA associated with neuropathological disease- were increased in Tat transgenic mice. Therefore, it could be concluded that dysregulation of neuronal functions by HIV-1 Tat protein might be miRNA-dependent [34].

10. IMMUNE MODULATION

It seems that the immune suppression resulting from HIV infection enhances the HCV and HBV pathogenesis, rather than impairing the viral clearance and chronicity of the infection [41]. Several studies have shown the direct correlation of higher hepatitis viral loads and lower CD4 counts [6, 13, 41]. In fact, the continuous activation of lymphocytes occurs during chronic viral hepatitis which leads to early activation of induced cell death and depletion of CD4+ cells population [6, 8]. Albeit this phenomena dysregulate the production of cytokines, causing enhanced HIV and HCV replication and increased pathogenesis [6].

Multiple studies have identified HIV Tat-mediated elevation of IP-10 (CXCL10) levels as a negative prognostic factor in HCV and HIV co-infection. It is thought that elevated IP-10 boosts HCV replication in hepatocytes and could recruit T cells within the liver, which ultimately leads to more tissue damages [46]. Extraordinary accumulation of cytotoxic CD8+ cells in the liver increases the inflammatory mediators in co-infected patients, and may increase tissue regeneration and promote fibrosis [39, 40].

Some studies also suggested the direct modulator effect of HCV proteins on immune system. The HCV E2, core, NS3 and NS5 proteins exert a variety of modulatory effects on innate or adaptive immune system [66, 67]. It was demonstrated that the NS3 protein with protease activity inhibits intracellular innate immunity by cleaving some key mediators like TRIF and MAVS proteins. On the other hand, impaired function of dendritic cells is another cause of HCV immune evasion. Recently, the contribution of core and NS3 in this impairment has been assessed *in vitro* [68], but its potential value in co-infection with HIV remains unclear [69]. The binding of NS5A to RNA dependent protein kinase R (PKR) *in vivo* inhibits its function that is an essential player for induction and transduction of the interferon-dependent antiviral response. Nonetheless, whether these kinds of interactions occur *in vivo* and how they influence immunity in HIV co-infected patients is still unclear.

Unsurprisingly, studies have demonstrated that HIV/HBV co-infection is associated with poor HBV-specific lymphocytes responses *in vitro* [70], which may be explained by programmed death-1 (PD-1) pathway during antigen presentation and immune suppression by regulatory T cells (Tregs) [71]. During HIV infection, PD-1L is up-regulated among the monocytes and dendritic cells that may increase HBV specific tolerance and viral persistence. If the role of PD-1 is adequately distinguished, specific blockade of PD-1 pathway would be a rational strategy to subvert HBV-specific tolerance [3]. Besides, other potential strategies would be targeting the Tregs as well as CCR5 receptor occupation on hepatocytes and HSCs, which seem as potential molecular therapeutic options for co-infected patients [72].

In contrast with previous reports, recent studies suggested that HBV may potentially impede HIV dissemination *via* preventing maturation of dendritic cells [3]. In fact, the HBV virion or HBsAg inhibits the maturation of dendritic cells and lead to immuno-tolerance to HBV [73]. Hence mature dendritic cells favor HIV transmission more competently than immature dendritic cells; this inhibitory effect may restrict HIV dissemination to its target cells.

In terms of HIV/GBV-C co-infection, the level of interferon activation in dendritic cells was significantly higher in HIV/GBV-C co-infected individuals. Specifically, active GBV-C infection reduces the level of activation markers CCR5 and CD38 on T cells that are induced in HIV infection [15, 74]. The multiple effects of GBV-C on immune cells can balance the chronic immune activation and appropriate induction of innate response, which would ultimately halt the progression of HIV infection [15].

11. CLINICAL MANAGEMENT OF HIV/HEPATITIS CO-INFECTION

It should be keep in mind that all HIV patients should be tested for HCV and HBV serologic markers first. After evaluation of HBsAg and Anti-HBc for HBV and Anti-HCV antibody for HCV infection, more confirmatory tests like PCR assay should be performed. Hence, regarding the primary testing, vaccination for HBV should be done and if the high risk behaviors are continued, HCV Antibody testing should be scheduled yearly.

The first step in the treatment of HCV infection is cessation of all hepatotoxic agents such as illegal drugs, alcohol, some medication (*i.e.* high dose acetaminophen) that tend to exacerbate liver fibrosis. Losing weight is the second important recommendation for obese patients. Recent studies have provided evidence that sooner initiation of the treatment in HCV infection leads to better and more sustainable responses, both in mono-infected and HIV/HCV co-infected patients. Overall 65% of patients respond to treatment in this situation regardless of the viral genotype. In fact, patient's response to therapy after 12 weeks of initiating the treatment can predict the outcome of treatment [75]. According to several studies, due to side effects of treatment in HIV co-infected patients, HCV treatment is recommended in CD4 cell>500; but in general, HCV treatment should be considered for all co-infected patients with good control of the HIV infection and when the HCV treatment is not contraindicated [76, 77]. Treatment of HCV infection might be contraindicated in certain conditions including [78]:

- The conditions related to interferon:
  - Decompensated liver disease
  - Severe poorly controlled psychological disorders, suicidal attempt
  - Solid organ transplantation
  - Untreated thyroid diseases
- And conditions that are related to ribavirin:
  - Probability of pregnancy (or any paternity plan for men and pregnancy plan for women)
  - Severe anemia (should be corrected before initiation of ribavirin)

Liver biopsy is the best guide for staging of liver disease and optimal timing of treatment; but it is not essential for starting the treatment, especially in genotype 2 and 3, acute infection and patients who are committed to treatment with any fibrosis score. Also, we can use serum biomarker tests like APRI (AST-to-platelet ratio) and FIB-4 (based on ALT, AST, platelet count and patient age) or fibroscan (transient elastography) taking into consideration their limitations and prices. Correspondingly, the severity of liver disease should be assessed in co-infected patients before starting HCV therapy by using biopsy or non-invasive methods.

The first-line treatment of chronic HCV in co-infected HIV/HCV is Pegylated-Interferon-alfa, administered weekly plus ribavirin daily (15mg/kg/day), as in mono-infected patients. In patients with CD4<200, it is strongly recommended to start the ART or continue the previous ART while HCV therapy should be postponed until the severely impairment of the immune system is corrected. It is noteworthy that during administration of Peg-Interferon plus ribavirin, some ARV drugs such as didanosine, zidovudine and stavudine should be avoided. The duration of HCV treatment is 48 weeks, regardless of HCV genotype (even 2 and 3) and longer duration (72 week) may be needed in genotype 1. Also, during the treatment, checking of HCV viral load in 1th and 3th months and end of treatment, monthly CBC and thyroid function test each three months are recommended. Recent studies showed that the level of vitamin D in patients, especially co-infected HIV/HCV, relates to the treatment outcome and patients with vitamin D deficiency tend to have poorer outcomes. Therefore, this finding should be considered in nutritional counseling of patients.

In the case of HBV [7, 79, 80], in patients with positive HBsAg, quantitative HBV DNA, HBeAg and liver enzymes should be checked. If HBV viral load is <2000 copies/mL especially when HBeAg is negative, only follow up measurement might be considered due to wide fluctuations in serum HBV DNA level. Decision for starting the treatment does not depend on result of liver biopsy in all patients. For example, when the patient has cirrhosis, CD4<350 or any indication of ARV therapy or in patients with elevated liver enzymes and with HBV DNA>2000 and/or HBeAg positive, treatment for HBV should be considered [81]. But if biopsy is performed in patient with HBV DNA<2000 and elevated ALT, treatment is indicated with Metavir score > A2 and/or >F2.

Two groups of drugs are available for the treatment in chronic hepatitis B including Interferon and nucleotide analogues (Adefovir, Entecavir, Emtricitabine, Lamivudine, Telbivudine and Tenofovir). Among the drugs for treatment of HIV/HBV co-infection, tenofovir is the first choice and should be considered as a part of ART regimen. In addition, it is recommended that tenofovir should be combined with another anti-HBV drug like lamivudine or emtricitabine [81].

Accordingly, in all patients with HIV/HBV co-infection eligible for HBV treatment, ART should be considered with a regimen that contains at least two drugs with good efficacy against HBV. On the other hand, in every co-infected HBV/HIV patient who needs HBV treatment without ART (for example CD4>350 and without clinical symptoms), ART should be considered with a regimen that contains at least two drugs with good efficacy against HBV. As a rule in co-infection, both infections should be treated [81].

12. CONCLUDING REMARKS AND FUTURE PERSPECTIVES

Although certain parts of the molecular interactions of HIV/hepatitis related viruses co-infection have been determined so far, many aspects still remain uncovered. Detailed description of the molecular pathways of HIV interactions with other viruses -particularly hepatitis related viruses- and identification of the possibly synergistic interactions can help us to better understand the mechanisms of molecular pathogenesis and developing novel therapeutic options that would target such pathways in co-infected patients. Future investigations are encouraged for designing possible anti-HIV miRNAs, production of novel blockers of the viral replication cycle, specific immune modulators, the use of novel strategies to down regulate the immune response (*i.e.* PD-1 blocker) and identifying new interfering agents such as the GBV-C NS5 peptide.

CONFLICT OF INTEREST

The authors confirm that they have no conflict of interest to declare for this publication.

ACKNOWLEDGEMENTS

Declared none.

REFERENCES

[1]   Crane M, Iser D, Lewin SR. Human immunodeficiency virus infection and the liver. World J Hepatol 2012; 4(3): 91-8.
        [http://dx.doi.org/10.4254/wjh.v4.i3.91] [PMID: 22489261]

[2]   Kim AY, Chung RT. Coinfection with HIV-1 and HCV--a one-two punch. Gastroenterology 2009; 137(3): 795-814.
        [http://dx.doi.org/10.1053/j.gastro.2009.06.040] [PMID: 19549523]

[3]   Li YJ, Wang HL, Li TS. Hepatitis B virus/human immunodeficiency virus coinfection: interaction among human immunodeficiency virus infection, chronic hepatitis B virus infection, and host

immunity. Chin Med J (Engl) 2012; 125(13): 2371-7.
[PMID: 22882864]

[4]   Roe B, Hall WW. Cellular and molecular interactions in coinfection with hepatitis C virus and human immunodeficiency virus. Expert Rev Mol Med 2008; 10: e30.
[http://dx.doi.org/10.1017/S1462399408000847] [PMID: 18928579]

[5]   Andreoni M, Giacometti A, Maida I, Meraviglia P, Ripamonti D, Sarmati L. HIV-HCV co-infection: epidemiology, pathogenesis and therapeutic implications. Eur Rev Med Pharmacol Sci 2012; 16(11): 1473-83.
[PMID: 23111959]

[6]   Operskalski EA, Kovacs A. HIV/HCV co-infection: pathogenesis, clinical complications, treatment, and new therapeutic technologies. Curr HIV/AIDS Rep 2011; 8(1): 12-22.
[http://dx.doi.org/10.1007/s11904-010-0071-3] [PMID: 21221855]

[7]   Fernández-Montero JV, Soriano V. Management of hepatitis C in HIV and/or HBV co-infected patients. Best Pract Res Clin Gastroenterol 2012; 26(4): 517-30.
[http://dx.doi.org/10.1016/j.bpg.2012.09.007] [PMID: 23199509]

[8]   Gonzalez VD, Falconer K, Blom KG, *et al.* High levels of chronic immune activation in the T-cell compartments of patients coinfected with hepatitis C virus and human immunodeficiency virus type 1 and on highly active antiretroviral therapy are reverted by alpha interferon and ribavirin treatment. J Virol 2009; 83(21): 11407-11.
[http://dx.doi.org/10.1128/JVI.01211-09] [PMID: 19710147]

[9]   Körner C, Tolksdorf F, Riesner K, *et al.* Hepatitis C coinfection enhances sensitization of CD4(+) T-cells towards Fas-induced apoptosis in viraemic and HAART-controlled HIV-1-positive patients. Antivir Ther (Lond) 2011; 16(7): 1047-55.
[http://dx.doi.org/10.3851/IMP1882] [PMID: 22024520]

[10]   Lin W, Weinberg EM, Chung RT. Pathogenesis of accelerated fibrosis in HIV/HCV co-infection. J Infect Dis 2013; 207 (Suppl. 1): S13-8.
[http://dx.doi.org/10.1093/infdis/jis926] [PMID: 23390300]

[11]   Lacombe K, Rockstroh J. HIV and viral hepatitis coinfections: advances and challenges. Gut 2012; 61 (Suppl. 1): i47-58.
[http://dx.doi.org/10.1136/gutjnl-2012-302062] [PMID: 22504919]

[12]   Hernandez MD, Sherman KE. HIV/hepatitis C coinfection natural history and disease progression. Curr Opin HIV AIDS 2011; 6(6): 478-82.
[http://dx.doi.org/10.1097/COH.0b013e32834bd365] [PMID: 22001892]

[13]   Sulkowski MS. Viral hepatitis and HIV coinfection. J Hepatol 2008; 48(2): 353-67.
[http://dx.doi.org/10.1016/j.jhep.2007.11.009] [PMID: 18155314]

[14]   Stapleton JT, Foung S, Muerhoff AS, Bukh J, Simmonds P. The GB viruses: a review and proposed classification of GBV-A, GBV-C (HGV), and GBV-D in genus Pegivirus within the family Flaviviridae. J Gen Virol 2011; 92(Pt 2): 233-46.
[http://dx.doi.org/10.1099/vir.0.027490-0] [PMID: 21084497]

[15]   Bhattarai N, Stapleton JT. GB virus C: the good boy virus? Trends Microbiol 2012; 20(3): 124-30.

[http://dx.doi.org/10.1016/j.tim.2012.01.004] [PMID: 22325031]

[16]   Tuyama AC, Hong F, Saiman Y, *et al*. Human immunodeficiency virus (HIV)-1 infects human hepatic stellate cells and promotes collagen I and monocyte chemoattractant protein-1 expression: implications for the pathogenesis of HIV/hepatitis C virus-induced liver fibrosis. Hepatology 2010; 52(2): 612-22.
[http://dx.doi.org/10.1002/hep.23679] [PMID: 20683959]

[17]   Blackard JT, Sherman KE. HCV/ HIV co-infection: time to re-evaluate the role of HIV in the liver? J Viral Hepat 2008; 15(5): 323-30.
[http://dx.doi.org/10.1111/j.1365-2893.2008.00970.x] [PMID: 18208497]

[18]   Vlahakis SR, Villasis-Keever A, Gomez TS, Bren GD, Paya CV. Human immunodeficiency virus-induced apoptosis of human hepatocytes *via* CXCR4. J Infect Dis 2003; 188(10): 1455-60.
[http://dx.doi.org/10.1086/379738] [PMID: 14624370]

[19]   Letendre S, Paulino AD, Rockenstein E, *et al*. HIV Neurobehavioral Research Center Group. Pathogenesis of hepatitis C virus coinfection in the brains of patients infected with HIV. J Infect Dis 2007; 196(3): 361-70.
[http://dx.doi.org/10.1086/519285] [PMID: 17597450]

[20]   Vivithanaporn P, Maingat F, Lin LT, *et al*. Hepatitis C virus core protein induces neuroimmune activation and potentiates Human Immunodeficiency Virus-1 neurotoxicity. PLoS One 2010; 5(9): e12856.
[http://dx.doi.org/10.1371/journal.pone.0012856] [PMID: 20877724]

[21]   Fletcher NF, Yang JP, Farquhar MJ, *et al*. Hepatitis C virus infection of neuroepithelioma cell lines. Gastroenterology 2010; 139(4): 1365-74.
[http://dx.doi.org/10.1053/j.gastro.2010.06.008] [PMID: 20538002]

[22]   Fletcher NF, Wilson GK, Murray J, Hu K, Lewis A, Reynolds GM. Hepatitis C virus infects the endothelial cells of the blood-brain barrie Gastroenterology 2010; 142(3): 634-643 e6.2011;
[PMID: 22138189]

[23]   Revie D, Salahuddin SZ. Human cell types important for hepatitis C virus replication *in vivo* and *in vitro*: old assertions and current evidence. Virol J 2011; 8: 346.
[http://dx.doi.org/10.1186/1743-422X-8-346] [PMID: 21745397]

[24]   Coffin CS, Mulrooney-Cousins PM, Peters MG, *et al*. Molecular characterization of intrahepatic and extrahepatic hepatitis B virus (HBV) reservoirs in patients on suppressive antiviral therapy. J Viral Hepat 2011; 18(6): 415-23.
[http://dx.doi.org/10.1111/j.1365-2893.2010.01321.x] [PMID: 20626626]

[25]   Blackard JT, Kemmer N, Sherman KE. Extrahepatic replication of HCV: insights into clinical manifestations and biological consequences. Hepatology 2006; 44(1): 15-22.
[http://dx.doi.org/10.1002/hep.21283] [PMID: 16799966]

[26]   Gong GZ, Lai LY, Jiang YF, He Y, Su XS. HCV replication in PBMC and its influence on interferon therapy. World J Gastroenterol 2003; 9(2): 291-4.
[http://dx.doi.org/10.3748/wjg.v9.i2.291] [PMID: 12532451]

[27]   Natarajan V, Kottilil S, Hazen A, *et al*. HCV in peripheral blood mononuclear cells are predominantly carried on the surface of cells in HIV/HCV co-infected individuals. J Med Virol 2010; 82(12): 2032-7.

[http://dx.doi.org/10.1002/jmv.21906] [PMID: 20981790]

[28] Iser DM, Warner N, Revill PA, *et al.* Coinfection of hepatic cell lines with human immunodeficiency virus and hepatitis B virus leads to an increase in intracellular hepatitis B surface antigen. J Virol 2010; 84(12): 5860-7.
[http://dx.doi.org/10.1128/JVI.02594-09] [PMID: 20357083]

[29] Kang L, Luo Z, Li Y, *et al.* Association of Vpu with hepatitis C virus NS3/4A stimulates transcription of type 1 human immunodeficiency virus. Virus Res 2012; 163(1): 74-81.
[http://dx.doi.org/10.1016/j.virusres.2011.08.011] [PMID: 21889553]

[30] Xiang J, George SL, Wünschmann S, Chang Q, Klinzman D, Stapleton JT. Inhibition of HIV-1 replication by GB virus C infection through increases in RANTES, MIP-1alpha, MIP-1beta, and SDF-1. Lancet 2004; 363(9426): 2040-6.
[http://dx.doi.org/10.1016/S0140-6736(04)16453-2] [PMID: 15207954]

[31] Spudich S, González-Scarano F. HIV-1-related central nervous system disease: current issues in pathogenesis, diagnosis, and treatment. Cold Spring Harb Perspect Med 2012; 2(6): a007120.
[http://dx.doi.org/10.1101/cshperspect.a007120] [PMID: 22675662]

[32] Jones G, Power C. Regulation of neural cell survival by HIV-1 infection. Neurobiol Dis 2006; 21(1): 1-17.
[http://dx.doi.org/10.1016/j.nbd.2005.07.018] [PMID: 16298136]

[33] Johnston JB, Zhang K, Silva C, *et al.* HIV-1 Tat neurotoxicity is prevented by matrix metalloproteinase inhibitors. Ann Neurol 2001; 49(2): 230-41.
[http://dx.doi.org/10.1002/1531-8249(20010201)49:2<230::AID-ANA43>3.0.CO;2-O] [PMID: 11220743]

[34] Chang JR, Mukerjee R, Bagashev A, *et al.* HIV-1 Tat protein promotes neuronal dysfunction through disruption of microRNAs. J Biol Chem 2011; 286(47): 41125-34.
[http://dx.doi.org/10.1074/jbc.M111.268466] [PMID: 21956116]

[35] Xu Y, Kulkosky J, Acheampong E, Nunnari G, Sullivan J, Pomerantz RJ. HIV-1-mediated apoptosis of neuronal cells: Proximal molecular mechanisms of HIV-1-induced encephalopathy. Proc Natl Acad Sci USA 2004; 101(18): 7070-5.
[http://dx.doi.org/10.1073/pnas.0304859101] [PMID: 15103018]

[36] Paulino AD, Ubhi K, Rockenstein E, *et al.* Neurotoxic effects of the HCV core protein are mediated by sustained activation of ERK *via* TLR2 signaling. J Neurovirol 2011; 17(4): 327-40.
[http://dx.doi.org/10.1007/s13365-011-0039-0] [PMID: 21660601]

[37] Wilkinson J, Radkowski M, Eschbacher JM, Laskus T. Activation of brain macrophages/microglia cells in hepatitis C infection. Gut 2010; 59(10): 1394-400.
[http://dx.doi.org/10.1136/gut.2009.199356] [PMID: 20675697]

[38] Cohen RA, de la Monte S, Gongvatana A, *et al.* Plasma cytokine concentrations associated with HIV/hepatitis C coinfection are related to attention, executive and psychomotor functioning. J Neuroimmunol 2011; 233(1-2): 204-10.
[http://dx.doi.org/10.1016/j.jneuroim.2010.11.006] [PMID: 21146232]

[39] Page EE, Nelson M, Kelleher P. HIV and hepatitis C coinfection: pathogenesis and microbial

translocation. Curr Opin HIV AIDS 2011; 6(6): 472-7.
[http://dx.doi.org/10.1097/COH.0b013e32834bbc71] [PMID: 21918438]

[40]   Letendre SL, Ellis RJ, Everall I, Ances B, Bharti A, McCutchan JA. Neurologic complications of HIV disease and their treatment. Top HIV Med 2009; 17(2): 46-56.
[PMID: 19401607]

[41]   Rotman Y, Liang TJ. Coinfection with hepatitis C virus and human immunodeficiency virus: virological, immunological, and clinical outcomes. J Virol 2009; 83(15): 7366-74.
[http://dx.doi.org/10.1128/JVI.00191-09] [PMID: 19420073]

[42]   Jang JY, Shao RX, Lin W, *et al.* HIV infection increases HCV-induced hepatocyte apoptosis. J Hepatol 2011; 54(4): 612-20.
[http://dx.doi.org/10.1016/j.jhep.2010.07.042] [PMID: 21146890]

[43]   Lin W, Weinberg EM, Tai AW, *et al.* HIV increases HCV replication in a TGF-beta1-dependent manner. Gastroenterology 2008; 134(3): 803-11.
[http://dx.doi.org/10.1053/j.gastro.2008.01.005] [PMID: 18325393]

[44]   Lin W, Wu G, Li S, *et al.* HIV and HCV cooperatively promote hepatic fibrogenesis via induction of reactive oxygen species and NFkappaB. J Biol Chem 2011; 286(4): 2665-74.
[http://dx.doi.org/10.1074/jbc.M110.168286] [PMID: 21098019]

[45]   Qu J, Yang Z, Zhang Q, *et al.* Human immunodeficiency virus-1 Rev protein activates hepatitis C virus gene expression by directly targeting the HCV 5'-untranslated region. FEBS Lett 2011; 585(24): 4002-9.
[http://dx.doi.org/10.1016/j.febslet.2011.11.008] [PMID: 22094166]

[46]   Rider PJ, Liu F. Crosstalk between HIV and hepatitis C virus during co-infection. BMC Med 2012; 10: 32.
[http://dx.doi.org/10.1186/1741-7015-10-32] [PMID: 22472061]

[47]   Gómez-Gonzalo M, Carretero M, Rullas J, *et al.* The hepatitis B virus X protein induces HIV-1 replication and transcription in synergy with T-cell activation signals: functional roles of NF-kappaB/NF-AT and SP1-binding sites in the HIV-1 long terminal repeat promoter. J Biol Chem 2001; 276(38): 35435-43.
[http://dx.doi.org/10.1074/jbc.M103020200] [PMID: 11457829]

[48]   Lu L, Zhang HY, Yueng YH, *et al.* Intracellular levels of hepatitis B virus DNA and pregenomic RNA in peripheral blood mononuclear cells of chronically infected patients. J Viral Hepat 2009; 16(2): 104-12.
[http://dx.doi.org/10.1111/j.1365-2893.2008.01054.x] [PMID: 19175882]

[49]   Iser DM, Lewin SR. The pathogenesis of liver disease in the setting of HIV-hepatitis B virus coinfection. Antivir Ther (Lond) 2009; 14(2): 155-64.
[PMID: 19430090]

[50]   Jung S, Eichenmüller M, Donhauser N, *et al.* HIV entry inhibition by the envelope 2 glycoprotein of GB virus C. AIDS 2007; 21(5): 645-7.
[http://dx.doi.org/10.1097/QAD.0b013e32803277c7] [PMID: 17314528]

[51]   Chang Q, McLinden JH, Stapleton JT, Sathar MA, Xiang J. Expression of GB virus C NS5A protein

from genotypes 1, 2, 3 and 5 and a 30 aa NS5A fragment inhibit human immunodeficiency virus type 1 replication in a CD4+ T-lymphocyte cell line. J Gen Virol 2007; 88(Pt 12): 3341-6.
[http://dx.doi.org/10.1099/vir.0.83198-0] [PMID: 18024904]

[52]   George SL, Varmaz D, Tavis JE, Chowdhury A. The GB virus C (GBV-C) NS3 serine protease inhibits HIV-1 replication in a CD4+ T lymphocyte cell line without decreasing HIV receptor expression. PLoS One 2012; 7(1): e30653.
[http://dx.doi.org/10.1371/journal.pone.0030653] [PMID: 22292009]

[53]   Cummins NW, Badley AD. Mechanisms of HIV-associated lymphocyte apoptosis: 2010. Cell Death Dis 2010; 1: e99.
[http://dx.doi.org/10.1038/cddis.2010.77] [PMID: 21368875]

[54]   Moenkemeyer M, Schmidt RE, Wedemeyer H, Tillmann HL, Heiken H. GBV-C coinfection is negatively correlated to Fas expression and Fas-mediated apoptosis in HIV-1 infected patients. J Med Virol 2008; 80(11): 1933-40.
[http://dx.doi.org/10.1002/jmv.21305] [PMID: 18814245]

[55]   Balasubramanian A, Koziel M, Groopman JE, Ganju RK. Molecular mechanism of hepatic injury in coinfection with hepatitis C virus and HIV. Clin Infect Dis 2005; 41 (Suppl. 1): S32-7.
[http://dx.doi.org/10.1086/429493] [PMID: 16265611]

[56]   Iser DM, Avihingsanon A, Wisedopas N, *et al.* Increased intrahepatic apoptosis but reduced immune activation in HIV-HBV co-infected patients with advanced immunosuppression. AIDS 2011; 25(2): 197-205.
[http://dx.doi.org/10.1097/QAD.0b013e3283410ccb] [PMID: 21076271]

[57]   Tang RX, Kong FY, Fan BF, *et al.* HBx activates FasL and mediates HepG2 cell apoptosis through MLK3-MKK7-JNKs signal module. World J Gastroenterol 2012; 18(13): 1485-95.
[http://dx.doi.org/10.3748/wjg.v18.i13.1485] [PMID: 22509080]

[58]   Liang X, Liu Y, Zhang Q, *et al.* Hepatitis B virus sensitizes hepatocytes to TRAIL-induced apoptosis through Bax. J Immunol 2007; 178(1): 503-10.
[http://dx.doi.org/10.4049/jimmunol.178.1.503] [PMID: 17182590]

[59]   Li LM, Hu ZB, Zhou ZX, *et al.* Serum microRNA profiles serve as novel biomarkers for HBV infection and diagnosis of HBV-positive hepatocarcinoma. Cancer Res 2010; 70(23): 9798-807.
[http://dx.doi.org/10.1158/0008-5472.CAN-10-1001] [PMID: 21098710]

[60]   Gupta A, Nagilla P, Le HS, *et al.* Comparative expression profile of miRNA and mRNA in primary peripheral blood mononuclear cells infected with human immunodeficiency virus (HIV-1). PLoS One 2011; 6(7): e22730.
[http://dx.doi.org/10.1371/journal.pone.0022730] [PMID: 21829495]

[61]   Gupta A, Swaminathan G, Martin-Garcia J, Navas-Martin S. MicroRNAs, hepatitis C virus, and HCV/HIV-1 co-infection: new insights in pathogenesis and therapy. Viruses 2012; 4(11): 2485-513.
[http://dx.doi.org/10.3390/v4112485] [PMID: 23202492]

[62]   Jopling CL, Yi M, Lancaster AM, Lemon SM, Sarnow P. Modulation of hepatitis C virus RNA abundance by a liver-specific MicroRNA. Science 2005; 309(5740): 1577-81.
[http://dx.doi.org/10.1126/science.1113329] [PMID: 16141076]

[63] Bandyopadhyay S, Friedman RC, Marquez RT, *et al.* Hepatitis C virus infection and hepatic stellate cell activation downregulate miR-29: miR-29 overexpression reduces hepatitis C viral abundance in culture. J Infect Dis 2011; 203(12): 1753-62.
[http://dx.doi.org/10.1093/infdis/jir186] [PMID: 21606534]

[64] Pegtel DM, van de Garde MD, Middeldorp JM. Viral miRNAs exploiting the endosomal-exosomal pathway for intercellular cross-talk and immune evasion. Biochim Biophys Acta 2011; 1809(11-12): 715-21.
[http://dx.doi.org/10.1016/j.bbagrm.2011.08.002] [PMID: 21855666]

[65] Wurdinger T, Gatson NN, Balaj L, Kaur B, Breakefield XO, Pegtel DM. Extracellular vesicles and their convergence with viral pathways. Adv Virol 2012; 2012: 767694.
[http://dx.doi.org/10.1155/2012/767694]

[66] Brenndörfer ED, Sällberg M. Hepatitis C virus-mediated modulation of cellular immunity. Arch Immunol Ther Exp (Warsz) 2012; 60(5): 315-29.
[http://dx.doi.org/10.1007/s00005-012-0184-z] [PMID: 22911132]

[67] Thimme R, Binder M, Bartenschlager R. Failure of innate and adaptive immune responses in controlling hepatitis C virus infection. FEMS Microbiol Rev 2012; 36(3): 663-83.
[http://dx.doi.org/10.1111/j.1574-6976.2011.00319.x] [PMID: 22142141]

[68] Tu Z, Hamalainen-Laanaya HK, Nishitani C, Kuroki Y, Crispe IN, Orloff MS. HCV core and NS3 proteins manipulate human blood-derived dendritic cell development and promote Th 17 differentiation. Int Immunol 2012; 24(2): 97-106.
[http://dx.doi.org/10.1093/intimm/dxr104] [PMID: 22190574]

[69] Hosseini SY, Sabahi F, Moazzeni SM, Modarressi MH, Saberi Firoozi M, Ravanshad M. Construction and preparation of three recombinant adenoviruses expressing truncated NS3 and core genes of hepatitis C virus for vaccine purposes. Hepat Mon 2012; 12(8): e6130.
[PMID: 23087750]

[70] Chang JJ, Wightman F, Bartholomeusz A, *et al.* Reduced hepatitis B virus (HBV)-specific CD4+ T-cell responses in human immunodeficiency virus type 1-HBV-coinfected individuals receiving HBV-active antiretroviral therapy. J Virol 2005; 79(5): 3038-51.
[http://dx.doi.org/10.1128/JVI.79.5.3038-3051.2005] [PMID: 15709024]

[71] Petrovas C, Casazza JP, Brenchley JM, *et al.* PD-1 is a regulator of virus-specific CD8+ T cell survival in HIV infection. J Exp Med 2006; 203(10): 2281-92.
[http://dx.doi.org/10.1084/jem.20061496] [PMID: 16954372]

[72] Wei C, Ni C, Song T, *et al.* The hepatitis B virus X protein disrupts innate immunity by downregulating mitochondrial antiviral signaling protein. J Immunol 2010; 185(2): 1158-68.
[http://dx.doi.org/10.4049/jimmunol.0903874] [PMID: 20554965]

[73] Op den Brouw ML, Binda RS, van Roosmalen MH, *et al.* Hepatitis B virus surface antigen impairs myeloid dendritic cell function: a possible immune escape mechanism of hepatitis B virus. Immunology 2009; 126(2): 280-9.
[http://dx.doi.org/10.1111/j.1365-2567.2008.02896.x] [PMID: 18624732]

[74] Capobianchi MR, Lalle E, Martini F, *et al.* Influence of GBV-C infection on the endogenous activation

of the IFN system in HIV-1 co-infected patients. Cell Mol Biol (Noisy-le-grand) 2006; 52(1): 3-8.
[PMID: 16914092]

[75] Cooper CL, Klein MB. HIV/hepatitis C virus coinfection management: changing guidelines and changing paradigms. HIV Med 2014; 15(10): 621-4.
[PMID: 24802099]

[76] Naggie S, Sulkowski MS. Management of patients coinfected with HCV and HIV: a close look at the role for direct-acting antivirals. Gastroenterology 2012; 142(6): 1324-34.
[http://dx.doi.org/10.1053/j.gastro.2012.02.012]

[77] Sulkowski MS. Current management of hepatitis C virus infection in patients with HIV co-infection. J Infect Dis 2013; 207 (Suppl. 1): S26-32.
[http://dx.doi.org/10.1093/infdis/jis764] [PMID: 23390302]

[78] European Association for Study of Liver. EASL Clinical Practice Guidelines: management of hepatitis C virus infection. J Hepatol 2014; 60(2): 392-420.
[http://dx.doi.org/10.1016/j.jhep.2013.11.003] [PMID: 24331294]

[79] European Association For The Study Of The Liver. EASL clinical practice guidelines: Management of chronic hepatitis B virus infection. J Hepatol 2012; 57(1): 167-85.
[http://dx.doi.org/10.1016/j.jhep.2012.02.010] [PMID: 22436845]

[80] Soriano V, Tuma P, Vispo E, *et al.* Hepatitis B in HIV patients: what is the current treatment and what are the challenges? J HIV Ther 2009; 14(1): 13-8.
[PMID: 19731560]

[81] Management of hepatitis B and HIV coinfection Europe [Accessed on: Oct 2010]; Available at: http://hivinsite.ucsf.edu/InSite?page=kb-05-03-04.

Testing for HIV Infection

Amin Farzanegan[1,*], **Seyed Hadi Razavi**[1] and **Asghar Abdoli**[2]

[1] *Faculty of Medical Sciences, Tarbiat Modares University, Tehran, Iran*

[2] *Department of Hepatitis and AIDS, Pasteur Institute of Iran, Tehran, Iran*

Abstract: An HIV test detects immunoglobulins against the virus or the genetic material (DNA or RNA) of HIV in the blood or specimen. P24 antigen, as a HIV core protein, momentarily becomes visible in the bloodstream during the ramp up phase when HIV-1 RNA concentration is increased up to 10,000 copies/mL.

Current rapid diagnostic tests possess high sensitivity and specificity (> 99%) and could be practical for screening individuals as they provide results in 20 minutes or less. A positive rapid HIV test results should be verified with using a supplemental test (namely, Western blot or RNA). The Western blot (an immunoblot test) detects antibodies to viral proteins and it is performed to confirm two positive ELISA tests. This confirmatory test is the gold standard among the diagnostic tests of HIV infection. ELISA is the most common HIV test performed to assay antibodies to HIV. One of the EIA-based tests is p24 antigen. New combined fourth-generation EIA antigen-antibody tests p24 antigen and anti-HIV-1/2 antibodies simultaneously. PCR is used for finding the DNA or RNA of HIV in white blood cells. This technique has high sensitivity and specificity and detects very small number of viral particles.

Keywords: DNA, Eclipse phase, ELISA, HIV, IFA, Immunoblot test, PCR, Rapid tests, RNA, Viremia, Western blot.

1. INTRODUCTION

The diagnosis of primary and incident HIV infections plays a major role in both prevention and treatment. In general, HIV test detects immunoglobulins to HIV or

* **Correspondence to Amin Farzanegan:** Faculty of Medical Sciences, Tarbiat Modares University, Tehran, Iran; Tel/Fax: +98 (21) 82883581; E-mail: amin_92f@yahoo.com.

SeyedAhmad SeyedAlinaghi (Ed.)

the genetic material (DNA or RNA) of HIV in the blood or other specimens. The test for HIV infection may be performed for a variety of reasons including detection of HIV infection in suspected individuals with risk factors or people with signs of HIV infection, screening of blood, blood products and organ donation as to prevent the transmission of HIV, HIV screening tests among pregnant women and for neonates who are born to a HIV-positive woman [1].

2. STAGES OF THE ACUTE PRIMARY HIV INFECTION: IMPLICATIONS FOR HIV TESTING

After transmission of HIV, an initial "eclipse phase" is produced. In this phase, infection can be identified in the local site of infection; however, dissemination is not yet available at detectable levels in the systemic circulation. The eclipse phase lasts as long as 10 days and later viral replication increases to peak levels when disseminated to lymphoid tissues and systemic circulation. In the next phase, ramp up phase of viremia or window period, HIV antibodies could not be detected. The period from infection with HIV to the point where antibodies to HIV are discovered in the bloodstream is referred as the window period or seroconversion . In this phase, an individual infected with HIV can transmit virus, even though an HIV test remains negative [1].

Fiebig *et al.*, categorized acute viremia and early seroconversion into six stages considering viral replication and evolving antibody responses [2]:

Stage I: Detection of HIV-1 RNA in the blood.

Stage II: After seven days, detection of p24 antigen, (a viral core protein, momentarily found in the bloodstream during the ramp up phase when HIV-1 RNA concentration is increased up to 10,000 copies/mL, and before the development of detectable HIV antibodies), intense inflammatory response described with high levels of cytokines and chemokines or "cytokine storm", appearance of a cellular immune response drawing escape mutants, symptoms of acute retroviral syndrome (*i.e.* fever, rash, night sweats, severe fatigue, headache, diarrhea, pharyngitis, arthralgia and myalgia) in some patients.

Stage III: Within ~five days after positive results obtained with p24 antigen test, detection of HIV-1 antibodies (IgM) with sensitive enzyme immunoassays (EIAs) (third-generation EIAs, 1-2 weeks after the appearance of primary retroviral signs).

Stage IV: About three days after positive results obtained with sensitive EIAs, a positive or negative Western blot test.

Stage V: The development of a positive Western blot about one month following the onset of infection (Western blot positive and P31 antigen negative).

Stage VI: Western blot positive, p31 antigen positive [2].

3. THE INITIAL DIAGNOSTIC TEST FOR HIV INFECTION

3.1. Rapid Diagnostic Tests

Current rapid diagnostic tests for HIV are generally antibody-based assays. They possess high sensitivity and specificity (> 99%) and could be practical for screening individuals as the results are generated in 20 minutes or less. Six FDA-approved rapid tests determine antibodies to HIV in blood, serum, or oral fluid samples. Before establishing the final diagnosis of HIV infection, a positive rapid HIV infection test should be verified using supplemental tests (namely, Western blot or PCR). If supplementary testing is negative or indeterminate, a testing should be performed on a blood sample gathered four weeks after the initial positive rapid HIV test. Six rapid tests are approved by the FDA for the diagnosis of HIV-1 and HIV-2 so that both can be discriminated. An increasing application of point-of-care leads to decreasing the number of early cases of HIV infection that are discovered by rapid HIV antibody tests for HIV screening. However, rapid HIV tests are considerably available in environments with limited resources and take benefits from same-day results [3 - 5].

3.2. Enzyme-linked Immunosorbent Assay (ELISA)

ELISA is the most common HIV test performed to assay antibodies to HIV. If antibodies to HIV are detected (positive), in order to confirm the diagnosis, the test is usually repeated. For negative ELISA, there is no need for supplementary tests. The drawbacks of such highly sensitive test are false positives, variation in the number and types of EIA assays and HIV prevalence in the population.

One of the EIA-based tests is p24 antigen. In some cases, P24 may be detectable before detection of HIV-antibody in patients with acute primary HIV infection. Also, P24 antigen would not be detected in all of patients in window period and even antigen may not be reliably found in individuals with HIV antibody-positive tests. Moreover, the p24 antigen emerges later than HIV RNA, and as antibodies are produced, it often disappears because they bind to the antigen. New combined fourth-generation EIA antigen-antibody tests are capable to detect p24 antigen and anti-HIV-1/2 antibodies simultaneously and to reduce the window period for the diagnosis of early HIV infection by four days on average (from two days to two weeks), in comparison with third generation EIAs. Although fourth-generation assays will miss fewer HIV infections due to the detection of p24 antigen (in antibody-negative cases), a window period will persist when only the HIV RNA become detectable [2, 6 - 9].

4. SUPPLEMENTARY TESTS FOR HIV INFECTION

4.1. Western Blot

The western blot (an immunoblot test) detects antibodies to viral proteins and it is performed to confirm two positive ELISA tests. This confirmatory test is the gold standard among the diagnostic tests of HIV infection. In this test, viral proteins (core and envelope) are disseminated based on molecular weight after a polyacrylamide gel electrophoresis and blotted on a nitrocellulose membrane. If antibodies to viral proteins are present in serum, they bind to antigens. After adding alkaline phosphatase labelled, anti-human immunoglobulin G conjugate and color development solution, a color band is produced. According to the manufacturer recommendations, the results of test are evaluated. If there is no band, the Western blot is considered as negative. A Western blot is positive when bands appear at the location of two or more HIV antigens: p24, gp41, or gp120/160. If there are bands but they have not the criteria for positivity (*i.e.* less than two of the latter bands are available), this western blot test are called indeterminate, and a follow-up sample one month after is needed [6, 10 - 13].

4.2. Indirect Immunofluorescence Assay (IFA)

The other confirmatory test for HIV infection is IFA. Although the performance of this test is simple, its interpretation needs an expert person [14].

4.3. Polymerase Chain Reaction (PCR)

PCR is used for finding the DNA or RNA of HIV in white blood cells. This technique has high sensitivity and specificity and detects very small number of viral particles. Due to the need of some technical skill and expensive equipment, this method is not performed on a routine basis as antibody testing. Despite the negative results of other tests, genetic material of HIV may be detected by PCR. The PCR test is thus helpful to identify incident infections.

With regard to exposure, HIV testing is usually performed at six weeks, three months, and six months after the exposure to understand whether a person has been infected with HIV or not [6, 15, 16].

5. HIV TEST RESULTS

The results of EIAs are generally provided in two to four days. Some other tests such as the Western blot or IFA require 1-2 weeks to obtain the results. Generally, the EIA results are categorized as reactive or non-reactive. A non-reactive result of the initial EIA is well thought-out HIV-negative. A reactive EIA test is repeated again. If the result of repeated test is reactive, a confirmatory test such as Western blot, IFA, or RNA test is requested. Correspondingly the negative and positive results of each test are interpreted as follows:

- No HIV antibodies (EIA) = Negative (Normal)
- No HIV antibodies in seroconversion period (EIA) = Repeat test
- No RNA or DNA of HIV(PCR) = Negative
- Not clear test results (Western blot) = Indeterminate
- Indeterminate results for six months or longer = Stable indeterminate results for six months or longer
- Positive HIV antibodies in a first assay = Abnormal
- Repeated positive HIV antibodies = Confirm with Western blot or IFA test
- Positive DNA or RNA= Positive [6]

- The factors affecting HIV test results cover the application of corticosteroids, indeterminate results during the seroconversion period (window period), autoimmune diseases, leukemia, syphilis and alcoholism, among others.

6. CD4 T CELL COUNT

It is well established that the progressive damage and functional deterioration of the CD4 memory/effectors T cell is the hallmark of HIV infection. Evaluation of immune system function in patients with HIV diagnosis is generally based on the CD4 count. In fact, a reduction of the CD4 count shows the effect of the HIV on the immune system function as the infection progresses toward AIDS. Thus, the reasons for performing CD4 counts are as following: monitoring the immune system status in patients with HIV, to settle a diagnosis of AIDS, to decide on initiation of antiretroviral therapy, assessing the risk of opportunistic infections and for deciding when to start the treatments to prevent opportunistic infections. The CD4 cell count is followed every three to six months, depending on the patients' health condition, preceding CD4 cell counts and whether the patient is under Highly Active Antiretroviral Therapy (HAART) or not [14].

CONFLICT OF INTEREST

The authors confirm that they have no conflict of interest to declare for this publication.

ACKNOWLEDGEMENTS

Declared none.

REFERENCES

[1]   Cohen MS, Gay CL, Busch MP, Hecht FM. The detection of acute HIV infection. J Infect Dis 2010; 202 (Suppl. 2): S270-7.
[http://dx.doi.org/10.1086/655651] [PMID: 20846033]

[2]   Fiebig EW, Wright DJ, Rawal BD, *et al.* Dynamics of HIV viremia and antibody seroconversion in plasma donors: implications for diagnosis and staging of primary HIV infection. AIDS 2003; 17(13): 1871-9.
[http://dx.doi.org/10.1097/00002030-200309050-00005] [PMID: 12960819]

[3]   Control CfD, Prevention. Immigrant and refugee health: screening for HIV infection during the refugee domestic medical examination 2012.

[4]   Control CfD. Prevention. Protocols for confirmation of reactive rapid HIV tests. MMWR 2004; 53(10): 221-2.
[PMID: 15717396]

[5]   Greenwald JL, Burstein GR, Pincus J, Branson B. A rapid review of rapid HIV antibody tests. Curr Infect Dis Rep 2006; 8(2): 125-31.
[http://dx.doi.org/10.1007/s11908-006-0008-6] [PMID: 16524549]

[6]   Fearon M. The laboratory diagnosis of HIV infections. Can J Infect Dis Med Microbiol 2005; 16(1): 26-30.
[PMID: 18159524]

[7]   Goudsmit J, de Wolf F, Paul DA, *et al.* Expression of human immunodeficiency virus antigen (HIV-Ag) in serum and cerebrospinal fluid during acute and chronic infection. Lancet 1986; 2(8500): 177-80.
[http://dx.doi.org/10.1016/S0140-6736(86)92485-2] [PMID: 2873436]

[8]   Schüpbach J, Tomasik Z, Knuchel M, *et al.* Swiss HIV Cohort Study, Swiss HIV Mother + Child Cohort Study. Optimized virus disruption improves detection of HIV-1 p24 in particles and uncovers a p24 reactivity in patients with undetectable HIV-1 RNA under long-term HAART. J Med Virol 2006; 78(8): 1003-10.
[http://dx.doi.org/10.1002/jmv.20655] [PMID: 16789014]

[9]   Masciotra S, McDougal JS, Feldman J, Sprinkle P, Wesolowski L, Owen SM. Evaluation of an alternative HIV diagnostic algorithm using specimens from seroconversion panels and persons with established HIV infections. J Clin Virol 2011; 52 (Suppl. 1): S17-22.
[http://dx.doi.org/10.1016/j.jcv.2011.09.011] [PMID: 21981983]

[10]   Nasrullah M, Ethridge SF, Delaney KP, *et al.* Comparison of alternative interpretive criteria for the HIV-1 Western blot and results of the Multispot HIV-1/HIV-2 Rapid Test for classifying HIV-1 and HIV-2 infections. J Clin Virol 2011; 52 (Suppl. 1): S23-7.
[http://dx.doi.org/10.1016/j.jcv.2011.09.020] [PMID: 21993309]

[11]   Centers for Disease Control and Prevention (CDC). Detection of acute HIV infection in two evaluations of a new HIV diagnostic testing algorithm - United States, 2011-2013. MMWR Morb Mortal Wkly Rep 2013; 62(24): 489-94.
[PMID: 23784012]

[12]   Styer LM, Sullivan TJ, Parker MM. Evaluation of an alternative supplemental testing strategy for HIV diagnosis by retrospective analysis of clinical HIV testing data. J Clin Virol 2011; 52 (Suppl. 1): S35-40.
[http://dx.doi.org/10.1016/j.jcv.2011.09.009] [PMID: 22018662]

[13]   Lodi S, Meyer L, Kelleher AD, *et al.* Immunovirologic control 24 months after interruption of antiretroviral therapy initiated close to HIV seroconversion. Arch Intern Med 2012; 172(16): 1252-5.
[http://dx.doi.org/10.1001/archinternmed.2012.2719] [PMID: 22826124]

[14]   Diagnostic, Monitoring, and Resistance Laboratory Tests for HIV Available at: http://www.hivguidelines.org/.

[15]   Keele BF, Giorgi EE, Salazar-Gonzalez JF, *et al.* Identification and characterization of transmitted and

early founder virus envelopes in primary HIV-1 infection. Proc Natl Acad Sci USA 2008; 105(21): 7552-7.
[http://dx.doi.org/10.1073/pnas.0802203105] [PMID: 18490657]

[16]   Fiebig EW, Heldebrant CM, Smith RI, Conrad AJ, Delwart EL, Busch MP. Intermittent low-level viremia in very early primary HIV-1 infection. J Acquir Immune Defic Syndr 2005; 39(2): 133-7.
[PMID: 15905727]

When to Start Antiretroviral Therapy

Behnam Farhoudi[*]

Islamic Azad University, Tehran Medical Sciences Branch, Iran

Abstract: Antiretroviral therapy (ART) has led to dramatical improvements in the prognosis of people living with HIV. ART suppresses viral replication, reconstitutes the immune system, decreases the possibility of many HIV-related complications, and lowers the risk of HIV acquisition. Despite of substantial health benefits of ART, it accompanies its own limits. ART does not cure HIV infection and needs taking several medicines simultaneously. It causes numerous adverse effects, it is expensive and efficacy requires complete adherence. Poor adherence leads to emergence of resistance virus and finally treatment failure.

However ART is now recommended for everyone with HIV regardless of CD4 count and stage of infection. Evidences in favor of earlier ART initiation include clinical trials, better understanding of viral dynamics, effect of inflammation on body organs, newer medications that are better tolerated, data derived from cohort studies, and public health benefits of ART in preventing HIV transmission. Concerns about early ART initiation include effect of long term ART toxicity, impact of possible ART non-adherence on viral resistance, and feasibility of implementing early ART.

Based on currently existing evidences, ART is recommended for all HIV-infected individuals. The suggestion is the strongest for people with lower counts of CD4 cells, or for those with pregnancy, history of AIDS-defining illness, any type of tuberculosis, acute opportunistic infections, HIV associated nephropathy, HBV co-infection and for all children <2 years old.

Keywords: Antiretroviral drugs, Antiretroviral therapy, ART benefits, ART feasibility, ART initiation, ART limitation, Early ART, Health benefits, Time of ART initiation, Viral suppression.

---

[*] **Correspondence to Behnam Farhoudi:** Islamic Azad University, Tehran Medical Sciences Branch, Shariati Street, Gholhak, Tehran, Iran; Tel/Fax: +98 (21) 22006660-7; E-mail: b_farhoudi@yahoo.com.

1. INTRODUCTION

Natural course of HIV infection is described by ongoing viral replication, continued depletion of CD4+ T lymphocytes that leads to unrelenting immune system destruction, development of opportunistic diseases and premature death. As well according to recent studies, HIV is accompanied with an increase in the risk of serious non-AIDS conditions like cardiovascular, renal and liver diseases as well as neurocognitive deficits and non-AIDS-defining cancers. Many of these effects can be mediated through continued activation of immune system and unremitting inflammation in various organ systems [1].

The introduction of powerful Antiretroviral Therapy (ART) has considerably improved the prognosis of people living with HIV. Today, HIV is not a fatal disease, and can be controlled through retaining adequate adherence to antiretroviral (ARV) drugs over the long term [2]. Potent combination ART, classically consisting of three or more ARVs, show pronounced improvement in the health and survival rates of HIV-infected subjects in those with access to ARVs. At present, more than 20 ARVs in six classes are accessible. It is possible to combine these in order to launch several effective regimens for initial and subsequent treatments. ART suppresses viral replication, reconstitutes the immune system, decreases the risk of numerous HIV-related and "non-AIDS" complications, and also reduces the risk of HIV acquisition [3].

Despite significant health benefits, ART has its own limits. It does not cure HIV infection and it needs taking several medicines for lifetime. ART is associated with diverse adverse effects (some severe), it is expensive, requires high adherence to be effective and to avoid the appearance of resistance, and occasionally fails (because of the patient's poor adherence or other factors). The absence of success in an ART regimen accompanied by drug resistance indicates that the succeeding regimens are less likely to suppress the virus [3].

Increasingly, gathering evidences state to the benefits of ART even for individuals with high counts of CD4. It seems that ART reduces immune system stimulation and protect against many of such morbidities through virologic suppression; nevertheless, it may cause dysfunction of immune system and may not fully reverse disease processes. The favorable effects of ART may be lessened for patients who start ART with lower counts of CD4 cell. Additionally, the risk of some ARV-related adverse events is greater for those starting ART at lower levels of CD4 [4].

The argument about 'When to Start' ART has raged since the introduction of zidovudine in 1987 [4] until recently when a clinical trial revealed offering ART to all HIV-infected people, regardless of CD4-cell count to improve outcome of PLWH [5].

2. EVIDENCES IN FAVOR OF EARLIER ART INITIATION

2.1. Evidences from Clinical Trials

A major international randomized clinical trial has showed that PLWH have a considerably decreased risk of developing AIDS or other serious illnesses if they start ART earlier, at the time of higher CD4+ T-cell, instead of waiting until the CD4+ cell count falls to lower levels. The study population was 4685 PLWH (treatment-naive adults) at 215 sites in 35 countries with an average follow-up of 3 years. In early 2015, the NIH released the study results early after an interim analysis revealed that, although the overall event rate was low (<3% over 3 years), the risk for serious illness or death was reduced by 53% in the early-treatment group. The reduction was greater for AIDS-related events than for non-AIDS events (70% and 33%, respectively).

2.2. Effect of Viral Dynamics

Viral dynamics studies demonstrated how fast rounds of *de novo* virus infection occur, producing 1 to 10 billion new viral copies per day [6]. With such large scale viral replication, both the viral life cycle and the half-life of infected CD4 T cells were estimated as short as one day or less with several million CD4 T cells being infected each day [7]. These findings indicate the great destructive effects of the viral replication cycles on the immune system even over the stage of "clinical latency" [6]. Therefore, it is necessary to onset impediment of the unremitting rounds of viral replication as soon as possible [4].

2.3. Effect of Inflammation on Body Organs

The continuous CD4 T cell stimulation and apoptosis are the basis of a continued inflammatory condition with high levels of inflammatory biomarkers [8]. The inflammation is associated with deleterious cardiovascular and metabolic consequences to the host [9]. Early therapy shows remarkable reduction in residual T cell activation *versus* individuals not on ART [10], which further supports the earlier ART initiation in order to lower the exposure duration to high inflammation levels [11].

2.4. Newer Medications are Better Tolerated

To date, ART regimens are less complex, generally better tolerated, less toxic and more potent; therefore, patients can stay on first-line therapy longer once it is started. Daily administrations of fixed-dose combination options obtained higher uniformity initiation of ART [4].

2.5. Data from Cohort Studies

Evolving clinical research continues to provide evidence in favor of earlier ART initiation. Data from the North America-AIDS Cohort Collaboration on Research and Design (NA-ACCORD) showed a statistically greater rate of adjusted mortality among the 6,935 patients postponed ART until their CD4 counts fell to <500 cells/µl compared to the 2,200 patients started ART with CD4 counts >500 cells/µl (risk ratio: 1.94, 95% CI: 1.37 to 2.79) [12]. Although large and representative of the PLWH in care in the United States, the study had restrictions intrinsic to its retrospective design, including the relatively small number of deaths and the potential for unmeasured confounders that might have influenced outcomes independent of treatment.

2.6. Public Health

High plasma HIV RNA is regarded as the main factor for HIV transmission risk and effective application of ART can lower viral load and therefore the transmission of HIV to sexual partners [13, 14]. Modeling studies indicate that the scaling up of ART may result in lower incidence and, eventually, prevalence of HIV [15]. So, a secondary by product of ART is to lower the risk of HIV transmission. It was suggested that early therapy is more effective in preventing HIV acquisition than all other behavioral and biomedical prevention interventions studied to date, including condom use, male circumcision, vaginal microbicides, HIV vaccination and pre-exposure prophylaxis [4].

The available information about early start of ART has showed the potential for a better CD4 cell count response and a more sustainable viral load response. The rationale is that when ART is started earlier, the patients have more bone marrow and lymphoid tissue reserve in general to mount a good CD4 response. Over the long term, the better CD4 cell response and viral load response that occurs with earlier therapy can reduce the risk for emergence of resistance to anti-HIV drugs [4, 16].

3. CONCERNS ABOUT EARLY ART INITIATION

3.1. Effect of Long Term ART Toxicity

Sooner initiation of ART increases probability of ARV adverse effects. For example, it was stated that cumulative exposure to some drugs of the Nucleoside Reverse Transcriptase Inhibitor (NRTIs) and Protease Inhibitors (PI) drug classes might be associated with increased incidence of Cardiovascular Diseases (CVD) [17, 18]. Also, continuous exposure to ART was associated with significantly greater loss of bone density compared with interruption or deferral of therapy [19]. Also, there may be unidentified complications linked to cumulative use of ARV drugs for many decades.

3.1.1. Effect of Early ART Initiation on Quality of Life

ART frequently causes an improvement in the quality of life for symptomatic patients. On the other hand, some side effects of ART may reduce quality of life for some persons, especially those asymptomatic at early therapy. For example, PIs may induce nausea or efavirenz may have disturbing neuropsychiatric side effects. These side effects can be very infuriating in an asymptomatic patient. Thereby, in spite of strong evidences on ART long term benefits, some people find that the inconvenience of taking medication every day outweighs the overall benefits of early ART and may select to defer treatment.

3.1.2. Impact of Possible ART Non-Adherence on Viral Resistance

At any CD4 count, adherence to ART shows a crucial role to reach viral suppresion and protect against the appearance of drug-resistance mutations. Clinicians must find areas for which further intervention is needed to improve adherence both before and after early therapy.

3.1.3. Feasibility of Implementing Early ART

Even in resource-rich settings, the magnitude of required resources is a limiting factor. Earlier ART means identifying those individuals who are HIV-infected earlier. Once people are tested and they know that they are infected from then on they should be linked to the healthcare to receive care. Then, once they have been established into care, the system should be able to pay for the medical service and for long-term ART. So, feasibility is really tied to whether the healthcare system can handle the number of patients that need to be on ART.

4. EVIDENCE-BASED TIMELY INITIATION OF ART

As stated earlier, ART recommended for all PLWH regardless of CD4 count, age and clinical condition; however, because of unmet need of resources it would not be provided for all PLWH. The following discussion may help to set priorities in the initiation of ART.

4.1. ART for Patients with a History of an AIDS-Defining Illness or CD4 Count <350 Cells/mm^3

PLWH with CD4 counts <200 cells/mm^3 are at greater risk of opportunistic diseases, non-AIDS morbidities and death. Randomized controlled trials in patients with CD4 counts <200 cells/mm^3 and/or a history of an AIDS-defining condition greatly support the positive impact of ART on improved survival and delay in disease progression in PLWH [20, 21]. In addition, comparative data from several observational cohort researches between earlier ART (*i.e.*, initiated at CD4 count >200 cells/mm^3) with later treatment (*i.e.*, initiated at CD4 count <200 cells/mm^3) showed robust evidence for these results [22, 23].

In patients with CD4 counts of 200 cells/mm^3 to 350 cells/mm^3 those who delayed

ART had a higher mortality rate compared to those who started therapy [24]. Together, these researches support the initiation of ART in patients with a history of an AIDS-defining illness or with a CD4 count <350 cells/mm^3.

4.2. ART for HIV-Associated Nephropathy (HIVAN)

HIVAN is virtually confined to black patients. It is very unusual in virologically suppressed patients [25]. ART in patients with HIVAN has been linked to both conserved renal function and prolonged survival [26]. So, ART should be initiated in all patients with HIVAN, irrespective of CD4 count, at the initial sign of renal dysfunction.

4.3. ART for Co-Infection with Hepatitis B Virus (HBV) and/or Hepatitis C Virus (HCV)

More rapid progression of viral hepatitis-related liver disease including cirrhosis, end-stage liver disease, hepatocellular carcinoma, and fatal hepatic failure is observed with HIV infection [27, 28]. In persons co-infected with HBV and/or HCV, ART may diminish liver disease progression through preserving or restoring immune function and reducing HIV-related immune activation and inflammation [29, 30]. Collectively, these data show that earlier treatment of HIV infection in persons co-infected with HBV (and likely HCV) may lower the progression risk of liver disease.

4.4. ART for Cardiovascular Diseases (CVD)

In HIV-infected patients, CVD is a key factor leading to morbidity and mortality, accounting for one-third of serious non-AIDS conditions and at least 10% of deaths [27]. Collectively, the increased risk of cardiovascular events with therapy interruption [19], the effects of ART on markers of inflammation and endothelial dysfunction [31], and the association between CVD and CD4 cell depletion [22] show that early control of HIV replication with ART can be applied as a strategy to lower the risk of CVD, particularly when avoided drugs with potential cardiovascular toxicity. However, no study is currently available about the prevention of CVD by the early onset of ART.

4.5. ART for Malignancies

Evidence states that initiating ART to reduce HIV replication and maintain counts of CD4 at levels > 350 to 500 cells/mm^3, reduce the overall incidence of AIDS-defining malignancies and may also lower the risk of non-AIDS-defining malignancies [32, 33]. The impact on incidence is most likely heterogeneous among different types of cancer [34].

4.6. ART for Neurological Diseases

ART when suppresses viral load, the incidence of HIV-associated Dementia (HAD) and severe Central Nervous System (CNS) Opportunistic Infections (OIs) are decreased dramatically and effectively [35]. In addition, the Peripheral Nervous System (PNS) is affected by HIV infection, and multiple types of neuropathies have been defined. The most common is HIV-associated polyneuropathy; which is a chronic, predominantly sensory and sometimes painful neuropathy. The impact of early treatment on this and other forms of neuropathy is not as clearly determined [36].

4.7. ART and Aging

The onset of treatment at an older age is constantly associated with a less robust CD4 count rise; hence initiating ART at a younger age may cause in better immunologic and possibly clinical outcomes [37].

4.8. ART for Prevention of Perinatal Transmission

ART prevents perinatal transmission of HIV. Suppression of HIV replication to the undetectable level is a major factor in this process. In the setting of ART initiation before 28 weeks gestation and an HIV RNA level <50 copies/mL near delivery, use of combination ART during pregnancy has lowered perinatal transmission rates of HIV from approximately 20%-30% to <0.5% [38]. Therefore, the initiation of ART is strongly recommended for all HIV-infected pregnant women.

4.9. ART for Prevention of Sexual Transmission

Researches provide strong support for the premise that treatment of the HIV-infected individual can considerably reduce sexual HIV transmission. In one of these studies, immediate treatment *versus* delayed therapy for the HIV-infected partner among HIV-serodiscordant couples, exhibited 96% decrease in transmission associated with early ART, (Hazard Ratio = 0.04; 95% confidence interval (CI): 0.01 to 0.27, $P<0.001$) [14]. Researches of HIV-serodiscordant heterosexual couples have stated a relationship between level of plasma viremia and risk of HIV transmission: Lower plasma HIV RNA levels associated with less risk of HIV transmission [39]. So, it is recommended that ART to be initiated in patients who may transmit HIV to their sexual partners. It should be stated that ART is not a substitute for consistent condom use, risky sexual activities should be avoided and ART does not avert other Sexually Transmitted Infections (STIs).

4.10. ART During Acute HIV Infection

Early initiation of ART decreases the severity of immune system destruction, lessens both the short-term and the long-term effects of HIV infection, and reduces the risk of HIV transmission. The DHHS Guidelines recommend ART to PLWH with early HIV infection. In this guideline, early HIV infection consisted of acute HIV infection (the phase of HIV disease immediately after infection during which anti-HIV antibodies are undetectable while HIV RNA or p24 antigen are present) and recent infection (considered the phase up to 6 months after infection during which anti-HIV antibodies are detectable) [40]. Recommendation of International AIDS Society in this regard is the same [41]. Its recommendation is based on studies suggesting reduction of proviral DNA and plasma viral load, lower viral set point, robust immune reconstitution, and CD4 cell count increases greater than 900/μL [41]. But none of the above benefits lasted for more than 24 months after treatment discontinuation. So discontinuation of ART after any duration of treatment is not recommended except in research situations [41].

4.11. ART Among Children

HIV infected Infants and young children have a remarkably high risk of poor outcomes. A study showed up to 52% of children born with HIV died before the age of two years in the lack of any intervention [42]. So, WHO recent guideline recommended that ART should be started among all children living with HIV, irrespective of clinical stage or level of CD4 cell count. In the setting of limited resources, it is stated that all children ≤2 years old or with WHO stage 3 or 4 or CD4 count ≤750 cells/mm³ or CD4 percentage <25% among children younger than 5 years and CD4 count ≤350 cells/mm³ among children 5 years and older are considered as priority [43].

4.12. ART for Elite Controller

Elite controllers suppress HIV viremia to below the limit of detection in the absence of ART. It seems that the size of the pool of HIV infected CD4 (+) T cells reduce considerably after starting ART and resurge to baseline upon interruption of treatment, suggesting that persistent viral replication occurs in untreated elite controllers even in the absence of detectable plasma viremia [44]; however, the evidence for the beginning of ART in these group of PLWH is stronger compared to the past, it is still insufficient to merit recommending routine treatment [41].

CONCLUSION

Based on present existing evidences, ART is recommended for all PLWH. This recommendation is the strongest for persons with lower CD4 cell counts, or for those with certain other conditions including following:

• Pregnancy
• History of AIDS-defining illness
• History of TB
• Acute opportunistic infections
• HIVAN
• HBV co-infection
• Acute HIV infection
• Children younger than 2 years old

In addition to CD4 count and patient clinical condition, the decision to onset ART should always focus any co-morbid conditions, the willingness and readiness of the patient to start therapy, and the availability of resources. For some patients, the potential risks of short- or long-term, drug-related complications and non-adherence to long-term therapy in asymptomatic patients may offset possible benefits of earlier initiation of therapy. In settings with unavailable resources to start ART in all patients, it is necessary to prioritize treatment for patients who benefit greater from treatment.

CONFLICT OF INTEREST

The author confirms that author has no conflict of interest to declare for this publication.

ACKNOWLEDGEMENTS

Declared none.

REFERENCES

[1]   Rodríguez B, Sethi AK, Cheruvu VK, *et al.* Predictive value of plasma HIV RNA level on rate of CD4 T-cell decline in untreated HIV infection. JAMA 2006; 296(12): 1498-506.
       [http://dx.doi.org/10.1001/jama.296.12.1498] [PMID: 17003398]

[2]   Volberding PA, Deeks SG. Antiretroviral therapy and management of HIV infection. Lancet 2010; 376(9734): 49-62.
       [http://dx.doi.org/10.1016/S0140-6736(10)60676-9] [PMID: 20609987]

[3]   Thompson MA, Aberg JA, Hoy JF, *et al.* Antiretroviral treatment of adult HIV infection: 2012 recommendations of the International Antiviral Society-USA panel. JAMA 2012; 308(4): 387-402.
       [http://dx.doi.org/10.1001/jama.2012.7961] [PMID: 22820792]

[4]   Franco RA, Saag MS. When to start antiretroviral therapy: as soon as possible. BMC Med 2013; 11: 147.
       [http://dx.doi.org/10.1186/1741-7015-11-147] [PMID: 23767762]

[5]   Danel C, Moh R. TEMPRANO ANRS 12136 Study Group. A Trial of Early Antiretrovirals and Isoniazid Preventive Therapy in Africa. N Engl J Med 2015; 373: 808-22.
       [http://dx.doi.org/10.1056/NEJMoa1507198]

[6]   Ho DD, Neumann AU, Perelson AS, Chen W, Leonard JM, Markowitz M. Rapid turnover of plasma virions and CD4 lymphocytes in HIV-1 infection. Nature 1995; 373(6510): 123-6.
       [http://dx.doi.org/10.1038/373123a0] [PMID: 7816094]

[7]   Wei X, Ghosh SK, Taylor ME, *et al.* Viral dynamics in human immunodeficiency virus type 1 infection. Nature 1995; 373(6510): 117-22.
       [http://dx.doi.org/10.1038/373117a0] [PMID: 7529365]

[8]   Neuhaus J, Jacobs DR Jr, Baker JV Jr, *et al.* Markers of inflammation, coagulation, and renal function

are elevated in adults with HIV infection. J Infect Dis 2010; 201(12): 1788-95.
[http://dx.doi.org/10.1086/652749] [PMID: 20446848]

[9]   Deeks SG. HIV infection, inflammation, immunosenescence, and aging. Annu Rev Med 2011; 62: 141-55.
[http://dx.doi.org/10.1146/annurev-med-042909-093756] [PMID: 21090961]

[10]   Jain V, Hartogensis W, Bacchetti P, *et al.* ART initiation during acute/early HIV infection compared to later ART initiation is associated with improved immunologic and virologic parameters during suppressive ART. Abstracts of the 18th Conference on Retroviruses and Opportunistic Infections. Feb 27 - Mar 2, 2011; Boston, MA. 2011.

[11]   Hunt PW, Martin JN, Sinclair E, *et al.* T cell activation is associated with lower CD4+ T cell gains in human immunodeficiency virus-infected patients with sustained viral suppression during antiretroviral therapy. J Infect Dis 2003; 187(10): 1534-43.
[http://dx.doi.org/10.1086/374786] [PMID: 12721933]

[12]   Kitahata MM, Gange SJ, Abraham AG, *et al.* NA-ACCORD Investigators. Effect of early *versus* deferred antiretroviral therapy for HIV on survival. N Engl J Med 2009; 360(18): 1815-26.
[http://dx.doi.org/10.1056/NEJMoa0807252] [PMID: 19339714]

[13]   Quinn TC, Wawer MJ, Sewankambo N, *et al.* Rakai Project Study Group. Viral load and heterosexual transmission of human immunodeficiency virus type 1. N Engl J Med 2000; 342(13): 921-9.
[http://dx.doi.org/10.1056/NEJM200003303421303] [PMID: 10738050]

[14]   Cohen MS, Chen YQ, McCauley M, *et al.* HPTN 052 Study Team. Prevention of HIV-1 infection with early antiretroviral therapy. N Engl J Med 2011; 365(6): 493-505.
[http://dx.doi.org/10.1056/NEJMoa1105243] [PMID: 21767103]

[15]   Granich RM, Gilks CF, Dye C, De Cock KM, Williams BG. Universal voluntary HIV testing with immediate antiretroviral therapy as a strategy for elimination of HIV transmission: a mathematical model. Lancet 2009; 373(9657): 48-57.
[http://dx.doi.org/10.1016/S0140-6736(08)61697-9] [PMID: 19038438]

[16]   NIAID. Starting Antiretroviral Treatment Early Improves Outcomes for HIV-Infected Individuals Strategic Timing of AntiRetroviral Treatment (START) study , [Accessed on: May 2015]; Available at: http://www.niaid.nih.gov/news/newsreleases/Archive/2011/Pages/START.aspx

[17]   Friis-Møller N, Reiss P, Sabin CA, *et al.* DAD Study Group. Class of antiretroviral drugs and the risk of myocardial infarction. N Engl J Med 2007; 356(17): 1723-35.
[http://dx.doi.org/10.1056/NEJMoa062744] [PMID: 17460226]

[18]   Worm SW, Sabin C, Weber R, *et al.* Risk of myocardial infarction in patients with HIV infection exposed to specific individual antiretroviral drugs from the 3 major drug classes: the data collection on adverse events of anti-HIV drugs (D:A:D) study. J Infect Dis 2010; 201(3): 318-30.
[http://dx.doi.org/10.1086/649897] [PMID: 20039804]

[19]   El-Sadr WM, Lundgren J, Neaton JD, *et al.* Strategies for Management of Antiretroviral Therapy (SMART) Study Group. CD4+ count-guided interruption of antiretroviral treatment. N Engl J Med 2006; 355(22): 2283-96.
[http://dx.doi.org/10.1056/NEJMoa062360] [PMID: 17135583]

[20]   Hammer SM, Squires KE, Hughes MD, *et al.* A controlled trial of two nucleoside analogues plus indinavir in persons with human immunodeficiency virus infection and CD4 cell counts of 200 per cubic millimeter or less. AIDS Clinical Trials Group 320 Study Team. N Engl J Med 1997; 337(11): 725-33.
[http://dx.doi.org/10.1056/NEJM199709113371101] [PMID: 9287227]

[21]   Zolopa A, Andersen J, Powderly W, *et al.* Early antiretroviral therapy reduces AIDS progression/death in individuals with acute opportunistic infections: a multicenter randomized strategy trial. PLoS One 2009; 4(5): e5575.
[http://dx.doi.org/10.1371/journal.pone.0005575] [PMID: 19440326]

[22]   Baker JV, Peng G, Rapkin J, *et al.* Terry Beirn Community Programs for Clinical Research on AIDS (CPCRA). CD4+ count and risk of non-AIDS diseases following initial treatment for HIV infection. AIDS 2008; 22(7): 841-8.
[http://dx.doi.org/10.1097/QAD.0b013e3282f7cb76] [PMID: 18427202]

[23]   Sterne JA, May M, Costagliola D, *et al.* When To Start Consortium. Timing of initiation of antiretroviral therapy in AIDS-free HIV-1-infected patients: a collaborative analysis of 18 HIV cohort studies. Lancet 2009; 373(9672): 1352-63.
[http://dx.doi.org/10.1016/S0140-6736(09)60612-7] [PMID: 19361855]

[24]   Severe P, Juste MA, Ambroise A, *et al.* Early *versus* standard antiretroviral therapy for HIV-infected adults in Haiti. N Engl J Med 2010; 363(3): 257-65.
[http://dx.doi.org/10.1056/NEJMoa0910370] [PMID: 20647201]

[25]   Estrella M, Fine DM, Gallant JE, *et al.* HIV type 1 RNA level as a clinical indicator of renal pathology in HIV-infected patients. Clin Infect Dis 2006; 43(3): 377-80.
[http://dx.doi.org/10.1086/505497] [PMID: 16804855]

[26]   Atta MG, Gallant JE, Rahman MH, *et al.* Antiretroviral therapy in the treatment of HIV-associated nephropathy. Nephrol Dial Transplant 2006; 21(10): 2809-13.
[http://dx.doi.org/10.1093/ndt/gfl337] [PMID: 16864598]

[27]   Weber R, Sabin CA, Friis-Møller N, *et al.* Liver-related deaths in persons infected with the human immunodeficiency virus: the D:A:D study. Arch Intern Med 2006; 166(15): 1632-41.
[http://dx.doi.org/10.1001/archinte.166.15.1632] [PMID: 16908797]

[28]   Balagopal A, Philp FH, Astemborski J, *et al.* Human immunodeficiency virus-related microbial translocation and progression of hepatitis C. Gastroenterology 2008; 135(1): 226-33.
[http://dx.doi.org/10.1053/j.gastro.2008.03.022] [PMID: 18457674]

[29]   Verma S, Goldin RD, Main J. Hepatic steatosis in patients with HIV-Hepatitis C Virus coinfection: is it associated with antiretroviral therapy and more advanced hepatic fibrosis? BMC Res Notes 2008; 1: 46.
[http://dx.doi.org/10.1186/1756-0500-1-46] [PMID: 18710499]

[30]   Ragni MV, Nalesnik MA, Schillo R, Dang Q. Highly active antiretroviral therapy improves ESLD-free survival in HIV-HCV co-infection. Haemophilia 2009; 15(2): 552-8.
[http://dx.doi.org/10.1111/j.1365-2516.2008.01935.x] [PMID: 19347994]

[31]   Ross AC, Armentrout R, O'Riordan MA, *et al.* Endothelial activation markers are linked to HIV status

and are independent of antiretroviral therapy and lipoatrophy. J Acquir Immune Defic Syndr 2008; 49(5): 499-506.
[http://dx.doi.org/10.1097/QAI.0b013e318189a794] [PMID: 18989230]

[32]   Bedimo RJ, McGinnis KA, Dunlap M, Rodriguez-Barradas MC, Justice AC. Incidence of non-AID-
       -defining malignancies in HIV-infected *versus* noninfected patients in the HAART era: impact of
       immunosuppression. J Acquir Immune Defic Syndr 2009; 52(2): 203-8.
       [http://dx.doi.org/10.1097/QAI.0b013e3181b033ab] [PMID: 19617846]

[33]   Bruyand M, Thiébaut R, Lawson-Ayayi S, *et al.* Groupe d'Epidémiologie Clinique du SIDA en
       Aquitaine (GECSA). Role of uncontrolled HIV RNA level and immunodeficiency in the occurrence of
       malignancy in HIV-infected patients during the combination antiretroviral therapy era: Agence
       Nationale de Recherche sur le Sida (ANRS) CO3 Aquitaine Cohort. Clin Infect Dis 2009; 49(7): 1109-
       16.
       [http://dx.doi.org/10.1086/605594] [PMID: 19705973]

[34]   Guiguet M, Boué F, Cadranel J, Lang JM, Rosenthal E, Costagliola D. Clinical Epidemiology Group
       of the FHDH-ANRS CO4 cohort. Effect of immunodeficiency, HIV viral load, and antiretroviral
       therapy on the risk of individual malignancies (FHDH-ANRS CO4): a prospective cohort study.
       Lancet Oncol 2009; 10(12): 1152-9.
       [http://dx.doi.org/10.1016/S1470-2045(09)70282-7] [PMID: 19818686]

[35]   Antinori A, Arendt G, Becker JT, *et al.* Updated research nosology for HIV-associated neurocognitive
       disorders. Neurology 2007; 69(18): 1789-99.
       [http://dx.doi.org/10.1212/01.WNL.0000287431.88658.8b] [PMID: 17914061]

[36]   Ellis RJ, Rosario D, Clifford DB, *et al.* CHARTER Study Group. Continued high prevalence and
       adverse clinical impact of human immunodeficiency virus-associated sensory neuropathy in the era of
       combination antiretroviral therapy: the CHARTER Study. Arch Neurol 2010; 67(5): 552-8.
       [http://dx.doi.org/10.1001/archneurol.2010.76] [PMID: 20457954]

[37]   Nogueras M, Navarro G, Antón E, *et al.* Epidemiological and clinical features, response to HAART,
       and survival in HIV-infected patients diagnosed at the age of 50 or more. BMC Infect Dis 2006; 6:
       159.
       [http://dx.doi.org/10.1186/1471-2334-6-159] [PMID: 17087819]

[38]   Tubiana R, Le Chenadec J, Rouzioux C, *et al.* Factors associated with mother-to-child transmission of
       HIV-1 despite a maternal viral load <500 copies/ml at delivery: a case-control study nested in the
       French perinatal cohort (EPF-ANRS CO1). Clin Infect Dis 2010; 50(4): 585-96.
       [http://dx.doi.org/10.1086/650005] [PMID: 20070234]

[39]   Tovanabutra S, Robison V, Wongtrakul J, *et al.* Male viral load and heterosexual transmission of HIV-
       1 subtype E in northern Thailand. J Acquir Immune Defic Syndr 2002; 29(3): 275-83.
       [http://dx.doi.org/10.1097/00126334-200203010-00008] [PMID: 11873077]

[40]   Panel on Antiretroviral Guidelines for Adult and Adolescents. Guideline for the use of antireriviral
       agents in HIV-1- infected Adult and Adolescents. Department of Health and Human Services 2014; 1-
       2. Available at: http://aidsinfo.nih.gov/ContentFiles/Adultand adulescentGL.pdf.

[41]   Günthard HF, Aberg JA, Eron JJ, *et al.* International Antiviral Society-USA Panel. Antiretroviral
       treatment of adult HIV infection: 2014 recommendations of the International Antiviral Society-USA

Panel. JAMA 2014; 312(4): 410-25.
[http://dx.doi.org/10.1001/jama.2014.8722] [PMID: 25038359]

[42]   Newell ML, Coovadia H, Cortina-Borja M, Rollins N, Gaillard P, Dabis F. Ghent International AIDS Society (IAS) Working Group on HIV Infection in Women and Children. Mortality of infected and uninfected infants born to HIV-infected mothers in Africa: a pooled analysis. Lancet 2004; 364(9441): 1236-43.
[http://dx.doi.org/10.1016/S0140-6736(04)17140-7] [PMID: 15464184]

[43]   World Health Organization. Guideline on when to start antiretroviral therapy and on pre-exposure prophylaxis for HIV. Accessed on: Sep 2015 Available at: http://www.who.int/hiv/pub/guidelines/earlyrelease-arv/en/.

[44]   Chun TW, Shawn Justement J, Murray D, *et al.* Effect of antiretroviral therapy on HIV reservoirs in elite controllers. J Infect Dis 2013; 208(9): 1443-7.
[http://dx.doi.org/10.1093/infdis/jit306] [PMID: 23847057]

CHAPTER 12

Antiretroviral Therapy (ART) in Pregnant Women

Holly Rawizza[*]

Brigham and Women's Hospital, Harvard Medical School, Boston, Massachusetts 02115, USA

Abstract: Interventions to prevent mother-to-child transmission (MTCT) of HIV have become increasingly efficacious over time. Furthermore, regimens and treatment protocols have become increasingly simplified to facilitate coverage at all levels of care and reduce time-to-initiation of prophylaxis regimens. Yet, a substantial number of HIV-infected pregnant women are still not being reached by PMTCT services globally. Although a challenging prospect, we have the tools to end the transmission of HIV from mothers to babies – now is the time for communities to redouble efforts to more effectively implement PMTCT strategies to reach this critical goal.

Keywords: Antiretroviral, Breastfeeding, Guidelines, HIV, Infant, Option B+, Perinatal, Maternal, Prevention of Mother-to-Child Transmission (PMTCT), Prophylaxis.

1. INTRODUCTION

With currently available antiretroviral regimens for the Prevention of Mother-to-Child Transmission (PMTCT) of HIV, perinatal transmission may be reduced from 20-45% without intervention to less than 2% [1, 2]. Based on considerable progress in the expansion of antiretroviral therapy (ART) and PMTCT services globally, as well as implementation of more efficacious PMTCT regimens as outlined in the 2010 and 2013 World Health Organization (WHO) guidelines [3, 4], the prospect of eliminating pediatric HIV is as close as ever [5].

The "Countdown to Zero" initiative announced by the Joint United Nations

[*] **Correspondence to Holly Rawizza:** Brigham and Women's Hospital, Harvard Medical School, Boston, Massachusetts 02115, USA; Tel: (617) 432-4686; Fax: (617) 432-3575; E-mail: hrawizza@hsph.harvard.edu.

SeyedAhmad SeyedAlinaghi (Ed.)

Programme on HIV/AIDS (UNAIDS) ambitiously aims to eliminate pediatric HIV infection by 2015 [6]. However, despite improved access to antiretrovirals (ARVs), PMTCT service utilization remains suboptimal. In 2012, just 62% of HIV-infected pregnant women received ARVs to reduce MTCT [7, 8], and, in 2011, only 35% of infants born to HIV-infected mothers underwent HIV testing in the first two months of life [8]. Although the number of children born with HIV infection has declined by 58% since 2002, an estimated 240,000 infants were born with HIV in 2013 [9, 10], falling far short of what can be achieved with available biomedical interventions.

Thus a comprehensive approach that includes treatment as prevention for women, access to family planning services, universal HIV testing in pregnancy, rapid linkage to care, increased retention of pregnant women, universal access to ART during pregnancy and breastfeeding, appropriate infant prophylaxis, among other comprehensive care interventions, is critically needed.

2. HISTORICAL OVERVIEW OF PMTCT

In 1982, approximately 18 months after the recognition of the first acquired immune deficiency syndrome (AIDS) cases among adults, the epidemic was recognized among among infants in the U.S. as well [11]. Soon after, awareness of the global extent of pediatric infection began to accumulate. One of the earliest reports estimated 11% prevalence among a small cohort of hospitalized children in Zaire [12].

While zidovudine (AZT, ZDV) was approved for use among adults in 1987, it took seven additional years to fully appreciate the potential for ARVs to reduce MTCT. The landmark study, PACTG 076, was first reported in 1994 after being stopped early by the study's Data Safety and Monitoring Board (DSMB) due to overwhelming success. The study found that transmission in the placebo group was 25.5% compared with 8.3% in the AZT group, a reduction in transmission of 67% [13]. This rapidly led to changes in guidelines for treatment of pregnant women with HIV. However, widespread implementation of intravenous AZT during labor and delivery was not felt to be feasible in many resource-constrained settings and thus multiple studies were subsequently performed to evaluate simplified oral regimens. In 1999, a study assessing short-course AZT in Thailand showed that transmission could be reduced by 50%, from 19% in the placebo group to 9% in the AZT group [14]. However, in a study from West Africa, follow-up of patients revealed a loss of efficacy over time due to high rates of HIV transmission during breastfeeding [15].

In 1999, the HIVNET 012 study found that a simple regimen of single-dose nevirapine (sdNVP) given during labor reduced the risk of transmission by nearly 50% [16]. However, enthusiasm for sdNVP quickly waned as high rates of NVP resistance were noted among mothers exposed to sdNVP. A meta-analysis of 10 studies showed that over a third of women developed NVP resistance [17]. However, the risk of NVP resistance was reduced by almost 90% if a 7-day "tail" of AZT/3TC was added after sdNVP [17].

Starting in 2010, a number of studies showed that maternal triple ARV prophylaxis was highly efficacious in reducing the risk of breastfeeding transmission. In the BAN (Breastfeeding, Antiretrovirals, and Nutrition) study, women were randomized to receive post-partum triple ARV prophylaxis, which reduced the rate of breastfeeding transmission to 3% by six months [2]. Two randomized trials, the Kesho Bora and Kisumu studies, which examined the efficacy of triple ARV prophylaxis starting late in pregnancy and continuing until rapid cessation of breastfeeding at six months, found similar rates of transmission of about 5% at 12 months of life [18, 19]. Finally, in the Mma Bana study carried out in Botswana, women were started on triple ARV prophylaxis starting between 26-34 weeks gestation and continued until weaning of breastfeeding at six months of life. Virologic suppression throughout breastfeeding was achieved by 93% of women and overall transmission was 1% through six months [1]. From a research perspective, studies have achieved near elimination of pediatric transmission utilizing simplified maternal and infant prophylaxis regimens. Yet achieving the goal globally will remain elusive unless all women are reached with these highly efficacious regimens.

3. THE GUIDELINES IN PRACTICE

3.1. When to Start

Early initiation of antiretroviral therapy is associated with improved HIV clinical outcomes and decreased HIV transmission. A number of observational studies and randomized controlled trials have shown that earlier initiation of ART is associated with decreased risk of progression to AIDS or death, while also reducing HIV transmission events [20 - 26]. As the body of evidence has grown to support earlier initiation of ART, guidelines have evolved to incorporate these findings. The 2010 WHO guidelines recommended ART initiation at a CD4+ cell count of 350 cells/mm³ or less [3]. Whereas the 2013 WHO Consolidated Guidelines recommend starting at CD4 counts of 500 cells/mm³ or less with priority for those <350 cells/mm³ [4]. Additionally, the 2013 guidelines recommend universal ART for special populations including HIV-infected individuals with TB disease, hepatitis B virus (HBV) coinfection with severe liver disease, all pregnant and breastfeeding women, all children 5 years and younger, and all HIV-infected individuals in serodiscordant relationships, regardless of CD4+ cell count. A comparison of the 2010 and 2013 guidelines is summarized in Table **1**.

Table 1. Comparison of 2010 and 2013 WHO guidelines for initiating ART [27].

	2010 Guidelines [3]	2013 Guidelines [4]
Adults and adolescents living with HIV	≤350 CD4 cells/mm³	≤500 CD4 cells/mm³
Children living with HIV	<24 months old: all 2-5 years old: <750 cells/mm³ or CD4% <25%	<5 years old: all
Pregnant women living with HIV	No specific provision	All
People coinfected with HIV and TB	All	All
People coinfected with HIV and hepatitis B virus	All with chronic active hepatitis	All with chronic severe liver disease
Serodiscordant couples	No specific provision	All

For pregnant HIV-infected women, the 2013 WHO guidelines represent a substantial change from those released in 2010. The 2013 WHO Consolidated

Guidelines recommend that all pregnant or breastfeeding women be initiated on triple ART regardless of WHO clinical stage or CD4+ cell count [4]. This is a significant change from the 2010 guidelines in which provision of ART for pregnant women depended on treatment eligibility status [3]. In the 2010 guidelines, lifelong ART was recommend for eligible women with CD4<350, while for non-eligible women the recommendation was to stop ART after breastfeeding cessation. Further, the 2013 guidelines recommend using the same triple antiretroviral regimen for all women regardless of CD4 count, while the programmatic decision focuses on whether to continue the regimen for life regardless of CD4 level (*i.e.* "Option B+") or discontinue ART after breastfeeding cessation (*i.e.* "Option B") for those with CD4 >500 cells/mm^3. These therapeutic options are discussed at length in the Section 3.2.

Another major change since the 2010 guidelines focuses on whether ART or ARV prophylaxis should be initiated during the first trimester. In the 2010 guidelines, gestational age did not impact timing of initiation among ART eligible women. However, for women who were not eligible based on their own health (*i.e.*, CD4 >350 cells/mm^3 in the 2010 guidelines), prophylaxis was recommended to start *after* 14 weeks gestation. Since then, studies have found no increased risk of birth defects with first trimester exposure to efavirenz [28, 29]. Thus, the 2013 guidelines recommend initiation of antiretrovirals as soon as possible during pregnancy regardless of gestational age. The current program options for ART in PMTCT are summarized in Table **2**.

Table 2. 2013 WHO programmatic options for management of pregnant women with HIV [4].

National PMTCT Strategy	Pregnant and Breast feeding women	
"Option B+" Use lifelong ART for all pregnant and breastfeeding women	Regardless of CD4+ cell count or clinical stage	
	Initiate ART and continue for life (do not stop after cessation of breastfeeding)	
"Option B" Lifelong ART only for eligible women	Eligible for treatment for own health (CD4 ≤500)	Not eligible for own health (CD4 >500)
	Initiate ART and maintain after delivery and cessation of breastfeeding	Initiate ART and stop after delivery and cessation of all breastfeeding

3.2. What to Start: Programmatic Options for PMTCT Care

At the same time that data suggest improved outcomes with earlier treatment, regimens have become less toxic, more convenient (one pill once a day), and more widely available. Simplified treatment regimens are critical for efforts to achieve global PMTCT goals of at least 90% coverage of pregnant women, where current coverage rates are about 62% [8]. As previously mentioned, the 2010 guidelines required CD4 staging prior to regimen selection. Whereas the 2013 guidelines are designed so that treatment may be initiated immediately, and access to baseline CD4 testing is not required. Although further research is needed to confirm the benefits of immediate treatment among pregnant women, this has the potential to reduce treatment delays and loss to follow-up.

The 2010 WHO PMTCT guidelines dichotomized treatment based on eligibility status with a CD4 threshold of 350 cells/mm^3. According to these guidelines, treatment for eligible pregnant women consisted of one of four ART regimens outlined in Table **3**. For non-eligible women with CD4>350, the 2010 guidelines recommended one of two prophylaxis regimens: "Option A" which consisted of zidovudine (AZT) during pregnancy, maternal single-dose NVP (sd-NVP) plus AZT and lamivudine (3TC) at delivery and for one week postpartum; or "Option B" which consisted of triple ARV drugs during pregnancy and throughout breastfeeding. However, the "Option B" regimens differed from those recommended for ART treatment given toxicity concerns surrounding nevirapine use among women with higher CD4 counts. The 2010 guidelines advised that national programs select an approach based on operational considerations.

In 2012, the WHO issued a programmatic update on the use of ARVs for preventing MTCT of HIV [30]. In this document, a third option (Option B+) was described which proposed use of a single triple ARV regimen (tenofovir/lamivudine/efavirenz; TDF/3TC/EFV) for all pregnant women regardless of CD4+ cell count and, importantly, that the regimen be continued for life. This strategy is thought to provide a number of advantages including "further simplification of regimen and service delivery and harmonization with ART programs, protection against mother-to-child transmission in future pregnancies, a continuing prevention benefit against sexual transmission to sero-discordant partners, and avoiding stopping and starting of ARV drugs" [30]. Notably, this strategy avoids the need for baseline CD4+ cell count enumeration prior to treatment stratification, thus decreasing delays as well as opportunities for patient loss between HIV diagnosis and ARV initiation. This may also overcome the challenges associated with provision of ART at the primary care level where laboratory facilities required to perform CD4+ cell count enumeration may not be available, thus reaching women in increasingly rural settings. Although the theoretical benefits of such a strategy are clear, whether utilization of Option B+ will result in improved retention, maternal health, and infant outcomes remains to be seen.

Table 3. Overview of 2010 WHO PMTCT guidelines: Programmatic options for treatment [3].

ART-eligible women CD4 ≤350 *or* stage 3 or 4 disease	ART non-eligible women CD4 >350 *and* asymptomatic	
	Option B (Triple ARV Prophylaxis)	**Option A** (Maternal AZT)
Maternal antepartum daily ART, starting as soon as possible irrespective of gestational age, and continued during pregnancy, delivery and thereafter. Recommended regimens include: AZT + 3TC + NVP or AZT + 3TC + EFV* or TDF + 3TC (or FTC) + NVP or TDF + 3TC (or FTC) + EFV*	Triple ARV prophylaxis starting as early as 14 weeks and continued until delivery, or, if breastfeeding until 1 week after all exposure to breast milk has ended. Recommended regimens include: AZT + 3TC + LVP/r or AZT + 3TC + EFV or TDF + 3TC (or FTC) + EFV or (AZT + 3TC + ABC)	Starting as early as 14 weeks of gestation: Twice-daily AZT At onset of labor: Single-dose NVP *plus* AZT/3TC twice daily (sdNVP can be omitted if AZT was given for >4 weeks)Post-partum: AZT/3TC twice daily for 7 days

The 2013 WHO Consolidated guidelines adopted the simplified regimen of TDF + 3TC (or FTC) + EFV as the preferred first-line regimen for all adults including pregnant women. Of particular note, this regimen is now recommended for women in the first trimester of pregnancy and women of childbearing age. Additionally, for the first time, the 2013 guidelines move away from the longstanding use of zidovudine in PMTCT regimens. Ever since landmark results were reported from the PACTG 076 trial in 1994 in which transmission was reduced by 67% [13], AZT has been a mainstay of PMTCT regimens. In fact, the 2010 WHO guidelines noted that AZT should be included in the regimen whenever possible, unless hemoglobin levels ≤ 8 g/dl or hematocrit < 24%.

However, non-AZT containing regimens have been shown to be equivalent or more effective in preventing transmission and thus the 2013 guidelines now recommend newer NRTI backbones to avoid toxicities. The 2013 WHO recommendations for first-line ART for adults including pregnant and breastfeeding women are summarized in Table **4**.

Table 4. Overview of 2013 WHO guidelines for first-line ART for adults including pregnant women [4].

ART Options	First-line ART for adults including pregnant women (and people with TB and HBV coinfection)
Preferred regimens	**TDF + 3TC (or FTC) + EFV**
Alternative regimens	AZT + 3TC + EFV (or NVP) TDF + 3TC (or FTC) + NVP
Special circumstances	Regimens containing ABC, d4T, and boosted PIs

3.3. ARVs in Special Populations of Pregnant Women

3.3.1. Hepatitis B Virus Co-Infection

In the 2010 WHO guidelines, hepatitis B virus (HBV) co-infection was considered an independent indication for ART initiation irrespective of CD4+ cell count or WHO clinical stage. The 2013 guidelines have slightly modified this recommendation for HIV/HBV coinfected patients who would not otherwise be eligible for ART (*i.e.* CD4>500). Specifically, they state that there is insufficient data to support initiating ART in all coinfected patients with CD4>500, and thus only those who have coexisting severe chronic liver disease should be initiated on treatment. That being said, since ART is recommended for all pregnant women regardless of CD4 count, those found to have coexisting HBV infection should be treated. The recommended regimen for HIV/HBV co-infected individuals includes two drugs that are also active against HBV, including TDF and 3TC or FTC. Given an increased risk for hepatotoxicity after ART initiation among coinfected individuals, close monitoring for elevation of liver transaminases and counseling regarding signs of liver toxicity is recommended. Once an HIV/HBV active triple ART regimen is started, HBV active agents should not be stopped given the risk for HBV flare, including, in rare cases, liver failure.

3.3.2. Women with Active Tuberculosis Infection

Similar to recommendations for adults with HIV/TB co-infection, pregnant women with active TB should start ART as soon as clinically possible, regardless of CD4+ cell count. Pregnant women with HIV infection are nearly ten times more likely to develop active TB than HIV negative counterparts [31]. Efavirenz is the preferred NNRTI for all patients with HIV/TB co-infection.

Table 5. Overview of 2010 WHO infant prophylaxis recommendations [3].

ART-eligible women CD4 ≤350 *or* stage 3 or 4 disease	ART non-eligible women CD4 >350 *and* asymptomatic	
	Option B (Triple ARV Prophylaxis)	Option A (Maternal AZT)
Infant Prophylaxis		
Daily NVP or twice-daily AZT from birth until 4 to 6 weeks of age (irrespective of mode of infant feeding)	*Irrespective of mode of infant feeding*: Daily NVP or twice-daily AZT from birth until 4 to 6 weeks of age	*For breastfeeding infants:* Daily NVP from birth until 1 week after all exposure to breast milk has ended (minimum of 4-6 weeks) *Infants receiving replacement feeding only:* Daily NVP or sd-NVP + AZT twice daily from birth until 4 to 6 weeks of age

4. INFANT ANTIRETROVIRAL PROPHYLAXIS

The guidelines for infant prophylaxis are similar in the 2010 and 2013 WHO guidelines. In the 2010 guidelines [3], the recommendations are again determined by the woman's ART eligibility status. For women who are on ART for their own health, a short duration of infant ARV prophylaxis consisting of either daily NVP or twice-daily AZT for 4-6 weeks is recommended regardless of infant feeding choice. As mentioned in Section 2, the Mma Bana study showed that successful maternal ART reduced the risk of infant transmission to 1%, with a rate of transmission during breastfeeding of only 0.3% [1]. Non-eligible women receiving triple ARV prophylaxis (Option B) should be continued until delivery, or, if breastfeeding, until one week after all exposure to breast milk has ended. Thus, the infant prophylaxis regimen is the same as that for women on ART, as is the case for countries that elect to start all pregnant women on triple ART for life (Option B+) regardless of CD4+ cell count. The duration of infant prophylaxis only varies if a woman receives maternal AZT as prophylaxis (Option A) and the infant is breastfeeding. In such cases, daily NVP should be continued from birth until at least one week after all exposure to breast milk has ended. However, Option A is no longer recommended. Tables **5** and **6** summarize the infant prophylaxis regimens from the 2010 [3] and 2013 [4] WHO guidelines, respectively.

Table 6. Overview of 2013 WHO infant prophylaxis recommendations [4].

National PMTCT Strategy	HIV-exposed infant	
"Option B+" Use lifelong ART for all pregnant and breastfeeding women	**Breastfeeding**	**Replacement feeding**
"Option B" Lifelong ART only for eligible women	6 weeks of infant prophylaxis with once-daily NVP	4-6 weeks of infant prophylaxis with once-daily NVP (or twice-daily AZT)

The recommendations for infant antiretroviral prophylaxis dosing have not changed between the 2010 and 2013 guidelines. See Table **7** for summary of dosing guidelines for infant prophylaxis.

Table 7. Recommended dosing for infant ARV prophylaxis and safety considerations.

Infant Prophylaxis	Dose	Safety Considerations
NVP	*From birth to 6 weeks of age* • Birth weight 2000-2499 gm: NVP 10 mg once daily • Birth weight ≥2500 gm: NVP 15 mg daily *>6 weeks to 6 months of age* • NVP 20 mg once daily *>6 months to 9 months of age* • NVP 30 mg once daily *>9 months to end of breastfeeding* • NVP 40 mg once daily	Risk of NVP resistance if infant becomes infected despite prophylaxis Potential for NVP toxicity if mother is also receiving NVP-based ART
AZT	*From birth to 6 weeks of age* • Birth weight <2500 gm: 10 mg twice daily • Birth weight ≥2500 gm: 15 mg twice daily	AZT-associated anemia

5. CHOICE OF ART REGIMEN FOR WOMEN WITH PRIOR EXPOSURE TO PMTCT PROPHYLAXIS

For women who subsequently become eligible for ART for their own health after recent exposure to PMTCT ARV prophylaxis, standard first-line ART regimens are recommended. Although less commonly encountered given the revised PMTCT guidelines, for women with single-dose NVP exposure less than 12 months prior to initiating ART for their own health, a Protease Inhibitor (PI)-based regimen is currently recommended. This is based on a number of studies documenting poor outcomes among women with sdNVP exposure who subsequently initiated NVP-based regimens within 12 months of exposure [32, 33].

In summary, the most recent WHO guidelines published in 2013 represent a substantial change in PMTCT care. The guidelines recommend earlier treatment of all HIV-infected individuals with CD4 cell counts <500 cells/mm^3 and universal ART for all pregnant and breastfeeding women. Further, the recommended regimen for ART-eligible and non-eligible women has been harmonized so that the same, simplified regimen is used in both cases. At the same time, the guidelines provide flexibility for countries to decide whether to implement lifelong ART *versus* prophylaxis regimens for pregnant women with CD4 counts >500. Although further research is needed to assess the true impact of these changes on maternal health, infant transmission, and infant mortality, the guidelines represent an important step toward the ultimate goal of eliminating perinatal HIV transmission.

CONFLICT OF INTEREST

The author confirms that author has no conflict of interest to declare for this publication.

ACKNOWLEDGEMENTS

Declared none.

REFERENCES

[1]   Shapiro RL, Hughes MD, Ogwu A, *et al*. Antiretroviral regimens in pregnancy and breast-feeding in Botswana. N Engl J Med 2010; 362(24): 2282-94.

[http://dx.doi.org/10.1056/NEJMoa0907736] [PMID: 20554983]

[2]   Chasela CS, Hudgens MG, Jamieson DJ, *et al.* BAN Study Group. Maternal or infant antiretroviral drugs to reduce HIV-1 transmission. N Engl J Med 2010; 362(24): 2271-81.
[http://dx.doi.org/10.1056/NEJMoa0911486] [PMID: 20554982]

[3]   World Health Organization. Antiretroviral drugs for treating pregnant women and preventing HIV infection in infants: recommendations for a public health approach; 2010 version. Geneva, Switzerland: WHO Press, World Health Organization 2010.

[4]   World Health Organization. Consolidated guidelines on the use of antiretroviral drugs for treating and preventing HIV infection: Recommendations for a public health approach June 2013. Geneva, Switzerland: WHO Press, World Health Organization 2013.

[5]   Mofenson LM. Protecting the next generation--eliminating perinatal HIV-1 infection. N Engl J Med 2010; 362(24): 2316-8.
[http://dx.doi.org/10.1056/NEJMe1004406] [PMID: 20554987]

[6]   Joint United Nations Programme on HIV/AIDS (UNAIDS). Countdown to zero: global plan for the elimination of new HIV infections among children by 2015 and keeping their mothers alive, 2011-2015. Geneva: UNAIDS 2011.

[7]   UNAIDS. Global report: UNAIDS report on the global AIDS epidemic 2012. WHO Library Cataloguing-in-Publication Data; UNAIDS/JC2417E 2012.

[8]   UNAIDS. Global report: UNAIDS report on the global AIDS epidemic 2013. WHO Library Cataloguing-in-Publication Data; UNAIDS/JC2502/1/E 2013.

[9]   UNAIDS. The Gap Report. [Accessed on: Jul 2014]; Available at: http://www.unaids.org/en/resources/ campaigns/2014/2014gapreport/gapreport/.

[10]   UNAIDS (2014, July). The Gap Report: Epi Slides. Available at: http://www.unaids.org /en/media/unaids/contentassets/documents/document/2014/2014gapreportslides/01_Epi_slides_2014July.pdf 2014.

[11]   Scott GB, Buck BE, Leterman JG, Bloom FL, Parks WP. Acquired immunodeficiency syndrome in infants. N Engl J Med 1984; 310(2): 76-81.
[http://dx.doi.org/10.1056/NEJM198401123100202] [PMID: 6606781]

[12]   Mann JM, Francis H, Davachi F, *et al.* Human immunodeficiency virus seroprevalence in pediatric patients 2 to 14 years of age at Mama Yemo Hospital, Kinshasa, Zaire. Pediatrics 1986; 78(4): 673-7.
[PMID: 3020492]

[13]   Connor EM, Sperling RS, Gelber R, *et al.* Reduction of maternal-infant transmission of human immunodeficiency virus type 1 with zidovudine treatment. Pediatric AIDS Clinical Trials Group Protocol 076 Study Group. N Engl J Med 1994; 331(18): 1173-80.
[http://dx.doi.org/10.1056/NEJM199411033311801] [PMID: 7935654]

[14]   Shaffer N, Chuachoowong R, Mock PA, *et al.* Bangkok Collaborative Perinatal HIV Transmission Study Group. Short-course zidovudine for perinatal HIV-1 transmission in Bangkok, Thailand: a randomised controlled trial. Lancet 1999; 353(9155): 773-80.
[http://dx.doi.org/10.1016/S0140-6736(98)10411-7] [PMID: 10459957]

[15]   Dabis F, Msellati P, Meda N, *et al.* 6-month efficacy, tolerance, and acceptability of a short regimen of oral zidovudine to reduce vertical transmission of HIV in breastfed children in Côte d'Ivoire and Burkina Faso: a double-blind placebo-controlled multicentre trial. DITRAME Study Group. DIminution de la Transmission Mère-Enfant. Lancet 1999; 353(9155): 786-92.
[http://dx.doi.org/10.1016/S0140-6736(98)11046-2] [PMID: 10459959]

[16]   Guay LA, Musoke P, Fleming T, *et al.* Intrapartum and neonatal single-dose nevirapine compared with zidovudine for prevention of mother-to-child transmission of HIV-1 in Kampala, Uganda: HIVNET 012 randomised trial. Lancet 1999; 354(9181): 795-802.
[http://dx.doi.org/10.1016/S0140-6736(99)80008-7] [PMID: 10485720]

[17]   Arrivé E, Newell ML, Ekouevi DK, *et al.* Ghent Group on HIV in Women and Children. Prevalence of resistance to nevirapine in mothers and children after single-dose exposure to prevent vertical transmission of HIV-1: a meta-analysis. Int J Epidemiol 2007; 36(5): 1009-21.
[http://dx.doi.org/10.1093/ije/dym104] [PMID: 17533166]

[18]   de Vincenzi I. Kesho Bora Study Group. Triple antiretroviral compared with zidovudine and single-dose nevirapine prophylaxis during pregnancy and breastfeeding for prevention of mother-to-child transmission of HIV-1 (Kesho Bora study): a randomised controlled trial. Lancet Infect Dis 2011; 11(3): 171-80.
[http://dx.doi.org/10.1016/S1473-3099(10)70288-7] [PMID: 21237718]

[19]   Thomas TK, Masaba R, Borkowf CB, *et al.* KiBS Study Team. Triple-antiretroviral prophylaxis to prevent mother-to-child HIV transmission through breastfeeding--the Kisumu Breastfeeding Study, Kenya: a clinical trial. PLoS Med 2011; 8(3): e1001015.
[http://dx.doi.org/10.1371/journal.pmed.1001015] [PMID: 21468300]

[20]   Emery S, Neuhaus JA, Phillips AN, *et al.* Strategies for Management of Antiretroviral Therapy (SMART) Study Group. Major clinical outcomes in antiretroviral therapy (ART)-naive participants and in those not receiving ART at baseline in the SMART study. J Infect Dis 2008; 197(8): 1133-44.
[http://dx.doi.org/10.1086/586713] [PMID: 18476292]

[21]   Sterne JA, May M, Costagliola D, *et al.* When To Start Consortium. Timing of initiation of antiretroviral therapy in AIDS-free HIV-1-infected patients: a collaborative analysis of 18 HIV cohort studies. Lancet 2009; 373(9672): 1352-63.
[http://dx.doi.org/10.1016/S0140-6736(09)60612-7] [PMID: 19361855]

[22]   Cohen MS, Chen YQ, McCauley M, *et al.* HPTN 052 Study Team. Prevention of HIV-1 infection with early antiretroviral therapy. N Engl J Med 2011; 365(6): 493-505.
[http://dx.doi.org/10.1056/NEJMoa1105243] [PMID: 21767103]

[23]   Ahdieh-Grant L, Yamashita TE, Phair JP, *et al.* When to initiate highly active antiretroviral therapy: a cohort approach. Am J Epidemiol 2003; 157(8): 738-46.
[http://dx.doi.org/10.1093/aje/kwg036] [PMID: 12697578]

[24]   Moore DM, Harris R, Lima V, *et al.* Antiretroviral Therapy Cohort Collaboration. Effect of baseline CD4 cell counts on the clinical significance of short-term immunologic response to antiretroviral therapy in individuals with virologic suppression. J Acquir Immune Defic Syndr 2009; 52(3): 357-63.
[http://dx.doi.org/10.1097/QAI.0b013e3181b62933] [PMID: 19668084]

[25]   Writing Committee for the CASCADE Collaboration. Timing of HAART initiation and clinical

outcomes in human immunodeficiency virus type 1 seroconverters. Arch Intern Med 2011; 171(17): 1560-9.
[http://dx.doi.org/10.1001/archinternmed.2011.401] [PMID: 21949165]

[26]   Kitahata MM, Gange SJ, Abraham AG, *et al.* NA-ACCORD Investigators. Effect of early *versus* deferred antiretroviral therapy for HIV on survival. N Engl J Med 2009; 360(18): 1815-26.
[http://dx.doi.org/10.1056/NEJMoa0807252] [PMID: 19339714]

[27]   WHO. Global update on HIV treatment 2013: Results, impact and opportunities. Who report in partnership with UNICEF and UNAIDS 2013. Available at: http://www.unaids.org/en/media /unaids/contentassets/documents/unaidspublication/2013/20130630_treatment_report_en.pdf

[28]   Ford N, Mofenson L, Kranzer K, *et al.* Safety of efavirenz in first-trimester of pregnancy: a systematic review and meta-analysis of outcomes from observational cohorts. AIDS 2010; 24(10): 1461-70.
[http://dx.doi.org/10.1097/QAD.0b013e32833a2a14] [PMID: 20479637]

[29]   Ford N, Calmy A, Mofenson L. Safety of efavirenz in the first trimester of pregnancy: an updated systematic review and meta-analysis. AIDS 2011; 25(18): 2301-4.
[http://dx.doi.org/10.1097/QAD.0b013e32834cdb71] [PMID: 21918421]

[30]   WHO. Programmatic Update: Use of Antiretroviral Drugs for Treating Pregnant Women and Preventing HIV Infection in Infants. Executive Summary 2012. Available from: http://www.who.int /hiv/pub/mtct/programmatic_update2012/en/

[31]   Pillay T, Khan M, Moodley J, Adhikari M, Coovadia H. Perinatal tuberculosis and HIV-1: considerations for resource-limited settings. Lancet Infect Dis 2004; 4(3): 155-65.
[http://dx.doi.org/10.1016/S1473-3099(04)00939-9] [PMID: 14998501]

[32]   Lockman S, Shapiro RL, Smeaton LM, *et al.* Response to antiretroviral therapy after a single, peripartum dose of nevirapine. N Engl J Med 2007; 356(2): 135-47.
[http://dx.doi.org/10.1056/NEJMoa062876] [PMID: 17215531]

[33]   Lockman S, Hughes MD, McIntyre J, *et al.* OCTANE A5208 Study Team. Antiretroviral therapies in women after single-dose nevirapine exposure. N Engl J Med 2010; 363(16): 1499-509.
[http://dx.doi.org/10.1056/NEJMoa0906626] [PMID: 20942666]

CHAPTER 13

HIV Drug Resistance

Hamid Emadi Koochak[1], Siavash Eskandari[1,2], Zeinab Najafi[1,2], Shooka Esmaeeli[1,2,*], Koosha Paydary[1,2], Sahra Emamzadeh Fard[3], Mona Mohammadi Firouzeh[1] and Shayan Tabe-Bordbar[4]

[1] *Iranian Research Center for HIV/AIDS, Iranian Institute for Reduction of High-Risk Behaviors, Tehran University of Medical Sciences, Iran*

[2] *Students' Scientific Research Center (SSRC), Tehran University of Medical Sciences (TUMS), Tehran, Iran*

[3] *Department of Radiology, Division of Interventional Radiology, Memorial Sloan-Kettering Cancer Center, New York, USA*

[4] *Department of Molecular and Integrative Physiology, University of Illinois at Urbana-Champaign, Illinois, USA*

Abstract: The ability of HIV to mutate and replicate in the presence of antiretroviral therapy (ART) drugs are called HIV drug resistance. There are many reasons for HIV drug resistance happening. Some determinants are related to virus such as infidel reverse transcriptase, error-prone replication, *etc*. The appearance of drug resistance mutations and viral evolution could be a result of continuing HIV-1 replication in ART among some infected subjects. A wide range of mechanisms has been described with difference characteristics for different classes of drugs and also for drugs of a given class. New antiretroviral (ARV) drugs which are often applied in treatment-experienced patients include the entry inhibitor (Enfuvirtide), protease inhibitors (PIs) (Darunavir and Tipranavir), a C-C chemokine receptor (CCR) type 5 antagonist (Maraviroc), an integrase inhibitor (Raltegravir) and a non-nucleoside reverse transcriptase inhibitor (NNRTI) (Etravirine). The overwhelming data presented in journals and at scientific meetings helps staying informed about current issues, but makes new developments a daunting task.

* **Correspondence to Shooka Esmaeeli:** Iranian Research Center for HIV/AIDS (IRCHA), Imam Khomeini Hospital, Keshavarz Blvd., Tehran, Iran; Tel/Fax: +98 (21) 66947984; E-mail: sh.esmaeeli@gmail.com.

SeyedAhmad SeyedAlinaghi (Ed.)

Keywords: Antiretroviral therapy, Determinants, Drug Resistance, Epidemiology, Guideline, HIV, Mechanism, Novel, Prevalence, Transmission, Treatment.

1. INTRODUCTION

HIV drug resistance is defined as the ability of HIV to mutate and replicate in the presence of antiretroviral (ARV) drugs. Drug resistance has become a universally challenging issue since the introduction of first ARV drugs for the treatment of Human Immunodeficiency Virus (HIV) infection [1]. ARV drug resistance is often observed in subjects with incomplete viral suppression and can limit both the scale and duration of the treatment response. As alternative great concern, the Transmitted Drug Resistance (TDR) to newly infected persons has been reported in almost all countries with access to Highly Active Antiretroviral Therapy (HAART) [1 - 11]. Although TDR has been recognized for more than a decade, the changes and the effects with respect to treatment's responses have not been defined yet [2].

The ARV resistance patterns among recently infected populations appear to reflect geographic trends with regard to the use of ARV medications worldwide. According to the worldwide surveillance program (WATCH), the resistance rate for any ARV drugs among treatment naive individuals was 5.5% in Africa, 7.4% in East Asia, 5.7 % in Southeast Asia, and 6.4 % in Latin America compared to higher levels in North America (11.4 %) and Europe (10.6 %) [3].

It has been previously implicated that the main reason for the emergence and spread of drug-resistant HIV strains might be inadequate adherence to therapy [4]. In fact, HIV replicates and mutates at high rates *in vivo* which leads to continuous production of genetically varying horde of viral strains [1].Although most of HIV-1 variation appears from the accumulation of point mutations, recombination can be also involved in the viral variations, since leaping in genetic evolution by merging two or more distinct beneficial mutations into a single genome.

It is necessary to maintain resistance surveillance programs throughout the developing countries and to report and analyze data in a consistent and timely manner. ARV resistance was especially common in persons who received mono- or dual- drug therapy before the application of HAART regimens that composed of Non-Nucleoside Reverse Transcriptase Inhibitors (NNRTIs) and Protease Inhibitors (PIs) [7].

2. GLOBAL EPIDEMIOLOGY OF TRANSMITTED DRUG RESISTANCE

Drug resistance to ARV agents has been documented since 1989. In fact, drug resistance is one of the most common reasons for HAART failure and is generally attributable to the patient's poor adherence or low potency of the therapeutic regimen [8].

Recent data suggest that HIV-1 resistance is decreasing in patients with antiretroviral regimens which are mainly the result of applying more potent drug combinations as therapy options. In the following section, we briefly describe the global epidemiology of TDR [10, 11].

2.1. TDR in The USA

The largest study that surveyed TDR in the USA enrolled 1082 recently infected patients from 10 cities and reported the prevalence of TDR to be about 8.3%. TDR was more common in Men who have Sex with Men (MSM), compared to heterosexual men and women (12%, 4.7% and 6.1% respectively) [12]. Furthermore, the prevalence of resistance mutants was reported to be 5.4% among African–American populations, and 13% in Caucasians. In another study in the USA, the prevalence of TDR was 25% in 2005 [13, 14]. Studies of newly infected patients showed intermediate rates of TDR in Canada (8% from 1997 until 2005). Finally, the reports gain different rates of TDR in the USA between 8.3% and 27.3%, based on the epidemiological situation [15].

2.2. TDR in Latin America

With regard to the lower availability of ART, a lower distribution of TDR in these countries are expected, however, some studies from Latin America (especially Brazil & Argentina) have reported a higher frequency of TDR in these countries. For example in Argentina, a sensible growth of TDR has been documented [16]: TDR prevalence was about 1% in 2001 and 12.9% in 2005 until 2007. However, the prevalence of TDR in other Latin American countries is relatively low. In Chile, Studies showed a 2.5% increase in TDR levels from 2000 to 2005 [17].

2.3. TDR in Europe

Two large European studies or investigations have addressed the frequency of TDR including CASCADE and SPREAD studies. In the CASCADE study, patients were analyzed from seven countries in Western Europe and Canada. Sample data was gathered from 438 treatment-naive patients, 45 (10.3%) harbor mutations involved in TDR [18]. In SPREAD, 2208 treatment-naive cases were analyzed and the overall spread of TDR was 10.4%. Also, as reported, TDR was higher in recently infected individuals *versus* patients with unknown date of infection (13.5% *vs.* 8.7%; $P < 0.01$) [19].

2.4. TDR in Africa & Asia

Many studies from Africa reported that although ART is not widely available in Africa, TDR does exist. The levels of TDR across sub-Saharan Africa differ from zero to 16.5% in chronically infected patients, and 2.1% to 11.5% in newly infected patients. Studies investigating TDR epidemiology in Asia are primarily originated in China, Japan, and Korea. In Asia, the prevalence of TDR has been reported between zero to 15% in chronically infected patients [2, 15, 20, 21].

2.5. TDR in Non-B Subtypes

In patients infected with the non-B subtype, lower levels of TDR have been reported. The CATCH study reported prevalence of TDR to be 4.8% in patients infected with non-B subtype strains compared with 12.9% in patients infected with B subtypes [19].

Conclusion

In terms of ART availability, higher prevalence of TDR was found in North America and Europe which have vast access to ART [15].

3. DETERMINANTS OF HIV DRUG RESISTANCE

3.1. Viral Determinants of Drug Resistance

There are many reasons for emerging HIV drug resistance. The infidel Reverse

Transcriptase (RT) and the error prone replication are the main viral determinants of HIV drug resistance. The appearance of drug resistance mutations and viral evolution could be a result of continuing HIV-1 replication during antiretroviral therapy (ART) in some patients [6, 22].

Many HIV-1 variations originate from the accumulation of point mutations, but recombination may affect viral evolution since this leaps in genetic evolution by merging two or more different beneficial mutations into a single genome. To occur recombination, different viruses must infect a host cell, each producing progeny RNAs. Then, various progeny RNAs must undergo bringing together in one virion. The next run of replication is accompanied by the shift of, the RT from one template to another, which leads to a chimeric molecule with sequences from the two distinct parental genomes [23, 24].

Viral genotype and phenotype reveal resistance patterns to antiretroviral agents. Genotype evaluates mutations in the virus's genetic material, whereas phenotype assesses the ability of the virus to grow in the presence of increasing concentrations of antiretroviral agents. Two key enzymes have been extensively studied with regard to their potential for development of resistance: RT and protease. Replication by the RT enzyme is highly susceptible to errors. Given that the HIV genome is approximately 10,000 nucleotides in length and that mutations *via* the RT enzyme occur approximately one in every 10,000 nucleotides copied, it has been estimated that a mutation occurs with every viral replication cycle. With up to 10 billion particles of virus being produced per day, the potential exists for 1,000 to 10,000 mutations occurring at each site in the HIV genome every day. Integrase resistance, including resistance mutations to Raltegravir exist, but has not yet been fully described, because its use is not widespread [25].

As mentioned previously, the viral genotype is an important aspect of drug resistance which is directly related to the occurring mutations. The viral replication may by impaired by many resistance mutations. Such mutations result in modified key viral proteins, having variable and deleterious impacts on protein functions. Of course, it is possible to relatively correct some deficits by compensatory mutations [26, 27]. In fact, viral strains in the context of developing higher levels of resistance under intense and continuous antiretroviral pressure usually show a significant impairment in their replication capacity [28]. The severity of replication impairment restricted to resistance mutations is remarkably variable. The most disabling mutations are related to resistance to protease inhibitors [29, 30], but significant replication defects are associated with mutations in reverse transcriptase that respond resistance to nucleoside analogs or non-nucleoside reverse transcriptase inhibitors, as well as envelope mutations associated with resistance to Enfuvirtide [31 - 33].

3.2. Host Factors

There are many factors related to host which may result in HIV drug resistance, among which genetic factors, adherence to ARV regimen and behavioral determinants are paramount. As an outcome of the incomplete suppression of HIV-1 replication by ARV drugs, resistance is a permanent threat for patients receiving ARV treatment, and transmission of resistant viral strains is a significant issue worldwide. Protection against resistance needs patient education about the risks of resistance and the application of improved drug regimens that ensure optimal tolerance, adherence, and potency [34].

Inadequate adherence to therapy has blunted advances in the treatment of HIV among some patients, and has been considered as a major barrier toward achieving satisfactory suppression of HIV viral load. Non- suppressed HIV viral load is involved in drug resistance, an increased risk of person-to-person HIV transmission and increased morbidity and mortality. For individuals failing HIV treatment due to poor adherence, becoming adherent to therapy might be a life-saving behavioral switch. In fact, increasing adherence to therapy is among the most important difficulties to succeed management of HIV infection. Various HIV-infected individuals are able to successfully gain prescribed ARV medications; about 37% of patients in developed countries face problems in maintaining proper rates of adherence. Although lower rates of poor adherence are reported in developing countries, recent researches indicate that inadequate adherence in an universal challenge toward management of patients [35, 36]. The ability of clinicians to predict adherence among their patients has been disappointing. The role the motivational readiness plays on an individual's ability to adhere to HIV treatment is the most important personal determinant. According to the 2011 DHHS (Department of Health & Human Services) guidelines, the 2010 International AIDS Society guidelines, and the current European AIDS Society guidelines for the use of antiretroviral agents in HIV-1 infected adults and adolescents, ARV treatment should be onset just when a patient is "ready" to adhere to ARV treatments. Readiness takes place when an individual with his or her own free will achieves a conscious awareness as a certain desired and beneficial behavior [37, 38]. Readiness has been identified as a critical component in a number of healthful behaviors such as cessation of excessive alcohol consumption [39] and adoption of asthma treatment strategies [40]. The presence of readiness has been shown to be an important predictor of ARV adherence [37].

Another important host factor is sexual behavior. Human sexuality and sexual behavior is crucial in determining the transmission and evolution of sexually transmitted microbial agents. In this regard, sex workers, HIV-discordant cohabiting couples, and men who have sex with men are in risk groups for contracting resistant HIV strains. Global change in sexual behavior including an increase in oral and anal sex, increased rate of homosexuality in some populations, changing age structures and unequal gender rates may affect the rate of TDR [41].

Another important host determinant is genetic differences between individuals. For example, some HIV-1–infected individuals, known as "elite suppressors" maintain viral loads of < 50 copies of HIV-1 RNA/mL of plasma and normal CD4+ T cell counts without receiving ART. The controlling mechanisms of viremia remain unclear among elite suppressors, but it seems that major histocompatibility complex class I allele group HLA-B*57 is over-expressed in elite suppressors, suggesting a role for the CD8+ T cells [42]. Interestingly, although some HLA-B*57–positive individuals suppress viremia early after infection, 10% of patients with progressive disease are HLA-B*57 positive. Control of viral replication in some HLA-B*57–positive individuals may involve host immune responses, characteristics of the infecting virus, or both. It is reported a case of virologic escape in a human leukocyte antigen (HLA)–B*57–positive patient shortly after seroconversion. The HLA-B57 Positive escape was associated with the development of mutations in two HLA-B*57–restricted CD8+ T cell Gag epitopes, reversion of the drug-resistance mutation M184V [43, 44].

4. MECHANISMS OF ANTI-RETROVIRAL DRUG RESISTANCE

A wide range of mechanisms have been defined in the context of resistance to different classes of ARV agents:

4.1. Resistance to Nucleoside and Nucleotide Analogues

Nucleoside and nucleotide analogues are precursors of the synthesis of viral DNA by reverse transcriptase. After phosphorylation by cellular kinases, reverse transcriptase merges these compounds into the nascent chain of viral DNA. Because of loss of 3' hydroxyl group in these analogues, no extra nucleotides can be attached which terminate the synthesis of viral DNA. Two different mechanisms are related to HIV resistance to these drugs: impairment of analogue incorporation into DNA and analogue elimination of prematurely terminated DNA chain [34].

Multiple mutations in reverse transcriptase can accord to resistance by impairing the capability of reverse transcriptase to incorporate an analogue into DNA. These mutations essentially cover the K65R mutation, the Q151M complex of mutations, and the M184V mutation. M184V is the basic mutation causing resistance to lamivudine, involving the substitution of Methionine by Valine at position 184 of the reverse transcriptase [45]. Methionine 184 is placed at the center of the catalytic site in reverse transcriptase, and its substitution by a Valine, which has a various side chain, prevents the proper positioning of lamivudine triphosphate within the catalytic site [46]. The M184V mutation induces very high levels of resistance to lamivudine. When lamivudine is used as mono-therapy, resistant strains will emerge in a few weeks [47] and when lamivudine is used as part of a failing regimen of HAART, the M184V mutation is almost always the first mutation to emerge [48].

The group of mutations known as the Q151M complex most often confers resistance to stavudine and didanosine. This pathway always begins with the Q151M substitution, a residue placed in the immediate vicinity of the nucleotide binding site of reverse transcriptase, and then the gradual accumulation of secondary mutations would occur that improve resistance and enhance the enzyme activity [49]. The Q151M complex is relatively rare in HIV-1 (fewer than 5% of all HIV strains with resistance to nucleoside analogues), but can accord to high level resistance to most, albeit not all (*e.g.*, lamivudine and tenofovir) analogues. Surprisingly, the Q151M complex is markedly more frequent in HIV-2 than in HIV-1. The K65R mutation exemplifies another mutation conferring resistance to nucleotide or nucleoside analogues, especially when the system includes tenofovir or abacavir. In fact this mutation emerges to confer resistance to most analogues, except zidovudine [50].

4.2. Resistance to NNRTIs

NNRTIs cover small molecules with great contribution to a hydrophobic pocket placed close to the catalytic domain of the reverse transcriptase. The flexibility of the enzyme is affected by inhibitors, so inhibitors would block its ability to synthesize DNA [48]. All mutations which cause resistance to NNRTIs affect the hydrophobic pocket [48 - 53]; on the other hand, the mutations that emerge most frequently are drug dependent. Resistance to nevirapine is often associated with the Y181C mutation, but other mutations such as Y188C, K103N, G190A, and V106A, also occur. Initial resistance to efavirenz is usually determined by the K103N mutation, but the Y188L mutation also emerges.

4.3. Resistance to PIs

The HIV protease enzyme cleaves large polypeptides to smaller structural proteins and enzymes that are necessary for the assembly of infectious viral particles. In the absence of a functional protease produced proteins will be immature. The protease has a central, symmetric active site. After discovering the exact and detailed shape of this site and the structure of substrates, efforts were undertaken to design effective inhibitors of the protease [51]. Such compounds demonstrate a strong affinity for the active site of the HIV protease and prevent the catalytic activity of the enzyme in a highly selective manner. Resistance to PIs is the consequence of amino acid substitutions appearing either inside the substrate linking domain of the enzyme or at distant sites. These substitutions change the counts and the nature of contact amino acid residues between inhibitors and protease, leading to lowered affinity for the enzyme [34]. Moreover, PIs have been designed to link the protease with maximal affinity and to occupy more space inside the active site cavity than natural substrates. Natural substrates have less affinity and looser binding to the active site of the enzyme. Resistance mutations in the protease, resulting in an overall enlargement of the catalytic site of the enzyme would show a heavy effect on the linking of inhibitors than the natural substrates. It is noteworthy that some mutations by causing specificities in the chemical structure of PIs can influence interaction with the substrate binding. However, a remarkable overlap is obvious between the combinations of mutations in HIV strains which exhibit resistance to PIs which explains the wide cross-resistance that is generally observed within this drug class [52, 53]. Remarkably, mutations in some natural viral substrates can also confer resistance to PIs. For example, amino acid substitutions near the cleavage sites of the gag polypeptide leads to increased level of resistance and replicative capacity of the virus by facilitating cleavage, when the amount of active enzyme is suboptimal through improved ability of mutant protease to interact with its substrate [54, 55].

4.4. Resistance to Fusion Inhibitors

For HIV-1 to enter its target cells a complex sequence of interactions between specific cell surface receptors and the HIV envelope glycoprotein (GP) complex (GP120–GP41) is required [56]. First step in this process provides GP41 an opportunity to interact with the cell membrane. Then, the target cell and membranes of the virus are brought into close proximity, strengthening their fusion through further rearrangement of GP41. In this step, HR2, a hydrophobic region of GP41, integrated into a more proximal hydrophobic region, HR1, effectively shortens the molecule. Enfuvirtide binds to HR1 and reduces stabilization of this process. Enfuvirtide viral resistance, usually results from mutations located in a stretch of 10 amino acids within HR1 [57, 58]. Cross resistance always occurs in agents within a given class of antiretroviral drugs, but all three classes of antiretroviral drugs are affected. Early evolution of resistance to nucleoside antiretroviral or protease inhibitors, viruses have low level of cross-resistance to alternative agents within each of those two classes of drugs. In patients infected with low levels of cross-resistance strains, rapid selection for highly resistant variants is involved with the shift to active alternative drugs, to the detriment of minimal evolutionary changes [34, 59].

5. GUIDELINES FOR TREATMENT OF FIRST-LINE TREATMENT RESISTANT INFECTIONS

About 25% of patients that receive HAART experience treatment failure within the first year of commencing therapy. Although the exact reasons for failure are still unknown, some factors such as history of low initial CD4 count, high initial viral load, and extensive use of ARV agents are assumed to be associated with higher risk of failure. Assessments of regimen failure are based on: (a) clinical symptoms, (b) surrogate marker data, and (c) regimen tolerability and adherence. The first sign of failure in many patients is a change in signs and symptoms. These changes can be mild (*e.g.*, increase in constitutional symptoms, new onset of oral thrush) or more severe (*e.g.*, new opportunistic infections) that indicate treatment failure and a need for changing ARV regimen. In order to change the regimen, some general rules are used to choose alternative ARV regimen such as:

1. If possible, the new regimen should contain ARV agents to which the patient has not been previously exposed to.
2. Alternative regimen should be initiated as soon as the previous regimen has failed. Prolonged treatment with a failing regimen would result in the accumulation of resistance mutations.
3. For selection of appropriate drug regimens, resistance testing is recommended. Optimally, genotype, phenotype, or virtual phenotype testing should occur while the patient is taking the failing regimen, or within four weeks of discontinuation to increase the likelihood of detecting resistant isolates [25].

Genotypic and phenotypic resistance assays are applied to select appropriate treatment tactics. Standard assays provide information on resistance to NRTIs, NNRTIs, and PIs. Testing for integrase and fusion inhibitor resistance can also be ordered from several commercial laboratories.

Whenever the application of a CCR5 antagonist is being considered, co-receptor tropism assays should be performed. Phenotypic co-receptor tropism assays have been applied in clinical practice and a genotypic assay to estimate co-receptor application is now commercially available [60].

4. One new drug should never be added to a failing regimen to prevent the development of resistance.

An exception to this rule is when the initial response to a first regimen has been inadequate. In this situation, some clinicians may intensify therapy with an additional agent provided that the viral load measurements were trending downward since initiation of therapy.

5. If possible, a regimen that has failed in the past should not be initiated again.
6. When treatment failure is a direct result of drug toxicity (rather than poor drug efficacy), the drug should be replaced with an alternative drug from a similar class, so potential for cross-resistance will decrease.
7. If a particular drug in a given regimen must be stopped, it is recommended that all agents in the regimen be stopped and restarted simultaneously to prevent the development of resistance.

Many alternative regimens are theoretical or have been recommended based on limited data. In addition, many potential options could not be used in some patients because of prior ARV regimen, toxicity, or past intolerances. Therefore, clinicians should carefully discuss these issues with the patient before changing the regimen [25].

New ARV drugs support short- and long-term tolerability, varying levels of enhanced activity against drug-resistant HIV strains, and dosing adjustability compared to previous agents. New ARV drugs which are commonly used in treatment-experienced patients include the entry inhibitors (enfuvirtide), some novel PIs (darunavir and tipranavir), a C-C chemokine receptor (CCR) type 5 antagonist (maraviroc), an integrase inhibitor (raltegravir) and a NNRTI (etravirine).

Generally, the proportion of viraemic subjects achieving viral suppression increases with the counts of active pharmacokinetically compatible ARV drugs in the regimen. Raltegravir plus a boosted PI is being investigated for second-line treatment in patients who are not responding to NNRTI-based first-line therapy in settings with limited resources. But low barrier against the resistance of raltegravir in this regimen is of some concern, while another issue of importance is the low penetration rate or coefficient of some PIs into the CNS.

In ARV experienced patients, new agents may be applied for simplification of the dosing schedule, reducing costs (such as by switching to boosted PI mono-therapy), lowering adverse effects or maintaining ARV drug options. For example, the shift of enfuvirtide to raltegravir removed painful injection-site reactions with no reduction in virological suppression. Two studies found different virological outcomes when patients were switched from lopinavir/ritonavir to raltegravir, but there was an improvement in the lipid profile. After reduction of plasma HIV RNA to <50 copies/mL, it is safe to use darunavir or ritonavir monotherapy which is more convenient. In fact, during this mono-therapy no emergence of resistance has been found, but long term data is needed to deliver a final conclusion. The initial suggestion that maraviroc may possess unique CD4+ T-cell boosting effects were not confirmed in several clinical trials [61].

CONCLUSION

The use of combination ARV therapy offers an effective method to maintain the prevalence of HIV infection and prolonging survival [62], but the development of drug resistance can compromise these benefits. Resistance is the consequence of mutations appearing in the viral proteins which are targeted by ARV agents. In the United States, as many as 50% of patients receiving ARV therapy are infected with viruses that show resistance to at least one of the available ARV drugs [34, 63, 64].

Factors involved in the development of drug resistance cover serial mono-therapy, lack of suppression of virus replication with suboptimal therapy strategies, difficult adherence to complex and toxic approaches, and delay in therapy initiation in the course of HIV infection [25, 65 - 67].

The efforts for controlling HIV infection continues to evolve. The overwhelming data presented in journals and at scientific meetings help to stay informed about current issues and new developments in the field. However, many clinicians, especially those who are actively caring for patients who are HIV infected, remain cautious and often confused regarding therapeutic options.

New technologies for the dissemination of medical information are constantly evolving. The Internet has allowed clinicians worldwide to exchange ideas, teach new concepts, and obtain access to limited resources. In addition, many research centers, patient advocacy groups, and academic institutions have posted sites on the Internet that have resulted in access to large amounts of high-quality medical information. However, this new technology has also allowed the dissemination of incomplete, misleading, or inaccurate information [25].

CONFLICT OF INTEREST

The authors confirm that they have no conflict of interest to declare for this publication.

ACKNOWLEDGEMENTS

Declared none.

REFERENCES

[1]   Ribeiro RM, Bonhoeffer S. Production of resistant HIV mutants during antiretroviral therapy. Proc Natl Acad Sci USA 2000; 97(14): 7681-6.
       [http://dx.doi.org/10.1073/pnas.97.14.7681] [PMID: 10884399]

[2]   Little SJ, Holte S, Routy JP, *et al.* Antiretroviral-drug resistance among patients recently infected with HIV. N Engl J Med 2002; 347(6): 385-94.
       [http://dx.doi.org/10.1056/NEJMoa013552] [PMID: 12167680]

[3]   Shekelle P, Maglione M, Geotz MB, *et al.* Antiretroviral (ARV) drug resistance in the developing world. Evid Rep Technol Assess (Full Rep) 2007; 156(156): 1-74.
       [PMID: 18088163]

[4]   Li JY, Li HP, Li L, *et al.* Prevalence and evolution of drug resistance HIV-1 variants in Henan, China. Cell Res 2005; 15(11-12): 843-9.
       [http://dx.doi.org/10.1038/sj.cr.7290356] [PMID: 16354557]

[5]   Kapoor A, Shapiro B, Shafer RW, Shulman N, Rhee SY, Delwart EL. Multiple independent origins of a protease inhibitor resistance mutation in salvage therapy patients. Retrovirology 2008; 5: 7.
       [http://dx.doi.org/10.1186/1742-4690-5-7] [PMID: 18221530]

[6]   Shi B, Kitchen C, Weiser B, *et al.* Evolution and recombination of genes encoding HIV-1 drug resistance and tropism during antiretroviral therapy. Virology 2010; 404(1): 5-20.
       [http://dx.doi.org/10.1016/j.virol.2010.04.008] [PMID: 20451945]

[7]   Minzi OM, Buma D, Kagashe GA. Self-initiation of antiretroviral therapy in the developing world: the involvement of private pharmacies in an HIV program. Drug Healthc Patient Saf 2012; 4: 27-31.
       [http://dx.doi.org/10.2147/DHPS.S23653] [PMID: 22570571]

[8]   Novak RM, Chen L, MacArthur RD, *et al.* Terry Beirn Community Programs for Clinical Research on AIDS 058 Study Team. s Prevalence of antiretroviral drug resistance mutations in chronically HIV-infected, treatment-naive patients: implications for routine resistance screening before initiation of antiretroviral therapy. Clin Infect Dis 2005; 40(3): 468-74.
[http://dx.doi.org/10.1086/427212] [PMID: 15668873]

[9]   Salomon H, Wainberg MA, Brenner B, *et al.* Prevalence of HIV-1 resistant to antiretroviral drugs in 81 individuals newly infected by sexual contact or injecting drug use. Investigators of the Quebec Primary Infection Study. AIDS 2000; 14(2): F17-23.
[http://dx.doi.org/10.1097/00002030-200001280-00003] [PMID: 10708278]

[10]   Scott P, Arnold E, Evans B, *et al.* Surveillance of HIV antiretroviral drug resistance in treated individuals in England: 1998-2000. J Antimicrob Chemother 2004; 53(3): 469-73.
[http://dx.doi.org/10.1093/jac/dkh102] [PMID: 14749345]

[11]   Richman DD, Morton SC, Wrin T, *et al.* The prevalence of antiretroviral drug resistance in the United States. AIDS 2004; 18(10): 1393-401.
[http://dx.doi.org/10.1097/01.aids.0000131310.52526.c7] [PMID: 15199315]

[12]   Weinstock HS, Zaidi I, Heneine W, *et al.* The epidemiology of antiretroviral drug resistance among drug-naive HIV-1-infected persons in 10 US cities. J Infect Dis 2004; 189(12): 2174-80.
[http://dx.doi.org/10.1086/420789] [PMID: 15181563]

[13]   de Mendoza C, Martín-Carbonero L, Gallego O, Corral A, González-Lahoz J, Soriano V. Relationship between drug resistance mutations, plasma viremia, and CD4+ T-cell counts in patients with chronic HIV infection. J Med Virol 2005; 76(1): 1-6.

[14]   Smith D, Moini N, Pesano R, *et al.* Clinical utility of HIV standard genotyping among antiretroviral-naive individuals with unknown duration of infection. Clin Infect Dis 2007; 44(3): 456-8.
[http://dx.doi.org/10.1086/510748] [PMID: 17205459]

[15]   Magiorkinis E, Detsika M, Hatzakis A, Paraskevis D. Monitoring HIV drug resistance in treatment-naive individuals: molecular indicators, epidemiology and clinical implications. Fut Med 2009; 3(4): 369-90.

[16]   Rodriguez-Rodrigues N, Duran A, Bouzas MB, *et al.* Increasing trends in primary NNRTI resistance among newly HIV-1-diagnosed individuals in Buenos Aires, Argentina. J Int AIDS Soc 2013; 16(1): 18519.
[http://dx.doi.org/10.7448/IAS.16.1.18519] [PMID: 24093951]

[17]   Ríos M, Delgado E, Pérez-Alvarez L, *et al.* Antiretroviral drug resistance and phylogenetic diversity of HIV-1 in Chile. J Med Virol 2007; 79(6): 647-56.
[http://dx.doi.org/10.1002/jmv.20881] [PMID: 17457921]

[18]   Masquelier B, Pereira E, Peytavin G, *et al.* APROCO/COPILOTE Study Group. Intermittent viremia during first-line, protease inhibitors-containing therapy: significance and relationship with drug resistance. J Clin Virol 2005; 33(1): 75-8.
[http://dx.doi.org/10.1016/j.jcv.2004.11.012] [PMID: 15797369]

[19]   Wensing AM, van de Vijver DA, Angarano G, *et al.* SPREAD Programme. Prevalence of drug-resistant HIV-1 variants in untreated individuals in Europe: implications for clinical management. J

Infect Dis 2005; 192(6): 958-66.
[http://dx.doi.org/10.1086/432916] [PMID: 16107947]

[20]   Sukasem C, Churdboonchart V, Sirisidthi K, *et al.* Genotypic resistance mutations in treatment-naïve and treatment-experienced patients under widespread use of antiretroviral drugs in Thailand: implications for further epidemiologic surveillance. Jpn J Infect Dis 2007; 60(5): 284-9.
[PMID: 17881868]

[21]   Yaotsè DA, Nicole V, Roch NF, Mireille PD, Eric D, Martine P. Genetic characterization of HIV-1 strains in Togo reveals a high genetic complexity and genotypic drug-resistance mutations in ARV naive patients. Infect Genet Evol 2009; 9(4): 646-52.
[http://dx.doi.org/10.1016/j.meegid.2009.04.002] [PMID: 19460333]

[22]   Rhee SY, Jordan MR, Raizes E, *et al.* HIV-1 drug resistance mutations: Potential applications for point-of-care genotypic resistance testing. PLoS One 2015; 10(12): e0145772.
[http://dx.doi.org/10.1371/journal.pone.0145772] [PMID: 26717411]

[23]   Jetzt AE, Yu H, Klarmann GJ, Ron Y, Preston BD, Dougherty JP. High rate of recombination throughout the human immunodeficiency virus type 1 genome. J Virol 2000; 74(3): 1234-40.
[http://dx.doi.org/10.1128/JVI.74.3.1234-1240.2000] [PMID: 10627533]

[24]   Zhuang J, Jetzt AE, Sun G, *et al.* Human immunodeficiency virus type 1 recombination: rate, fidelity, and putative hot spots. J Virol 2002; 76(22): 11273-82.
[http://dx.doi.org/10.1128/JVI.76.22.11273-11282.2002] [PMID: 12388687]

[25]   Koda-Kimble MA, Young LY. Applied therapeutics: the clinical use of drugs. In: Adams JL, Dumond JB, Kashuba AD, Eds. Pharmacotherapy of Human Immunodeficiency Virus Infection. 10th ed. Philadelphia, PA: Lippincott Williams, & Wilkins 2013; pp. 1707-15.

[26]   Borman AM, Paulous S, Clavel F. Resistance of human immunodeficiency virus type 1 to protease inhibitors: selection of resistance mutations in the presence and absence of the drug. J Gen Virol 1996; 77(Pt 3): 419-26.
[http://dx.doi.org/10.1099/0022-1317-77-3-419] [PMID: 8601776]

[27]   Nijhuis M, Schuurman R, de Jong D, *et al.* Increased fitness of drug resistant HIV-1 protease as a result of acquisition of compensatory mutations during suboptimal therapy. AIDS 1999; 13(17): 2349-59.
[http://dx.doi.org/10.1097/00002030-199912030-00006] [PMID: 10597776]

[28]   Barbour JD, Wrin T, Grant RM, *et al.* Evolution of phenotypic drug susceptibility and viral replication capacity during long-term virologic failure of protease inhibitor therapy in human immunodeficiency virus-infected adults. J Virol 2002; 76(21): 11104-12.
[http://dx.doi.org/10.1128/JVI.76.21.11104-11112.2002] [PMID: 12368352]

[29]   Malet I, Roquebert B, Dalban C, *et al.* Association of Gag cleavage sites to protease mutations and to virological response in HIV-1 treated patients. J Infect 2007; 54(4): 367-74.
[http://dx.doi.org/10.1016/j.jinf.2006.06.012] [PMID: 16875739]

[30]   Martinez-Picado J, Savara AV, Sutton L, D'Aquila RT. Replicative fitness of protease inhibitor-resistant mutants of human immunodeficiency virus type 1. J Virol 1999; 73(5): 3744-52.
[PMID: 10196268]

[31] Back NK, Nijhuis M, Keulen W, *et al.* Reduced replication of 3TC-resistant HIV-1 variants in primary cells due to a processivity defect of the reverse transcriptase enzyme. EMBO J 1996; 15(15): 4040-9. [PMID: 8670908]

[32] Bleiber G, Munoz M, Ciuffi A, Meylan P, Telenti A. Individual contributions of mutant protease and reverse transcriptase to viral infectivity, replication, and protein maturation of antiretroviral drug-resistant human immunodeficiency virus type 1. J Virol 2001; 75(7): 3291-300. [http://dx.doi.org/10.1128/JVI.75.7.3291-3300.2001] [PMID: 11238855]

[33] Fun A, Wensing AM, Verheyen J, Nijhuis M. Human Immunodeficiency Virus Gag and protease: partners in resistance. Retrovirology 2012; 9: 63. [http://dx.doi.org/10.1186/1742-4690-9-63] [PMID: 22867298]

[34] Clavel F, Hance AJ. HIV drug resistance. N Engl J Med 2004; 350(10): 1023-35. [http://dx.doi.org/10.1056/NEJMra025195] [PMID: 14999114]

[35] Bonolo PdeF, Machado CJ, César CC, Ceccato Md, Guimarães MD. BonoloPde F. Vulnerability and non-adherence to antiretroviral therapy among HIV patients, Minas Gerais State, Brazil. Cad Saude Publica 2008; 24(11): 2603-13. [http://dx.doi.org/10.1590/S0102-311X2008001100015] [PMID: 19009140]

[36] Uzochukwu BS, Onwujekwe OE, Onoka AC, Okoli C, Uguru NP, Chukwuogo OI. Determinants of non-adherence to subsidized anti-retroviral treatment in southeast Nigeria. Health Policy Plan 2009; 24(3): 189-96. [http://dx.doi.org/10.1093/heapol/czp006] [PMID: 19276155]

[37] Enriquez M, McKinsey DS. Strategies to improve HIV treatment adherence in developed countries: clinical management at the individual level. HIV AIDS (Auckl) 2011; 3: 45-51. [http://dx.doi.org/10.2147/HIV.S8993] [PMID: 22096406]

[38] Glikman D, Walsh L, Valkenburg J, Mangat PD, Marcinak JF. Hospital-based directly observed therapy for HIV-infected children and adolescents to assess adherence to antiretroviral medications. Pediatrics 2007; 119(5): e1142-8. [http://dx.doi.org/10.1542/peds.2006-2614] [PMID: 17452493]

[39] Stein LA, Minugh PA, Longabaugh R, *et al.* Readiness to change as a mediator of the effect of a brief motivational intervention on posttreatment alcohol-related consequences of injured emergency department hazardous drinkers. Psychol Addict Behav 2009; 23(2): 185-95. [http://dx.doi.org/10.1037/a0015648] [PMID: 19586135]

[40] Fisher EB, Strunk RC, Highstein GR, *et al.* A randomized controlled evaluation of the effect of community health workers on hospitalization for asthma: the asthma coach. Arch Pediatr Adolesc Med 2009; 163(3): 225-32. [http://dx.doi.org/10.1001/archpediatrics.2008.577] [PMID: 19255389]

[41] Nahmias SB, Nahmias D. Society, sex, and STIs: human behavior and the evolution of sexually transmitted diseases and their agents. Ann N Y Acad Sci 2011; 1230: 59-73. [http://dx.doi.org/10.1111/j.1749-6632.2011.06079.x] [PMID: 21824166]

[42] Migueles SA, Sabbaghian MS, Shupert WL, *et al.* HLA B*5701 is highly associated with restriction of virus replication in a subgroup of HIV-infected long term nonprogressors. Proc Natl Acad Sci USA

2000; 97(6): 2709-14.
[http://dx.doi.org/10.1073/pnas.050567397] [PMID: 10694578]

[43]   Bailey JR, Zhang H, Wegweiser BW, *et al.* Evolution of HIV-1 in an HLA-B*57-positive patient during virologic escape. J Infect Dis 2007; 196(1): 50-5.
[http://dx.doi.org/10.1086/518515] [PMID: 17538883]

[44]   Bailey JR, Brennan TP, O'Connell KA, Siliciano RF, Blankson JN. Evidence of CD8+ T-cel-
-mediated selective pressure on human immunodeficiency virus type 1 nef in HLA-B*57+ elite suppressors. J Virol 2009; 83(1): 88-97.
[http://dx.doi.org/10.1128/JVI.01958-08] [PMID: 18945771]

[45]   Boucher CA, Cammack N, Schipper P, *et al.* High-level resistance to (-) enantiomeric 2'-deoxy--
'-thiacytidine *in vitro* is due to one amino acid substitution in the catalytic site of human immunodeficiency virus type 1 reverse transcriptase. Antimicrob Agents Chemother 1993; 37(10): 2231-4.
[http://dx.doi.org/10.1128/AAC.37.10.2231] [PMID: 7504909]

[46]   Sarafianos SG, Das K, Clark AD Jr, *et al.* Lamivudine (3TC) resistance in HIV-1 reverse transcriptase involves steric hindrance with beta-branched amino acids. Proc Natl Acad Sci USA 1999; 96(18): 10027-32.
[http://dx.doi.org/10.1073/pnas.96.18.10027] [PMID: 10468556]

[47]   Foudraine NA, de Jong JJ, Jan Weverling G, *et al.* An open randomized controlled trial of zidovudine plus lamivudine *versus* stavudine plus lamivudine. AIDS 1998; 12(12): 1513-9.
[http://dx.doi.org/10.1097/00002030-199812000-00014] [PMID: 9727573]

[48]   Descamps D, Flandre P, Calvez V, *et al.* Mechanisms of virologic failure in previously untreated HIV-infected patients from a trial of induction-maintenance therapy. Trilège (Agence Nationale de Recherches sur le SIDA 072) Study Team). JAMA 2000; 283(2): 205-11.
[http://dx.doi.org/10.1001/jama.283.2.205] [PMID: 10634336]

[49]   Matsumi S, Kosalaraksa P, Tsang H, Kavlick MF, Harada S, Mitsuya H. Pathways for the emergence of multi-dideoxynucleoside-resistant HIV-1 variants. AIDS 2003; 17(8): 1127-37.
[http://dx.doi.org/10.1097/00002030-200305230-00003] [PMID: 12819513]

[50]   Iversen AK, Shafer RW, Wehrly K, *et al.* Multidrug-resistant human immunodeficiency virus type 1 strains resulting from combination antiretroviral therapy. J Virol 1996; 70(2): 1086-90.
[PMID: 8551567]

[51]   Roberts NA, Martin JA, Kinchington D, *et al.* Rational design of peptide-based HIV proteinase inhibitors. Science 1990; 248(4953): 358-61.
[http://dx.doi.org/10.1126/science.2183354] [PMID: 2183354]

[52]   Hertogs K, Bloor S, Kemp SD, *et al.* Phenotypic and genotypic analysis of clinical HIV-1 isolates reveals extensive protease inhibitor cross-resistance: a survey of over 6000 samples. AIDS 2000; 14(9): 1203-10.
[http://dx.doi.org/10.1097/00002030-200006160-00018] [PMID: 10894285]

[53]   Race E, Dam E, Obry V, Paulous S, Clavel F. Analysis of HIV cross-resistance to protease inhibitors using a rapid single-cycle recombinant virus assay for patients failing on combination therapies. AIDS 1999; 13(15): 2061-8.

[http://dx.doi.org/10.1097/00002030-199910220-00008] [PMID: 10546858]

[54]   Zhang YM, Imamichi H, Imamichi T, *et al.* Drug resistance during indinavir therapy is caused by mutations in the protease gene and in its Gag substrate cleavage sites. J Virol 1997; 71(9): 6662-70. [PMID: 9261388]

[55]   Doyon L, Croteau G, Thibeault D, Poulin F, Pilote L, Lamarre D. Second locus involved in human immunodeficiency virus type 1 resistance to protease inhibitors. J Virol 1996; 70(6): 3763-9. [PMID: 8648711]

[56]   Kilby JM, Eron JJ. Novel therapies based on mechanisms of HIV-1 cell entry. N Engl J Med 2003; 348(22): 2228-38. [http://dx.doi.org/10.1056/NEJMra022812] [PMID: 12773651]

[57]   Lohrengel S, Hermann F, Hagmann I, *et al.* Determinants of human immunodeficiency virus type 1 resistance to membrane-anchored gp41-derived peptides. J Virol 2005; 79(16): 10237-46. [http://dx.doi.org/10.1128/JVI.79.16.10237-10246.2005] [PMID: 16051817]

[58]   Ray N, Harrison JE, Blackburn LA, Martin JN, Deeks SG, Doms RW. Clinical resistance to enfuvirtide does not affect susceptibility of human immunodeficiency virus type 1 to other classes of entry inhibitors. J Virol 2007; 81(7): 3240-50. [http://dx.doi.org/10.1128/JVI.02413-06] [PMID: 17251281]

[59]   Dulioust A, Paulous S, Guillemot L, Delavalle AM, Boué F, Clavel F. Constrained evolution of human immunodeficiency virus type 1 protease during sequential therapy with two distinct protease inhibitors. J Virol 1999; 73(1): 850-4. [PMID: 9847401]

[60]   Guidelines for the Use of Antiretroviral Agents in HIV-1-Infected Adults and Adolescents. Section Drug-Resistance Testing , [Accessed on: Jan 2016]; Available at: https://aidsinfo.nih.gov/guidelines/html/1/adult-and-adolescent-treatment-guidelines/0.

[61]   Taiwo B, Murphy RL, Katlama C. Novel antiretroviral combinations in treatment-experienced patients with HIV infection: rationale and results. Drugs 2010; 70(13): 1629-42. [http://dx.doi.org/10.2165/11538020-000000000-00000] [PMID: 20731472]

[62]   Palella FJ Jr, Delaney KM, Moorman AC, *et al.* HIV Outpatient Study Investigators. Declining morbidity and mortality among patients with advanced human immunodeficiency virus infection. N Engl J Med 1998; 338(13): 853-60. [http://dx.doi.org/10.1056/NEJM199803263381301] [PMID: 9516219]

[63]   DeGruttola V, Dix L, D'Aquila R, *et al.* The relation between baseline HIV drug resistance and response to antiretroviral therapy: re-analysis of retrospective and prospective studies using a standardized data analysis plan. Antivir Ther (Lond) 2000; 5(1): 41-8. [PMID: 10846592]

[64]   Onafuwa-Nuga A, Telesnitsky A. The remarkable frequency of human immunodeficiency virus type 1 genetic recombination. Microbiol Mol Biol Rev 2009; 73(3): 451-80. [http://dx.doi.org/10.1128/MMBR.00012-09] [PMID: 19721086]

[65]   Iqbal HS, Solomon SS, Saravanan S, *et al.* HIV-1 drug resistance among newly HIV-1 infected individuals attending tertiary referral center in Chennai, India. Indian J Med Sci 2011; 65(11): 488-96.

[http://dx.doi.org/10.4103/0019-5359.109538] [PMID: 23525026]

[66]   Boden D, Hurley A, Zhang L, *et al.* HIV-1 drug resistance in newly infected individuals. JAMA 1999; 282(12): 1135-41.
[http://dx.doi.org/10.1001/jama.282.12.1135] [PMID: 10501116]

[67]   Paydary K, Esmaeeli S, SeyedAlinaghi S, Rouzrokh P, Emamzadeh-Fard S. Emerging HIV drug resistance in the resource-poor world: challenges and strategies. J AIDS Clin Res 2013; 5: 2.

CHAPTER 14

Serodiscordant Couples and Fertility Management

Koosha Paydary[1,2]**, Shooka Esmaeeli**[1,2]**, Siavash Eskandari**[1,2]**, Zeinab Najafi**[1,2]**, Alireza Hosseini**[1,2]**, Hamid Emadi Koochak**[1]**, Shayan Tabe Bordbar**[3] **and SeyedAhmad SeyedAlinaghi**[1,*]

[1] *Iranian Research Center for HIV/AIDS, Iranian Institute for Reduction of High-Risk Behaviors, Tehran University of Medical Sciences, Iran*

[2] *Students' Scientific Research Center (SSRC), Tehran University of Medical Sciences, Iran*

[3] *Physiology Department, University of Illinois at Urbana-Champaign (UIUC), USA*

Abstract: HIV spread in many developing countries is high as a result of homosexual, heterosexual intercourses and drug abusing. Most HIV infected individuals are attributable to heterosexual intercourse. There are several biologic and behavioral risk factors lead switching a discordant couple to concordant one such as having a high HIV viral load, living together, being uncircumcised for men, and reporting a Sexually Transmitted Disease (STD) within the six months before the beginning of consensual sex intercourse for women. Strategies on prevention includes the use of condom, abstinence and bed separation, contractual agreements for outside sexual partners, and cessation of relationships for any couple, providing early sexually transmitted disease diagnosis and treatment, antiretroviral therapy (ART), and specially designed counseling to HIV discordant couples in stable relationship. ART can protect against the HIV transmission from an infected sexual partner to an uninfected one by reducing viral replication.

Keywords: Antiretroviral therapy, Behavior and attitude, Counseling, Epidemiology, HIV serodiscordant, Pregnancy, Preventing routes, Processed semen.

---

* **Correspondence to SeyedAhmad SeyedAlinaghi:** Iranian Research Center for HIV/AIDS (IRCHA), Imam Khomeini Hospital, Keshavarz Blvd., Tehran, Iran; Tel/Fax: +98 (21) 66947984; E-mail: s_a_alinaghi@yahoo.com.

1. INTRODUCTION

Many discordant couples have shown strong desires for having a biological child. Studies showed having their own child has positive psychological effects on quality of life (QOL) of discordant couples [1].

The risk of HIV transmission during a single episode of unprotected sexual intercourse should be explained to serodiscordant couples before any decision [2, 3]. Table **1** shows the most substantial factors that have effects on HIV transmission risk.

Table 1. The most important variables that affect transmission risk.

Stage of the disease (viral load*, CD4 count, AIDS defining symptoms)
Use of antiretroviral therapy
Source of infection
Stability and length of relationship
Anal intercourse
Genital tract lesion or infection
Circumcision of male partner
Time of menstrual cycle (maximum risk during menstruation)
Frequency of intercourse

*HIV levels in plasma and semen are not well correlated [4, 5].

Reproductive Counselors have an important responsibility regarding serodiscordant couples. Reviews and studies in African and non-African settings have investigated the efficacy of VCT (Voluntary HIV Counseling and Testing) in lowering risk behaviors and occasionally rate of HIV sero-conversion in VCT recipients. Most HIV infections in Sub-Saharan countries occur during hetero-sexual intercourses between serodiscordant couples [6]. In a previous report, 95 serodiscordant couples were studied in which a male partner was sero-positive and maintained sexual unprotected intercourse during the period of follow up. Seven months later, four women sero-converted (two of them sero-converted postpartum) [2]. Hence, we should emphasize the importance of the "Reproductive Counseling" and "Assisted Reproduction method by using sperm washing" for serodiscordant couples [2]. Since 1989, assisted reproductions using sperm washing method were done in many discordant couples. Finally, all pregnancies without any case of female sero-conversion or pediatric infection were achieved [2, 7].

2. INSEMINATION OF HIV NEGATIVE WOMEN WITH PROCESSED SEMEN OF HIV POSITIVE PARTNERS

Processing semen from HIV positive men can reduce HIV-1 levels to undetectable levels [5, 8]. The processing method that was first described by Semprini *et al.*, consists of gradient centrifugation and repeated washing followed by swim up procedure to isolate motile and virus-free spermatozoa [8] (see Table **2**). Sperms do not describe remarkable rates of HIV receptors (CD4, CCR5, and CXCR4); as a result they are less likely to be key targets for HIV infection [4, 5]. To date, several studies have tried assisted conception explained above and all babies born to mothers using this method remain sero-negative [2 - 4, 8]. There are several techniques to assess the HIV levels after processing such as "immune fluorescence" or "detecting HIV-1 RNA copies per mL using nucleic acid based sequence amplification (NASBA)". Immune fluorescence method is not as sensitive as NASBA and hence, is not recommended nowadays [9]. We should consider that these procedures do not always remove detectable HIV-RNA. Consequently, it is strongly recommended that all samples for insemination are to be tested before insemination using NASBA or a similar sensitive assay and that only samples in which HIV cannot be detected be used [3, 9].

Table 2. Summary of studies on the safety and effectiveness of the "Sperm-washing" method.

Semprini *et al.*, [8]	• Women were inseminated with the processed semen (using sperm washing method) of their HIV positive partners during a timed insemination course and none of them sero-converted. Ten babies born to these mothers remained sero-negative.
Chrystie *et al.*, [9]	• Treatment of semen from HIV-infected men using standard procedures can reduce HIV-1 RNA concentration in the final sample to undetectable levels and this reduction is more efficiently performed using Percoll rather than Ficol gradients. • An experience of over 1000 insemination without any subsequent sero-conversion

(Table 2) contd.....

Kim *et al.*, [5]	• Spermatozoa are unlikely to be major targets for HIV infections. • Purifying spermatozoa reduces the level of HIV RNA and proviral DNA to below the detection limit of assays irrespective of the amount of virus present in the unfractionated semen.
Gilling-Smith C [3]	• Treating 53 HIV serodiscordant couples with the sperm-washing method resulted in the birth of 15 children. • To date there have been no sero-conversion in uninfected partner or child.
Ohl *et al.*, [4]	• 39 serodiscordant couples were treated though 54 assisted reproduction technique attempts and 14 children were already born for 12 couples. • No sero-conversion has occurred through the use of treated sperm.
Bojan *et al.*,[7]	• This was the first multi-center retrospective study of assisted reproduction following sperm-washing. This study demonstrates that the method is effective and significantly reduces HIV-1 transmission risk of uninfected female partner (no sero-conversion occurred in 50 pregnancies).

3. HIV STATUS IN DISCORDANT COUPLES

Some studies have reported data on HIV discordant heterosexual couples (couples in which one member is HIV positive and the other is HIV negative) [3, 4, 10].

The proportion of serodiscordance resulting from infection before couples got together *versus* infections introduced into the stable relationships through outside partners is unknown. Discordant couples are at a critical risk. Annually risk of infection for a partner of a HIV positive person is about 10%, reducing the number of new infections entering a relationship is the main target of strategies at decreasing new HIV infections [11].

Prevention strategies cover the application of condom, abstinence and bed separation, contractual agreements for outside sexual partners, relationship cessation for any couple [11] and offering early sexually transmitted disease (STD) diagnosis and treatment, antiretroviral therapy, and specially designed counseling to HIV discordant couples in stable relationship [12].

There are several biologic and behavioral risk factors lead switching a discordant couple to concordant one including high HIV loads, living together, being uncircumcised for men, and reporting STD within the six months before the beginning of consensual sex intercourse for women. Increased frequency of sexual contact and relationship duration exert a direct influence on the risk of shifting to concordant couple, as a result, living together would increase the risk. One of the difficulties with HIV discordant couples is that the stable relationship increases the risk of infection rather than having outside sexual partners. As a result, HIV discordant couples should know that being in a monogamous stable relationship does not mean that partners are not at risk for HIV transmission. Voluntary HIV counseling and testing (VCT) for couples, including married couples, is a critical component of prevention activities. There are many studies about different aspects of HIV discordant couples. Here we indicate some of them.

A study in Ugandan population investigated the role of men and women as sources of HIV transmission in discordant couples and found that men are predominant source of new infections in rural villages. Risk factors and preventive behaviors vary in men and women and sero-conversion rates are similar in both sexes [13].

Another study in Sub-Saharan Africa investigated serodiscordance in resistant relationships to create a gender balance of index-case infections. Most couples in this region live in serodiscordant situation in stable relationships and men are thought to be the index case in most cases. As suggested this systemic study, HIV prevention strategies are required to focus on both sexes, including promotion of condom use and mitigation of risk behaviors [14].

Another study investigated serodiscordant couples in five African countries: Cameroon, Kenya, Tanzania, Burkina Faso and Ghana. This study was about implications for prevention strategies. It shows that in this five African countries, at least two-thirds of HIV-infected couples are serodiscordant. Consequently, it is very important to inform these couples about prevention methods as well as joining to voluntary counseling and testing might be useful. The second finding is that a sizable proportion of HIV-infected couples are serodiscordant couples in which only the woman is infected. Nevertheless, women have low self-reported levels of extramarital sex. It is in contradiction with the common perception that unfaithful males are the most important source of transmission of HIV from high risk groups to population. Either extramarital sex is more common than reported, or if it is not frequent, women are highly vulnerable to infection during extramarital sex. So, extramarital sex by women seems to be a serious route through which HIV is transmitted, and it is important as much as extramarital sex among men, in preventive efforts [15].

4. HIV-1 SUBTYPES PATHOGENICITY IN HETEROSEXUAL COUPLES

The HIV type 1 (HIV-1) has various sub-subtypes and inter-subtype recombinant forms which differ in viral fitness, pathogenicity, syncytium-forming properties, and chemokine co-receptor usage. Evidence of subtype differences in HIV is increasing, but data on heterosexual HIV-1 transmission by subtype are limited. Information on subtype differences in transmission is important for HIV vaccine development.

Here are some studies about differences between subtypes:

Result of a study in Thailand shows a higher rate of heterosexual transmission for CRF01_AE (formerly subtype E) compared to subtype B [16].

One Ugandan study demonstrates no significant differences in distribution of subtypes among infected individuals during follow-up over a decade. However, this research did not directly investigate infectivity by HIV subtype [13].

Another study in Rakaia, Uganda, among HIV-1-discordant couples found that subtype A viruses have a significantly higher rate of heterosexual transmission than subtype D viruses. Previously subtype D was found to cause quicker rate of disease progression than subtype A. Ultimately, these findings confirm the observed increased proportion of infections due to subtype A, compared to the decreased proportion of infections due to subtype D [17]. A recent study of population-level changes in HIV-1 subtype distribution over an 8-year interval in Rakaia also supports this hypothesis. A remarkable reduction in proportion of subtype D viruses from 71 to 63% and an increase in subtype A viruses from 15 to 20% were observed [18]. Why heterosexual HIV-1 transmission differs by infecting viral subtype? It is not yet clear [17].

5. NEW CASES OF HIV POSITIVE PATIENTS IN MARRIED OR COHABITING COUPLES

In Sub-Saharan Africa about 7% of married couples are in serodiscordant marriages and about half of married HIV-positive individuals have HIV-negative spouses [19]. Sub-Saharan Africa has a high rate of HIV infection. The transmission of HIV-1 infection occurs mainly in heterosexual couples in which the presence of other STDs acts synergistically. Some studies from there suggest that women were at higher risk of contracting HIV in a marital relationship [19].

Chance of bring HIV infection to marital relationship for men is twice as women and that is because of extramarital sexual activities of men. Studies from the United States and Europe have shown that rate of HIV transmission male-to-female was higher than female-to-male [20, 21]. In some studies from Northern California this rate of transmission from male-to-female was approximately 7-9 times more than female-to-male. In fact, women are infected more than men in serodiscordant relationship because of increased biological susceptibility [22, 23].

6. RATE OF HIV TRANSMISSION PER COITAL ACT

Estimating the rate of HIV infection transmission per coital act among couples has been marvel of HIV epidemiology. There are some intangible elements which vary this estimation between developed and developing countries and different studies (see Table. 3). These factors are: male-to-female transmission (approximately eight times more in female per coital act), stage of infection of the positive partner, the effect of behavioral characteristics (*e.g.* alcohol and drug use), non safe sex practices (*e.g.* non condom use and anal sex), STDs co-infection, antiretroviral therapy, counseling and VCTs, uncircumcised male partner, younger age (<30 years), HIV-1 subtype (subtype E) and disclosure of HIV sero-positive result. Doubtless these estimations are needed for modeling the epidemic and for projecting the effects of prevention strategies, but for the time being, the estimates of the probability of transmission per coital act, mostly derived from empirical studies on HIV discordant couples, which vary problematically in results [16, 23 - 26].

People living with HIV (PLHIV) have to face stigma, depression and oppression to have a sexual life. Demonstrating the rate of transmission per coital act plus the effect of antiretroviral therapy to reduce it and other protective ways in preventing programs worldwide could have a significant effect on QOL of PLHIV universally [27].

To date, there is some empirical evidence that men with acute HIV-1 infection are more infectious because of increased genital shedding of HIV. In other words, the high levels of HIV viruses in plasma lead to increase amount of it in genital shedding, as a result increase rate of transmission to partner. Also, it is remarkable that the predicted rate of transmission increase impressively when one of the partners is infected with STD. This has implications for HIV prevention and for projecting the effects of antiretroviral treatment on HIV transmission and co-infection of HIV and STDs in public health scale [22, 28, 29].

The overall probability of HIV transmission per coital act is 0.001 which increase in acute infection up to 0.008/coital act (See Table **3** for more statistical data). Men are twice as likely as women to bring HIV infection into a couple, probably through extramarital sexual behavior. Within serodiscordant couples, women become infected twice as fast as men, because of increased biological susceptibility. Married women, with HIV-positive partners are at very high risk of HIV infection. Discordant couples should be encouraged to attend HIV counseling together so that they can be identified and advised accordingly. There are some modifying risk factors to reduce the rate of transmission like condom use and reduction in the HIV RNA level and for the uninfected partner STDs like herpes simplex virus type two, trichomonas vaginitis or cervicitis, genital ulcers and male circumcision which can be used in counseling programs [18, 22, 30].

Table 3. HIV transmission rate per coital act.

Country	Transmission route	Transmission probability
Uganda [31]	Heterosexual	**0.0001** when viral load < 1700 copies/ml to **0.0023** when viral load > 38500 copies/ml
Uganda [29]	-	**0.0082** within ~2.5 months after seroconversion of the index partner **0.0015** within 6-15 months after seroconversion of the index partner **0.0007** among HIV-prevalent index partners
Europe [20]	-	**0.0005–0.001**

(Table 3) contd.....

Country	Transmission route	Transmission probability
Europe [21]	-	**0.0011 - 0.0001** if the viral load is less than 1700 copies/ml
USA [20]	Male-to-female	**0.0008–0.001**
Thailand [20]	-	**0.002**
Africa [32]	-	9 per 100 person years
USA [20]	Female-to-male	**0.001**
Africa [32]	-	4 per 100 person years

7. PREVENTING ROUTES

7.1. Condom Use

The application of condom is a key element in a comprehensive, effective, and sustainable approach to HIV prevention and treatment. Prevention is regarded as the most essential part of the response to AIDS. Consistent use of male condoms continues to be advocated for primary prevention of HIV. Consistent use is defined as using a condom for all acts of penetrative vaginal intercourse. It is important to note, however, that use of condoms can reduce the risk of HIV transmission, but it is not as effective as choosing partner from low risk group or someone who is known to be negative for HIV antibody. Although the correct use of condoms is known to reduce the risk of HIV transmission, it cannot eliminate the risk completely [33 - 36]. Moreover, we should be concerned about the spread of other sexually transmitted infections (STIs) if condoms are not used. This can lead to HIV and other STIs co-infection which increases the risk of transmission [37, 38].

Condom effectiveness is 80-95% [39]. In spite of the above mentioned positive effects of using condoms, we cannot be sure that condoms really reduce the HIV incidence by 80-95%. Some studies show its true effectiveness of risk reduction maybe as low as 46-69% [33]. It is important to note that in these studies the investigators have not examined type of condom, sexual behavior and correct use of it. Some other mentioned about influence of other important points on this amount of risk reduction. It may be, for example, that some people who always use condoms, also practice safe sex, have fewer partners and are adherent to their therapies, thereby reducing their HIV risk [33, 35, 40].

As mentioned before, condoms do not eliminate the risk of HIV transmission, because they may leak HIV, also HIV may be transmitted through urogenital and anal routes. Consequently, condom use may have some negative outcomes as general population may understand the avoidance of HIV transmission instead of reduction in the risk of transmission. Also, lack of information about using condoms may lead to an elevated transmission risk. In counseling and advising patients, it is very important to mention: To achieve the maximum protective effect, condoms must be used both consistently and correctly [33, 35, 37, 41]. VCTs and counseling have an important role on increasing condom usage worldwide. In a study in Rwanda, the proportion of discordant couples using condoms increased from 4% to 57% after one year of follow up by VCTs. This data indicate that HIV sero-testing with counseling can cause a large increase in condom use and is associated with a lower rate of new HIV infections and transmissions mostly among serodiscordant couples [32].

To conclude, condoms use have contributed in reducing HIV infection rates worldwide and to control the HIV epidemic mostly in countries that have heterosexual epidemics. Condoms have also encouraged safer sexual behavior between couples all over the world. In other words, condoms are the single, most efficient, available technology to reduce the sexual transmission of HIV and other STIs. Therefore, condoms must be available universally, either free or at low cost, and should be promoted by different programs worldwide. Unfortunately, based on UNFPA estimation, current supply of condoms in low- and middle- income nations is too less than what is required [42, 43].

7.2. Male Circumcision

Male circumcision has been performed on boys for a long time. Initially it was just for religious and cultural reasons but in our day male circumcision has become one of the preventing programs for HIV. It has now become clear that medical male circumcision lowers the risk of female-to-male sexual HIV transmission about 60-70%. Because of this, since 2007 voluntary medical male circumcision has become one of the preventing programs worldwide [44, 45].

Male circumcision is usual between Muslims and Jews. Maybe the high effect of pre-pubertal circumcision in protecting HIV is related to the religious behaviors and safer sex behaviors, but certainly circumcision which is a onetime procedure, either post pubertal or pre-pubertal can act as a partial preventer of HIV transmission for men long life [46].

As estimated, 50 million persons have HIV infection worldwide, about half are men, and mostly are infected sexually via their penises. The inner shell of the foreskin and frenulum has many HIV receptors. Trauma and other STIs could usually happen in these two places. As a result, they are common sites of primary HIV infection entrance in men. The use of condom is the first option to protect against sexual transmission of HIV. Nevertheless, no consistent or correct use may break the condoms during sexual intercourse leaking HIV. Circumcision at puberty, as practiced by many Muslim countries, is an effective measure to reduce HIV infection rates since it can be done before young men start their sexually active life [47].

Male circumcision provides 60-70% of protection against HIV infection, equivalent to what a vaccine of moderate efficacy would have achieved. This process is recommended for countries with high HIV prevalence, generalized heterosexual HIV epidemics and low level of men circumcision to have the greatest public health impact. It is remarkable that this procedure is a partial preventer so it is recommended for discordant couples, mostly for those that the female partner is HIV positive, alongside other preventing programs [44, 46, 48]. Male circumcision may pave the ground to decrease the prevalence of HIV infection in Sub-Saharan Africa [49].

7.3. Voluntary Counseling and Testing (VCT) for Couples

Over 20 years, client-initiated HIV testing and counseling, called as voluntary counseling and testing (VCT), has informed millions of people from their HIV status and acted as a prevention method. VCT is an important and essential gateway to HIV prevention, treatment, care and support services. The benefits of VCT for HIV are well established with evidence of reducing risky behavior. Moreover, VCTs bring early knowledge of one's positive HIV status, which can maximize opportunities for the PLHIV to access treatment, thereby lowering

HIV-related morbidity and mortality significantly. Furthermore, being on effective treatment reduces the risk of HIV transmission impressively. More than that, for HIV negative people there are plans like evidence-based prevention methods programs, such as safe sex practices, condom use, male circumcision, safe injecting equipment and reduced number of sex partners [2, 50, 51].

To discuss VCT for couples, we face the time when one of the partners of a couple realizes that only one have been infected with HIV, at this time the need of VCT for couples becomes more obvious. For most men who shared their results with their partners the process of disclosure, was not very bothersome. On the other hand, the reaction that women seemed to fear the most was abandonment. Negative reactions, mostly abandonment, were a reality for some women who chose to share test results to partners as an affirmation of their fear [52, 53]. In this context, VCT for couples have an important role to help people manage their fears of result disclosure, by achieving sensitization meetings, individual-level counseling to gain agreement from the HIV-infected partner and finally opening disclosure of results by the couple [53]. Also, VCTs for couples have an important duty which is addressing barriers to HIV prevention programs among couples [50].

Furthermore, there are many people who are a part of discordant couples but they are not aware of that. Up to 50 percent of PLHIV who are in relationships are estimated to be part of discordant couples [54]. Provision of VCT for family members of people known as HIV positives, is an important intervention for both finding new cases and protection against HIV acquisition. Providing couples with HIV testing and counseling, can reduce the prevalence of HIV universally. There are many PLHIV who do not use safe sex practices because they believe that their couple has become infected too, but there is some evidences that about half of the spouses of HIV infected married patients are HIV negative [55, 56].

After HIV testing and counseling, discordant couples reduce their unprotected intercourses and increase condom use. Couples who regularly attend VCTs are more likely to report 100% condom use. The results reveal VCT as an effective secondary program of HIV prevention; because, participants who know their HIV-positive status usually lower their sexual risk behavior, their risk of subsequent reinfection and their risk of infecting others. However, participants receiving a negative HIV test result usually did not modify their sexual risk behavior similar to individuals who did not participate in VCT. Hence, it seems that VCT is not an effective primary prevention strategy [32, 54, 56, 57].

To date, HIV testing and counseling approaches have largely focused on individuals, despite the fact that many people cohabiting and married get infected with HIV and many of them are expecting to have children. Clearly, important opportunities are being lost for preventing HIV acquisition, by heterosexual transmission or mother-to-child HIV transmission by mothers who have been infected by their partners [2].

According to the ever-increasing HIV/AIDS epidemic in Sub-Saharan Africa, and considering that most new HIV infections in Africa now occur in cohabiting couples, the expansion of VCT as an important part of HIV prevention programs is needed. It is necessary to rely on promotion campaigns to have an idea of the perceived benefits and barriers to HIV-1 testing. Merging of family in VCT programs on a routine basis as a part of HIV care and treatment programs will plays a great role in public health efforts to control the HIV epidemic and it will impact on a longer life expectancy and higher QOL for PLHIV [2, 32, 52, 56].

7.4. Serodiscordant Couples Behavior and Attitude

Understanding that a partner of a couple is HIV positive, known as sero status notification, can cause dramatic changes in the relationship, acts and sexual behaviors of the couple as we know it. First of all, in the serodiscordant couples (F+/M-), which is less prevalent, there will be changes in men sexual behavior. Such men start to have more extramarriage sex practices but with consistently condom use. Secondly, since the risk of HIV transmission is much higher while unprotected penetrative vaginal sex practices are done, desiring a child could become a dream for these couples. While having almost always protected sex by using condom, and just having unprotected sex during woman's perceived fertile period, can help them experience pregnancy with either low risk of transmission and HIV-infected child. Changes in sexual behaviors could also be responsible for altered living patterns. Relationship problems, such as divorce, will happen mostly among (F+/M-) couple. Interestingly, divorce prevalence is not higher between serodiscordant couples and most of these couples can stay together [58].

For some time now, it has been noted an alarming high prevalence of HIV transmission to uninfected partner among serodiscordant couples. It has been found that the presence of some factors causes more prevalent unprotected sex, a condition which eventually leads to increase amount of transmission. Age, religion and beliefs, economic situation and alcohol use are the factors which are significantly related to unprotected sex and the only one that can be modified is alcohol use, which is more prevalent among men. The alcohol intoxication, however slight, led to increased desire for unprotected sex, often seen as more pleasurable, or a minimization of the perceived risk that unprotected sex presented to themselves and their partners. Due to the fact that alcohol use usually is followed by unprotected sex practices, counseling about it should be a part of HIV protection programs, specially among those found to be serodiscordant couples [59].

VCTs and counseling can have an important role on the serodiscordant couples behavior and attitude. Mostly, couples who have a longer history of union and have more than two children attend to counseling regularly. For having a successful intervention on the sexual behavior regarding sero status notification, it is important for VCTs to attract young, illiterate, and unemployed couples who believe in less sexual equality [60]. HIV discordant couples are an important target population for protection, because of the high transmission rate when they are unaware of their HIV status. Disclosure problems which are mostly a result of fear and stigma can be reduced by VCTs. Increased access to counseling and testing services can help identification of HIV-1 discordant couples for prevention interventions and enrollment into HIV prevention trials. Considering the public health benefits, it is important to enhance the number of serodiscordant couples to be tested for HIV-1 as couples rather than as individuals, and extend training of counselors and counseling messages about serodiscordant couples [61].

8. PRE EXPOSURE PROPHYLAXIS (PrEP) FOR A SAFE CONCEPTION

As mentioned before many HIV discordant couples wish to have a child. Because of that the procedure of intrauterine insemination (IUI) with processed semen has been introduced to decrease the risk of HIV transmission in discordant couples in which male partner is infected [62, 63].

Unfortunately, studies in Europe showed that most of the male partners only accept the artificial insemination procedure with processed semen. This method is cumbersome and the rate of pregnancy in each cycle rich only 15%. Furthermore, the effect on risk reduction of the IUI practice in patients treated with Highly Active Antiretroviral Therapy (HAART) cannot be determined exactly [62, 63]. Indeed, since the introduction of HAART, there is not a documented study published about transmission rate under stable HAART.

There is other method to conceive a child with a safe condition, that is timed intercourse with PrEP (PrEP is usage of antiretroviral drug). The method of timed intercourse and PrEP became the principal method that physicians proposed. The following guidelines were indicated to decrease the risk of HIV transmission by unprotected conception with timed intercourse:

1. Male partner has been completely treated with undetectable HIV-RNA in plasma (<50 copies/ml).
2. No unprotected sex with other partners and no report of any symptoms of genital infections.
3. Determine the optimal time of conception with LH-test in the urine (36 hours after LH-peak).
4. Administration of PrEP with Tenofovir: First dose at LH peak and second dose one day later.
5. After six unsuccessful attempts, a fertility test is suggested.

Timed intercourse with PrEP provides an easier approach to lower the HIV-transmission risk. The pregnancy rate in timed intercourse with PrEP was much higher than previously reported for IUI with processed semen. Eventually, the method proposed here to reduce the theoretically risk of HIV transmission and have a healthy child is timed intercourse and PrEP and it can be considered as a psychological support for the couples to cope with their anxiety [62, 64].

9. ANTIVIRAL AGENTS' EFFECTIVENESS (PARTNERSHIP INTERVENTIONS)

Given the impact of successful antiretroviral treatment on dramatical reduction of viremia and the reduction of HIV transmission risk in discordant heterosexual couples, a consensus statement by the Swiss National AIDS Commission advised that after six months' treatment, if the virus is undetectable in the plasma and in the absence of another sexually transmitted infection, the risk of transmitting HIV is negligible [37].

The effect of ART on sexual risk behavior is unknown. However, it may protect against HIV transmission because of lowered infectivity. By the way, cell-associated genital HIV transmission may occur in people with low plasma HIV viral load [65].

ART can protect against HIV transmission from an infected sexual partner to an uninfected one, through lowering viral replication. In discordant couples in which the infected partner receives antiretroviral drugs, the risk of transmission becomes more than three-times less than in couples their infected partner was not receiving treatment. Although the World Health Organization (WHO) already suggests ART for all patients with ≤350 CD4 cells/μL, in serodiscordant couples for HIV-positive partners with CD4 count higher than 350 cells/μL, ART should be offered to decrease HIV transmission to uninfected partners [66].

The efficiency of ART in lowering viral loads and ART programs in reducing sexual risk behavior will determine HIV transmission in discordant couple. Some research on homosexual, heterosexual and injecting drug user populations in the United States have exhibited that risky sexual behaviors and STI incidence are higher among HIV-infected patients on ART compared to the lack of treatment [20, 21]. In contrast, other studies, including several from Europe, have shown significantly lower rates of risky sex among those on ART [20, 21]. Aggregated data from 16 studies from industrialized countries showed that prevalence of unprotected sex was no higher among those receiving ART than those not on ART [21].

While ART has been shown to reduce viral load and mortality in Africa, its effect on risky sexual behavior has not been investigated in a prospective cohort. A study in Uganda assessed sexual behavior before and six months after onset of ART, consisting of: 1. factors involved in sexual activity; 2. changes in desire and frequency of sexual behavior after six months of ART; and 3. changes in estimated risk of HIV transmission based on viral load, risky sex, and established condom failure rates. The results demonstrate that integrated ART and prevention programs can lower HIV incidence among uninfected sexual partners of persons on therapy in Africa. Moreover, minimizing the transmission of HIV by taking ART will help to reduce primary infections with drug-resistant strains of HIV and help to extend the utility of less expensive first-line regimens in Africa. Randomized efficacy evaluations of simple prevention interventions that can be implemented in ART clinical settings are needed. Given the extremely high cost of ART, even for generic formulations, the added investment by ART programs for a strong prevention component would be marginal while the potential gains in lowering the transmission of HIV could be significant [65].

As mentioned above one important way to break chains of transmission is the intervention with ART in sexual partnerships which in turn will lower the transmission risk from the infected person (often called the index case) to the uninfected partner or fetus [67].

Efficacy of antiretroviral drugs in the prevention of mother-to-child transmission of HIV is proven and may affect the prevention of HIV transmission in discordant couples. Viral load is the major predictor controlling the risk of sexual transmission in discordant couples and hence, effective ART should remarkably decrease the rate of transmission [68].

CONFLICT OF INTEREST

The authors confirm that they have no conflict of interest to declare for this publication.

ACKNOWLEDGEMENTS

Declared none.

REFERENCES

[1]   Semprini AE, Fiore S, Pardi G. Reproductive counselling for HIV-discordant couples. Lancet 1997; 349(9062): 1401-2.
[http://dx.doi.org/10.1016/S0140-6736(05)63250-3] [PMID: 9149735]

[2]   Painter TM. Voluntary counseling and testing for couples: a high-leverage intervention for HIV/AIDS prevention in sub-Saharan Africa. Soc Sci Med 2001; 53(11): 1397-411.
[http://dx.doi.org/10.1016/S0277-9536(00)00427-5] [PMID: 11710416]

[3]   Gilling-Smith C. Fertility management of HIV-discordant couples Carole. Curr Obstet Gynaecol 2003; 13: 307-13.
[http://dx.doi.org/10.1016/S0957-5847(03)00045-3]

[4]   Ohl J, Partisani M, Wittemer C, *et al.* Assisted reproduction techniques for HIV serodiscordant couples: 18 months of experience. Hum Reprod 2003; 18(6): 1244-9.
[http://dx.doi.org/10.1093/humrep/deg258] [PMID: 12773453]

[5]   Kim LU, Johnson MR, Barton S, *et al.* Evaluation of sperm washing as a potential method of reducing HIV transmission in HIV-discordant couples wishing to have children. AIDS 1999; 13(6): 645-51.
[http://dx.doi.org/10.1097/00002030-199904160-00004] [PMID: 10397558]

[6]   Sunderam S, Hollander L, Macaluso M, *et al.* Safe conception for HIV discordant couples through sperm-washing: experience and perceptions of patients in Milan, Italy. Reprod Health Matters 2008; 16(31): 211-9.
[http://dx.doi.org/10.1016/S0968-8080(08)31342-1] [PMID: 18513622]

[7]   Bujan L, Hollander L, Coudert M, *et al.* CREAThE network. Safety and efficacy of sperm washing in HIV-1-serodiscordant couples where the male is infected: results from the European CREAThE network. AIDS 2007; 21(14): 1909-14.
[http://dx.doi.org/10.1097/QAD.0b013e3282703879] [PMID: 17721098]

[8]   Semprini AE, Levi-Setti P, Bozzo M, *et al.* Insemination of HIV-negative women with processed semen of HIV-positive partners. Lancet 1992; 340(8831): 1317-9.
[http://dx.doi.org/10.1016/0140-6736(92)92495-2] [PMID: 1360037]

[9]   Chrystie IL, Mullen JE, Braude PR, *et al.* Assisted conception in HIV discordant couples: evaluation of semen processing techniques in reducing HIV viral load. J Reprod Immunol 1998; 41(1-2): 301-6.
[http://dx.doi.org/10.1016/S0165-0378(98)00066-7] [PMID: 10213318]

[10] Feldblum PJ. Results from prospective studies of HIV-discordant couples. AIDS 1991; 5(10): 1265-6.
[http://dx.doi.org/10.1097/00002030-199110000-00020] [PMID: 1786156]

[11] Bunnell RE, Nassozi J, Marum E, *et al.* Living with discordance: knowledge, challenges, and prevention strategies of HIV-discordant couples in Uganda. AIDS Care 2005; 17(8): 999-1012.
[http://dx.doi.org/10.1080/09540120500100718] [PMID: 16176896]

[12] Malamba SS, Mermin JH, Bunnell R, *et al.* Couples at risk: HIV-1 concordance and discordance among sexual partners receiving voluntary counseling and testing in Uganda. J Acquir Immune Defic Syndr 2005; 39(5): 576-80.
[PMID: 16044010]

[13]   Serwadda D, Gray RH, Wawer MJ, *et al.* The social dynamics of HIV transmission as reflected through discordant couples in rural Uganda. AIDS 1995; 9(7): 745-50.
[http://dx.doi.org/10.1097/00002030-199507000-00012] [PMID: 7546420]

[14]   Eyawo O, de Walque D, Ford N, Gakii G, Lester RT, Mills EJ. HIV status in discordant couples in sub-Saharan Africa: a systematic review and meta-analysis. Lancet Infect Dis 2010; 10(11): 770-7.
[http://dx.doi.org/10.1016/S1473-3099(10)70189-4] [PMID: 20926347]

[15]   de Bruyn G, Magaret A, Baeten JM, *et al.* Partners in Prevention HSV/HIV Transmission Study Team. Mortality in members of HIV-1 serodiscordant couples in Africa and implications for antiretroviral therapy initiation: results of analyses from a multicenter randomized trial. BMC Infect Dis 2012; 12: 277.
[http://dx.doi.org/10.1186/1471-2334-12-277] [PMID: 23130818]

[16]   Nelson KE, Rungruengthanakit K, Margolick J, *et al.* High rates of transmission of subtype E human immunodeficiency virus type 1 among heterosexual couples in Northern Thailand: role of sexually transmitted diseases and immune compromise. J Infect Dis 1999; 180(2): 337-43.
[http://dx.doi.org/10.1086/314882] [PMID: 10395847]

[17]   Kiwanuka N, Laeyendecker O, Quinn TC, *et al.* HIV-1 subtypes and differences in heterosexual HIV transmission among HIV-discordant couples in Rakai, Uganda. AIDS 2009; 23(18): 2479-84.
[http://dx.doi.org/10.1097/QAD.0b013e328330cc08] [PMID: 19841572]

[18]   Gray RH, Wawer MJ, Brookmeyer R, *et al.* Rakai Project Team. Probability of HIV-1 transmission per coital act in monogamous, heterosexual, HIV-1-discordant couples in Rakai, Uganda. Lancet 2001; 357(9263): 1149-53.
[http://dx.doi.org/10.1016/S0140-6736(00)04331-2] [PMID: 11323041]

[19]   Dunkle KL, Stephenson R, Karita E, *et al.* New heterosexually transmitted HIV infections in married or cohabiting couples in urban Zambia and Rwanda: an analysis of survey and clinical data. Lancet 2008; 371(9631): 2183-91.
[http://dx.doi.org/10.1016/S0140-6736(08)60953-8] [PMID: 18586173]

[20]   Hansasuta P, Rowland-Jones SL. HIV-1 transmission and acute HIV-1 infection. Br Med Bull 2001; 58: 109-27.
[http://dx.doi.org/10.1093/bmb/58.1.109] [PMID: 11714627]

[21]   Vandermaelen A, Englert Y. Human immunodeficiency virus serodiscordant couples on highly active antiretroviral therapies with undetectable viral load: conception by unprotected sexual intercourse or by assisted reproduction techniques? Hum Reprod 2010; 25(2): 374-9.
[http://dx.doi.org/10.1093/humrep/dep412] [PMID: 19945963]

[22]   Carpenter LM, Kamali A, Ruberantwari A, Malamba SS, Whitworth JA. Rates of HIV-1 transmission within marriage in rural Uganda in relation to the HIV sero-status of the partners. AIDS 1999; 13(9): 1083-9.
[http://dx.doi.org/10.1097/00002030-199906180-00012] [PMID: 10397539]

[23]   Padian NS, Shiboski SC, Glass SO, Vittinghoff E. Heterosexual transmission of human immunodeficiency virus (HIV) in northern California: results from a ten-year study. Am J Epidemiol 1997; 146(4): 350-7.
[http://dx.doi.org/10.1093/oxfordjournals.aje.a009276] [PMID: 9270414]

[24]   Gray RH, Wawer MJ. Probability of heterosexual HIV-1 transmission per coital act in sub-Saharan Africa. J Infect Dis 2012; 205(3): 351-2.
[http://dx.doi.org/10.1093/infdis/jir751] [PMID: 22241799]

[25]   Padian NS, Shiboski SC, Jewell NP. Female-to-male transmission of human immunodeficiency virus. JAMA 1991; 266(12): 1664-7.
[http://dx.doi.org/10.1001/jama.1991.03470120066034] [PMID: 1886189]

[26]   Skurnick JH, Kennedy CA, Perez G, *et al.* Behavioral and demographic risk factors for transmission of human immunodeficiency virus type 1 in heterosexual couples: report from the Heterosexual HIV Transmission Study. Clin Infect Dis 1998; 26(4): 855-64.
[http://dx.doi.org/10.1086/513929] [PMID: 9564464]

[27]   Shapiro K, Ray S. Sexual health for people living with HIV. Reproductive health matters 2007; 15(29): 67-92.
[http://dx.doi.org/10.1016/S0968-8080(07)29034-2]

[28]   Pilcher CD, Tien HC, Eron JJ Jr, *et al.* Quest Study, Duke-UNC-Emory Acute HIV Consortium. Brief but efficient: acute HIV infection and the sexual transmission of HIV. J Infect Dis 2004; 189(10): 1785-92.
[http://dx.doi.org/10.1086/386333] [PMID: 15122514]

[29]   Wawer MJ, Gray RH, Sewankambo NK, *et al.* Rates of HIV-1 transmission per coital act, by stage of HIV-1 infection, in Rakai, Uganda. J Infect Dis 2005; 191(9): 1403-9.
[http://dx.doi.org/10.1086/429411] [PMID: 15809897]

[30]   Hughes JP, Baeten JM, Lingappa JR, *et al.* Partners in Prevention HSV/HIV Transmission Study Team. Determinants of per-coital-act HIV-1 infectivity among African HIV-1-serodiscordant couples. J Infect Dis 2012; 205(3): 358-65.
[http://dx.doi.org/10.1093/infdis/jir747] [PMID: 22241800]

[31]   Attia S, Egger M, Müller M, Zwahlen M, Low N. Sexual transmission of HIV according to viral load and antiretroviral therapy: systematic review and meta-analysis. AIDS 2009; 23(11): 1397-404.
[http://dx.doi.org/10.1097/QAD.0b013e32832b7dca] [PMID: 19381076]

[32]   Allen S, Tice J, Van de Perre P, *et al.* Effect of serotesting with counselling on condom use and seroconversion among HIV discordant couples in Africa. BMJ 1992; 304(6842): 1605-9.
[http://dx.doi.org/10.1136/bmj.304.6842.1605] [PMID: 1628088]

[33]   Weller SC. A meta-analysis of condom effectiveness in reducing sexually transmitted HIV. Soc Sci Med 1993; 36(12): 1635-44.
[http://dx.doi.org/10.1016/0277-9536(93)90352-5] [PMID: 8327927]

[34]   World Health Organization (WHO). Condoms for HIV prevention [Accessed on: Mar 2009]; Available from: www.who.int/hiv/topics/condoms/en.

[35]   Weller S, Davis K. Condom effectiveness in reducing heterosexual HIV transmission. Cochrane Database Syst Rev 2002; 1(1): CD003255. [Review].
[PMID: 11869658]

[36]   Varghese B, Maher JE, Peterman TA, Branson BM, Steketee RW. Reducing the risk of sexual HIV transmission: quantifying the per-act risk for HIV on the basis of choice of partner, sex act, and

condom use. Sex Transm Dis 2002; 29(1): 38-43.
[http://dx.doi.org/10.1097/00007435-200201000-00007] [PMID: 11773877]

[37]   Garnett GP, Gazzard B. Risk of HIV transmission in discordant couples. Lancet 2008; 372(9635): 270-1.
[http://dx.doi.org/10.1016/S0140-6736(08)61089-2] [PMID: 18657692]

[38]   Holmes KK, Levine R, Weaver M. Effectiveness of condoms in preventing sexually transmitted infections. Bull World Health Organ 2004; 82(6): 454-61.
[PMID: 15356939]

[39]   Weller SC, Davis-Beaty K. Condom effectiveness in reducing heterosexual HIV transmission. The Cochrane Collaboration library. John Wiley & Sons 2007.(4): New Jersey, United States. Avaible at: http://apps.who.int/rhl/reviews/langs/CD003255.pdf
[PMID: 11869658]

[40]   Wilkinson D. Condom effectiveness in reducing heterosexual HIV transmission: RHL commentary 2002.The WHO Reproductive Health LibraryGeneva: World Health Organization [Accessed on: Nov 2002]; Avaible at: http://apps.who.int/rhl/hiv_aids/dwguide/en/

[41]   Ahmed S, Lutalo T, Wawer M, *et al.* HIV incidence and sexually transmitted disease prevalence associated with condom use: a population study in Rakai, Uganda. AIDS 2001; 15(16): 2171-9.
[http://dx.doi.org/10.1097/00002030-200111090-00013] [PMID: 11684937]

[42]   World Health Organization (WHO) revised position statement on condoms and HIV prevention. 2009. Available from: www.who.int/hiv/pub/condoms/20090318_position_condoms.pdf.

[43]   UNFPA. Report on donor support for contraceptive and condoms for STI/HIV prevention 2007; 30-1. Available from: http://www.unfpa.org/publications /donor-support-contraceptives-and-con-oms-stihiv-prevention-2010

[44]   World Health Organization (WHO). Available from: www.who.int/hi/topics/ malecircumcision/fact__ sheet/en/.

[45]   Addanki KC, Pace DG, Bagasra O. A practice for all seasons: male circumcision and the prevention of HIV transmission. J Infect Dev Ctries 2008; 2(5): 328-34.
[PMID: 19745498]

[46]   Gray RH, Kiwanuka N, Quinn TC, *et al.* Rakai Project Team. Male circumcision and HIV acquisition and transmission: cohort studies in Rakai, Uganda. AIDS 2000; 14(15): 2371-81.
[http://dx.doi.org/10.1097/00002030-200010200-00019] [PMID: 11089626]

[47]   Szabo R, Short RV. How does male circumcision protect against HIV infection? BMJ 2000; 320(7249): 1592-4.
[http://dx.doi.org/10.1136/bmj.320.7249.1592] [PMID: 10845974]

[48]   Auvert B, Taljaard D, Lagarde E, Sobngwi-Tambekou J, Sitta R, Puren A. Randomized, controlled intervention trial of male circumcision for reduction of HIV infection risk: the ANRS 1265 Trial. PLoS Med 2005; 2(11): e298.
[http://dx.doi.org/10.1371/journal.pmed.0020298] [PMID: 16231970]

[49]   Gray RH, Kigozi G, Serwadda D, *et al.* Male circumcision for HIV prevention in men in Rakai, Uganda: a randomised trial. Lancet 2007; 369(9562): 657-66.

[http://dx.doi.org/10.1016/S0140-6736(07)60313-4] [PMID: 17321311]

[50]   UNAIDS/WHO policy statement on HIV testing. [Accessed on: Jun 2004]; Available from: www.who.int/hiv/pub/vct/en/ hivtestingpolicy04.pdf

[51]   Namazzi JA. Determinants of Using Voluntary Counseling and Testing for HIV/AIDS in Kenya. Journal of Management Policy and Practice 2010; 11(5): 89-96.

[52]   Maman S, Mbwambo J, Hogan NM, Kilonzo GP, Sweat M. Women's barriers to HIV-1 testing and disclosure: challenges for HIV-1 voluntary counselling and testing. AIDS Care 2001; 13(5): 595-603. [http://dx.doi.org/10.1080/09540120120063223] [PMID: 11571006]

[53]   Kairania R, Gray RH, Kiwanuka N, *et al.* Disclosure of HIV results among discordant couples in Rakai, Uganda: a facilitated couple counselling approach. AIDS Care 2010; 22(9): 1041-51. [http://dx.doi.org/10.1080/09540121003602226] [PMID: 20824557]

[54]   World Health Organization (WHO). Experts to discuss HIV testing and counselling for discordant couples. [Accessed on: Feb 2011]; Available from: www.who.int/hiv/events/testing_counselling/en/.

[55]   Were WA, Mermin JH, Wamai N, *et al.* Undiagnosed HIV infection and couple HIV discordance among household members of HIV-infected people receiving antiretroviral therapy in Uganda. J Acquir Immune Defic Syndr 2006; 43(1): 91-5. [http://dx.doi.org/10.1097/01.qai.0000225021.81384.28] [PMID: 16885775]

[56]   Allen S, Meinzen-Derr J, Kautzman M, *et al.* Sexual behavior of HIV discordant couples after HIV counseling and testing. AIDS 2003; 17(5): 733-40. [http://dx.doi.org/10.1097/00002030-200303280-00012] [PMID: 12646797]

[57]   Weinhardt LS, Carey MP, Johnson BT, Bickham NL. Effects of HIV counseling and testing on sexual risk behavior: a meta-analytic review of published research, 1985-1997. Am J Public Health 1999; 89(9): 1397-405. [http://dx.doi.org/10.2105/AJPH.89.9.1397] [PMID: 10474559]

[58]   Ryder RW, Kamenga C, Jingu M, Mbuyi N, Mbu L, Behets F. Pregnancy and HIV-1 incidence in 178 married couples with discordant HIV-1 serostatus: additional experience at an HIV-1 counselling centre in the Democratic Republic of the Congo. Trop Med Int Health 2000; 5(7): 482-7. [http://dx.doi.org/10.1046/j.1365-3156.2000.00582.x] [PMID: 10964270]

[59]   Coldiron ME, Stephenson R, Chomba E, *et al.* The relationship between alcohol consumption and unprotected sex among known HIV-discordant couples in Rwanda and Zambia. AIDS Behav 2008; 12(4): 594-603. [http://dx.doi.org/10.1007/s10461-007-9304-x] [PMID: 17705032]

[60]   Kempf MC, Allen S, Zulu I, *et al.* Rwanda Zambia HIV Research Group. Enrollment and retention of HIV discordant couples in Lusaka, Zambia. J Acquir Immune Defic Syndr 2008; 47(1): 116-25. [http://dx.doi.org/10.1097/QAI.0b013e31815d2f3f] [PMID: 18030162]

[61]   Lingappa JR, Lambdin B, Bukusi EA, *et al.* Partners in Prevention HSV-2/HIV Transmission Study Group. Regional differences in prevalence of HIV-1 discordance in Africa and enrollment of HIV-1 discordant couples into an HIV-1 prevention trial. PLoS One 2008; 3(1): e1411. [http://dx.doi.org/10.1371/journal.pone.0001411] [PMID: 18183292]

[62]   Vernazza PL, Graf I, Sonnenberg-Schwan U, Geit M, Meurer A. Preexposure prophylaxis and timed

intercourse for HIV-discordant couples willing to conceive a child. AIDS 2011; 25(16): 2005-8.
[http://dx.doi.org/10.1097/QAD.0b013e32834a36d0] [PMID: 21716070]

[63]   Semprini AE, Bujan L, Englert Y, *et al*. Establishing the safety profile of sperm washing followed by ART for the treatment of HIV discordant couples wishing to conceive. Hum Reprod 2007; 22(10): 2793-4.
[http://dx.doi.org/10.1093/humrep/dem197] [PMID: 17609245]

[64]   Vernazza PL, Hollander L, Semprini AE, *et al*. HIV-discordant couples and parenthood: how are we dealing with the risk of transmission? AIDS 2006; 20(4): 635-6.
[PMID: 16470136]

[65]   Bunnell R, Ekwaru JP, Solberg P, *et al*. Changes in sexual behavior and risk of HIV transmission after antiretroviral therapy and prevention interventions in rural Uganda. AIDS 2006; 20(1): 85-92.
[http://dx.doi.org/10.1097/01.aids.0000196566.40702.28] [PMID: 16327323]

[66]   Guidance On Couples Hiv Testing And Counselling Including Antiretroviral Therapy For Treatment And Prevention In Serodiscordant Couples. Recommendations for a public health approach , [Accessed on: Apr 2012]; Available at: http://apps.who.int/iris/bitstream/10665/44646/1/9789241501972_eng.pdf?ua=1.

[67]   Low N, Broutet N, Adu-Sarkodie Y, Barton P, Hossain M, Hawkes S. Global control of sexually transmitted infections. Lancet 2006; 368(9551): 2001-16.
[http://dx.doi.org/10.1016/S0140-6736(06)69482-8] [PMID: 17141708]

[68]   Reynolds SJ, Makumbi F, Nakigozi G, *et al*. HIV-1 transmission among HIV-1 discordant couples before and after the introduction of antiretroviral therapy. AIDS 2011; 25(4): 473-7.
[http://dx.doi.org/10.1097/QAD.0b013e3283437c2b] [PMID: 21160416]

CHAPTER 15

Aging in People Living with HIV

Katayoun Tayeri*

Iranian Research Center for HIV/AIDS, Iranian Institute for Reduction of High Risk Behaviors, Tehran University of Medical Sciences, Tehran, Iran

Abstract: The invention and administration of novel antiretroviral therapies (ART) has led to the increased lifespan of People Living with HIV (PLHIV) especially in the developed world and thus, we are facing with increased number of HIV infected people over the age of 50 years. It seems that HIV infection may accelerate the aging process by accelerating the shortening of telomeres. Several adverse habits such as smoking and drug abuse as well as co-infection with other pathogens are more common among PLHIV. So, by increasing the age, inappropriate lifestyle and adverse habits such as cigarette smoking, drinking a lot of coffee, being physically inactive or inappropriate activity, opium and drug abuse and alcoholism put people in higher risk of osteoporosis. Several issues should be considered about aging like osteoporosis, neurocognitive impairment, cardiovascular disorders, and impairment of liver function along with the especial consideration about ART in elderly. There are several recommendations for slowing down the aging process in PLHIV. The cessation of cigarette smoking is the main step to prevent undesirable complications such as lung diseases and cancer, increased risk of heart attacks and strokes, bone mineral loss, muscle wasting and memory disorders. Drug abuse, especially some newer drugs like amphetamines and "crystal" may lead to several memory and behavioral impairment, depression and suicide. Regular exercise is another health habit that should be promoted among older PLHIV.

Keywords: Aging, ART, Cardiovascular disorders, CD4 cells, Drug abuse, Lipodystrophy, Neurocognitive impairment, Osteoporosis, PLHIV, Smoking.

* **Correspondence to Katayoun Tayeri:** Iranian Research Center for HIV/AIDS (IRCHA), Imam Khomeini Hospital, Keshavarz Blvd., Tehran, Iran; Tel/Fax: +98 (21) 66947984; E-mail: katayon_tayeri@yahoo.com.

SeyedAhmad SeyedAlinaghi (Ed.)

1. INTRODUCTION

Considering the improvements in the total health globally, the numbers of old people have increased throughout the world; therefore, specific health conditions that are related to older age would be of more importance in this age group, including HIV infection. In fact, the invention and administration of novel antiretroviral therapies (ART) has led to the increased lifespan of People Living with HIV especially in the developed world and thus, we are facing with increased number of HIV infected people over the age of 50. According to recent studies *it is estimated that by 2015, over half of all PLHIV in US will be over 50 years of age or older* [1].

On the other hand, wider educational programs throughout the world have resulted in wider HIV testing among all age groups which should be regarded as another reason for increasing numbers of known HIV infected people especially in age 50 and older [2]. Evidently, certain health conditions may require further clinical care among elderly PLHIV *i.e.*, neurological and cardiovascular disorders, osteoporosis and hypogonadism. Also, in the elderly there are some particularities regarding the diagnosis, pre exposure prophylaxis, rate of progression toward AIDS, varying pharmacokinetics of ART agents, treatment adherence and drug interactions in older age groups.

According to a report on aging *"there is gender difference related to sexual activity and it was found that 71% of men and 51% of women aged 60 and older continue to engage in sexual activity"* [3]. But due to several reasons, aged people would not be likely to use condoms (*i.e.* not being afraid of pregnancy). Also, atrophic vaginitis in women and impotency and arousal difficulties in men tend to further reduce the use of condom [3]. Such reasons put older people at higher risk for Sexually Transmitted Infections (STIs) including HIV. Therefore, it is very important to discuss the proper use of barrier methods with the elderly [4]. On the other hand, the prevalence of persons aged over 50 who have a positive history of IV drug use has also increased significantly in the last several years [5]. Thereby, needle sharing that is one of the main routes of HIV transmission among youth should be considered in elderly too.

2. THE PROCESS OF AGING

There are several genetic, environmental and biological factors that are pivotal in senescence. It is important to keep in mind that senescence also occurs at the cellular level. The replication capacity of cells is related to the small fragments at the end of the chromosomes, called telomeres. The length of telomeres is associated to cell age. During life, cells reproduce hundreds or thousands of times from original cells and in each division, telomeres become shorter and shorter. When telomere is long enough, cells are young with normal function. Following the shortening of telomeres, cellular activities deteriorate and cellular division would not be possible afterward. At the end of this process, the weakening of several body systems like musculoskeletal system occurs.

It seems that HIV infection may accelerate the aging process by accelerating the shortening of telomeres [6]. Several adverse habits such as smoking and drug abuse as well as co-infection with other pathogens are more common among PLHIV. In addition, certain organic disorders tend to be more prevalent among PLHIV such as:

- Cardiovascular diseases
- Renal diseases
- Muscles weakness and weakened bones
- Lipodystrophies
- Liver diseases

Some of the above conditions may result from ART. Organic disorders may also be due to direct effect of HIV, such as HIV nephropathy, HIV cardiomyopathy and HIV enteropathy, or be the consequence of other factors such as cervical cancer due to HPV infection, heart attack and lung cancer due to smoking, and liver failure due to HCV and HBV co-infections.

3. AGING OF THE IMMUNE SYSTEM

Aging has been associated with decreased production of some cytokines like IL-2 that is important in cellular immunity and impaired production of this cytokine promotes dysfunction of T cells. When older patients are chronically infected with

HIV, CD4 T cell depletion is more prominent compared to younger HIV infected patients [7, 8].

As people age, their immune functions typically decline. This is in part related to the atrophy of the thymus gland, where newly produced T-cells mature. In addition, T cell function seems to decrease over time, a phenomenon known as immune-senescence. Also, studies suggest that this cellular aging occurs more rapidly in the presence of HIV infection. An important finding related to the rapid progression of immuno-senescence among PLHIV is the decreased expression of CD28 on CD4 and CD8 T cells. Decreased CD28 expression is accompanied with decreased length and activity of telomerase that leads to impaired proliferation capacity. These phenomena eventually lead to faster progression of aging in PLHIV [9]. In addition, chronic inflammation in PLHIV directly disturbs the normal function of internal organs and exacerbates the co-morbidities. According to a report in January 2009, differentiation stage of T cells reflects the aging of T cells and expression of several markers on them can explain the aging process [9]. Such observations may explain the accelerated aging process in PLHIV. It is noteworthy that adherence to a healthy lifestyle and proper control of HIV infection *via* appropriate ART can reduce the speed of aging among PLHIV.

4. SPECIAL ASPECT OF AGING AND HIV INFECTION

4.1. Osteoporosis

Inappropriate lifestyle and adverse habits such as cigarette smoking, drinking a lot of coffee, being physically inactive or inappropriate activity, opium and drug abuse and alcoholism put people in higher risk of osteoporosis. Also, hormonal deficiency during menopause and hypogonadism and low testosterone level, calcium and vitamin D insufficiency, depression and inadequate physical activities, co-infections such as HCV result in accelerated bone damage. Some of the ART agents such as tenofovir tend to reduce the bone mineral density. Such conditions are more frequently observed in HIV infected people, especially older age groups that would eventually lead to osteoporosis [10 - 12]. Due to inadequate use of dairy products and milk especially among PLHIV with opiate addiction, osteoporosis may develop as a result of lower calcium intake. On the other hand, poor nutrition, as a consequence of gender inequality, can be more common in women and in addition to hormonal disturbance and menopause more severe skeletal disorders are anticipated in women. Some studies have shown that Asian HIV infected women are at higher risk of osteoporosis [12].

4.2. Neurocognitive Impairment

There are quite limited numbers of studies that have emphasized on the role of aging as a significant predictor of neurocognitive disorders [13]. Other risk factors for developing HIV-associated neurocognitive disorders in the elderly include female gender, high viral load and advanced disease, history of drug use especially cocaine and other mood elevators, co-infections with viruses like CMV, HH6 and JC virus [4, 14]. There is a spectrum of symptoms in HIV-associated neurocognitive disorders form minor cognitive motor disorder -that may remain hidden from the physicians- to real HIV-associated dementia with prominent symptoms of cognitive, motor and behavioral disturbances including progressive impairment of concentration, memory loss and behavioral changes [4, 14].

4.3. Cardiovascular Disorders

As a result of effective ARTs and consequently increased survival of PLHIV, the prevalence of cardiovascular diseases, hypertension, diabetes mellitus and dyslipidemia have increased. Although many of the above conditions are associated with older age, HIV infection increases the total risk by metabolic toxicities or direct endothelial damage that is induced by HIV itself [15 - 21]. Cardiovascular diseases that result from prolonged use of ART are among the main causes of mortality in PLHIV worldwide. Unsurprisingly, special drug classes of ARTs lead to heart conditions and ART-related obesity is another cause of cardiovascular diseases among PLHIV [22]. Consecutively, all HIV infected old patients should be regularly monitored for cardiovascular disorders.

4.4. Impairment of Liver Function

In addition to cardiovascular diseases, liver diseases are among the leading causes of mortality in PLHIV throughout the world [23]. In the case of positive history of liver poor conditions such as hepatitis B and/or C co-infection, management of patients would be more complicated. Drug interaction and side effects are a major concern in this situation. On the other hand, HIV itself and ARV drugs affect the hepatocytes [24]. Some of important ARV drugs cause liver toxicity (drug hepatitis). A study has shown that the immune system of HIV/HCV co-infected patients is at least 10 years older than mono infected patients with HCV [25]. Overall, main risk factors of liver toxicity in HIV patients are:

- Co-infection with hepatitis B/C
- Obesity
- Female gender
- Alcohol and drug use
- Older age [25]

Therefore, physicians should be aware about the patients' risk factors and start the ART with caution.

4.5. ART in the Elderly

It is important to note that generally the metabolism of ARV drugs is diminished in older age which can lead to more side effects [26]. Prolong use of ARV drugs lead to lipodystrophy and increases serum cholesterol level and also heart attack that is more prominent in older age. Correspondingly, more careful selection of ARV drugs and close monitoring are recommended in elderly [27].

There are several studies that indicate the differences between treatment in older and younger HIV infected people. A French prospective cohort study assessed clinical outcomes in 3015 treatment-naive patients, 401 of whom were over age 50. After six months of ART, older patients significantly had better viral suppression but they showed more AIDS-defining illnesses [28]. Most importantly, ARV drugs are eliminated from kidney and/or liver. Since in older age there is some impairment in organic function, the possibility of drugs accumulation and side effects could be increased [29].This situation is more important with protease inhibitors (PIs). On the hand, older people usually use several drugs, sometimes over-the-counter for several reasons like pain relief, laxative and herbal drugs [25] that may interact with ARVs or increase their side effects.In EuroSida cohort, time need to reach the sustained CD4>200 was longer in older compared with younger patients [30]. So, this finding can show that long-term treatment with prophylactic medication is needed in the elderly.

Adherence to ART is another key factor in obtaining appropriate result from ART. There are several factors that can affect the patient's adherence, some of which are more important in older ages like high pill burden, illiteracy, forgetfulness, isolation and not having treatment supporter, depression and other neurocognitive impairments. All of such factors can reduce the treatment adherence and lead to treatment failure and drug resistance. However, several studies confirmed higher adherence to treatment in older patients compared to younger PLHIV [31]. It seems that physicians can have an important role in maintaining good adherence and assessing it by appropriate counseling, discontinuation of unnecessary drugs, use of adherence tools like pill boxes and daily calendar and regularly visiting the patients.

It is noteworthy that there are no specific differences in the dose of ARV drugs between older and younger PLHIV, unless in the presence of liver or kidney impairment [32]. Another reason for increased drug–related toxicities among older patients can be due to decreased albumin level and changes in the activity of cytochrome p450 enzyme system. Therefore, regular patients' treatment monitoring and evaluation of side effects symptoms should be done in all patients, especially in the elderly [33].

5. STIGMA AND SOCIAL SUPPORT IN OLDER PLHIV

In general, older PLHIV seem to be more socially isolated than younger patients [34]. HIV stigma is an important barrier in access to care in PLHIV and in older ages, it can be worse, especially in some countries. Elderly population is mainly considered as the reference in society. Therefore, being infected with HIV is more stigmatized in elders and may further make them isolated. On the other hand, the main supporters of HIV infected patients are their parents, especially mothers. But in age >50, the patients may not usually receive good support from their parents [35]. As a result, older patients usually experience more stigma and discrimination. Several studies showed that being socially active and in connection with other people, especially peer groups would help PLHIV to live healthier and longer. Isolation can be more harmful in elderly because in several situations they need others to overcome their complains. In this regard, certain supportive foundations can help them to be more socially active and effective.

6. RECOMMENDATIONS FOR SLOWING DOWN THE PROCESS OF AGING AMONG PLHIV

Cessation of cigarette smoking is the main step to prevent undesirable complications like lung diseases and cancer, increased risk of heart attacks and strokes, bone mineral loss, muscle wasting and memory problems [6]. Drug abuse, especially some newer drugs like amphetamines and "crystal" may lead to several memory and behavioral impairment, depression and suicide. Regular exercise is another health habit that should be promoted among older PLHIV. In this regard, 30-60 minutes daily brisk walking would be a good recommendation. Moreover, appropriate nutrition is an inseparable issue throughout all stages of the HIV infection. Before starting ART, appropriate nutrition improves immune status and reduces the rate of HIV progression [36]. After starting ART, good nutrition decreases drug side effects and metabolic changes and increases adherence to treatment. In HIV/TB co-infection, appropriate nutrition can be very important and enough vitamin D supplementation is advised [37]. Using some herbal remedies that are usual in old age sometimes would reduce the ART efficacy or interact with it like garlic tablets, licorice, valerian, oxtongue and ginkobilia [36]. Additionally, one of the old complains of elders is constipation and can be controlled with increasing amount of liquid and fiber intake in daily regimen. Wheat bran, whole grain, vegetables and fruits are very useful [36]. Also fibers can reduce the risk of heart diseases, hyperlipidemia, hypertension and diabetes mellitus in elders. In this regard, away from consumption of too much sugar and processed and fried foods, unhealthy fats and red meat should be preferably avoided [38].

CONFLICT OF INTEREST

The author confirms that author has no conflict of interest to declare for this publication.

ACKNOWLEDGEMENTS

Declared none.

REFERENCES

[1]   Effros RB, Fletcher CV, Gebo K, *et al.* Aging and infectious diseases: workshop on HIV infection and aging: what is known and future research directions. Clin Infect Dis 2008; 47(4): 542-53.
[http://dx.doi.org/10.1086/590150] [PMID: 18627268]

[2]   Levy JA, Ory MG, Crystal S. HIV/AIDS interventions for midlife and older adults: current status and challenges. J Acquir Immune Defic Syndr 2003; 33 (Suppl. 2): S59-67.
[http://dx.doi.org/10.1097/00126334-200306012-00002] [PMID: 12853854]

[3]   Levy BR, Ding L, Lakra D, Kosteas J, Niccolai L. Older persons' exclusion from sexually transmitted disease risk-reduction clinical trials. Sex Transm Dis 2007; 34(8): 541-4.
[PMID: 17297381]

[4]   Guide for HIV/AIDS Clinical Care. HRSA HIV/AIDS Bureau 2012. Available at: http://hab.hrsa.gov/

[5]   Zablotsky D, Kennedy M. Risk factors and HIV transmission to midlife and older women: knowledge, options, and the initiation of safer sexual practices. J Acquir Immune Defic Syndr 2003; 33 (Suppl. 2): S122-30.
[http://dx.doi.org/10.1097/00126334-200306012-00009] [PMID: 12853861]

[6]   Youle M, Murphy G. Coming of age, a guide to aging well with HIV. 2010. Available at: www.hivdent.org/_medical_/2010/coming_of_age_book.pdf

[7]   Negoro S, Hara H, Miyata S, *et al.* Mechanisms of age-related decline in antigen-specific T cell proliferative response: IL-2 receptor expression and recombinant IL-2 induced proliferative response of purified Tac-positive T cells. Mech Ageing Dev 1986; 36(3): 223-41.
[http://dx.doi.org/10.1016/0047-6374(86)90089-8] [PMID: 3099104]

[8]   Lederman MM, McKinnis R, Kelleher D, *et al.* Cellular restoration in HIV infected persons treated with abacavir and a protease inhibitor: age inversely predicts naive CD4 cell count increase. AIDS 2000; 14(17): 2635-42.
[http://dx.doi.org/10.1097/00002030-200012010-00002] [PMID: 11125881]

[9]   Cao W, Jamieson BD, Hultin LE, Hultin PM, Effros RB, Detels R. Premature aging of T cells is associated with faster HIV-1 disease progression. J Acquir Immune Defic Syndr 2009; 50(2): 137-47.
[http://dx.doi.org/10.1097/QAI.0b013e3181926c28] [PMID: 19131896]

[10]   Arnsten JH, Freeman R, Howard AA, Floris-Moore M, Lo Y, Klein RS. Decreased bone mineral density and increased fracture risk in aging men with or at risk for HIV infection. AIDS 2007; 21(5): 617-23.
[http://dx.doi.org/10.1097/QAD.0b013e3280148c05] [PMID: 17314524]

[11]   Klein RS, Lo Y, Santoro N, Dobs AS. Androgen levels in older men who have or who are at risk of acquiring HIV infection. Clin Infect Dis 2005; 41(12): 1794-803.
[http://dx.doi.org/10.1086/498311] [PMID: 16288406]

[12]   Osteoporosis. Fact sheet number 557, The AIDS InfoNet. Available at: http://www.aidsinfonet.org/

fact_sheets/view/557 [Last date of access: June 13, 2014]

[13]   Wilkie FL, Goodkin K, Khamis I, *et al.* Cognitive functioning in younger and older HIV-1-infected adults. J Acquir Immune Defic Syndr 2003; 33 (Suppl. 2): S93-S105.
       [http://dx.doi.org/10.1097/00126334-200306012-00006] [PMID: 12853858]

[14]   Sacktor N, Skolasky RL, Seaberg E, *et al.* Prevalence of HIV-associated neurocognitive disorders in the Multicenter AIDS Cohort Study. Neurology 2015; pii. [Epub ahead of print]
       [http://dx.doi.org/10.1212/WNL.0000000000002277] [PMID: 26718568]

[15]   Centers for disease control and prevention. HIV/AIDS Surveillance Report 1993; 5(1): 11. Available at: http://www.cdc.gov/hiv/library/reports/surveillance/.

[16]   Behrens G, Schmidt H, Meyer D, Stoll M, Schmidt RE. Vascular complications associated with use of HIV protease inhibitors. Lancet 1998; 351(9120): 1958.
       [http://dx.doi.org/10.1016/S0140-6736(98)26026-0] [PMID: 9654284]

[17]   Gallet B, Pulik M, Genet P, Chedin P, Hiltgen M. Vascular complications associated with use of HIV protease inhibitors. Lancet 1998; 351(9120): 1958-9.
       [http://dx.doi.org/10.1016/S0140-6736(05)78643-8] [PMID: 9654285]

[18]   Vittecoq D, Escaut L, Monsuez JJ. Vascular complications associated with use of HIV protease inhibitors. Lancet 1998; 351(9120): 1959.
       [http://dx.doi.org/10.1016/S0140-6736(05)78644-X] [PMID: 9654286]

[19]   Huang MB, Hunter M, Bond VC. Effect of extracellular human immunodeficiency virus type 1 glycoprotein 120 on primary human vascular endothelial cell cultures. AIDS Res Hum Retroviruses 1999; 15(14): 1265-77.
       [http://dx.doi.org/10.1089/088922299310160] [PMID: 10505675]

[20]   Huang MB, Khan M, Garcia-Barrio M, Powell M, Bond VC. Apoptotic effects in primary human umbilical vein endothelial cell cultures caused by exposure to virion-associated and cell membrane-associated HIV-1 gp120. J Acquir Immune Defic Syndr 2001; 27(3): 213-21.
       [http://dx.doi.org/10.1097/00126334-200107010-00001] [PMID: 11464139]

[21]   Park IW, Ullrich CK, Schoenberger E, Ganju RK, Groopman JE. HIV-1 Tat induces microvascular endothelial apoptosis through caspase activation. J Immunol 2001; 167(5): 2766-71.
       [http://dx.doi.org/10.4049/jimmunol.167.5.2766] [PMID: 11509621]

[22]   Deeks SG, Phillips AN. HIV infection, antiretroviral treatment, ageing, and non-AIDS related morbidity. BMJ 2009; 338(7689): a3172.
       [http://dx.doi.org/10.1136/bmj.a3172] [PMID: 19171560]

[23]   Knobel H, Guelar A, Valldecillo G, *et al.* Response to highly active antiretroviral therapy in HIV-infected patients aged 60 years or older after 24 months follow-up. AIDS 2001; 15(12): 1591-3.
       [http://dx.doi.org/10.1097/00002030-200108170-00025] [PMID: 11505000]

[24]   Kirk JB, Goetz MB. Human immunodeficiency virus in an aging population, a complication of success. J Am Geriatr Soc 2009; 57(11): 2129-38.
       [http://dx.doi.org/10.1111/j.1532-5415.2009.02494.x] [PMID: 19793157]

[25]   Sitar DS. Aging issues in drug disposition and efficacy. Proc West Pharmacol Soc 2007; 50: 16-20.
       [PMID: 18605223]

[26] Uphold CR, Shehan CL, Bender JM, Bender BS. Emotional bonds and social support exchange between men living with HIV infection and their mothers. Am J Men Health 2012; 6(2): 97-107.
[http://dx.doi.org/10.1177/1557988311413118] [PMID: 21816862]

[27] Gebo KA. HIV and aging: implications for patient management. Drugs Aging 2006; 23(11): 897-913.
[http://dx.doi.org/10.2165/00002512-200623110-00005] [PMID: 17109568]

[28] Simone MJ, Appelbaum J. HIV in older adults. Geriatrics 2008; 63(12): 6-12.
[PMID: 19061274]

[29] Tumbarello M, Rabagliati R, de Gaetano Donati K, *et al.* Older age does not influence CD4 cell recovery in HIV-1 infected patients receiving highly active antiretroviral therapy. BMC Infect Dis 2004; 4: 46.
[http://dx.doi.org/10.1186/1471-2334-4-46] [PMID: 15530169]

[30] Steinman MA, Hanlon JT. Managing medications in clinically complex elders: "There's got to be a happy medium". JAMA 2010; 304(14): 1592-601.
[http://dx.doi.org/10.1001/jama.2010.1482] [PMID: 20940385]

[31] Viard JP, Mocroft A, Chiesi A, *et al.* EuroSIDA Study Group. Influence of age on CD4 cell recovery in human immunodeficiency virus-infected patients receiving highly active antiretroviral therapy: evidence from the EuroSIDA study. J Infect Dis 2001; 183(8): 1290-4.
[http://dx.doi.org/10.1086/319678] [PMID: 11262215]

[32] Wellons MF, Sanders L, Edwards LJ, Bartlett JA, Heald AE, Schmader KE. HIV infection: treatment outcomes in older and younger adults. J Am Geriatr Soc 2002; 50(4): 603-7.
[http://dx.doi.org/10.1046/j.1532-5415.2002.50152.x] [PMID: 11982658]

[33] Sotaniemi EA, Arranto AJ, Pelkonen O, Pasanen M. Age and cytochrome P450-linked drug metabolism in humans: an analysis of 226 subjects with equal histopathologic conditions. Clin Pharmacol Ther 1997; 61(3): 331-9.
[http://dx.doi.org/10.1016/S0009-9236(97)90166-1] [PMID: 9091249]

[34] Puoti M, Nasta P, Gatti F, *et al.* HIV-related liver disease: ARV drugs, coinfection, and other risk factors. J Int Assoc Physicians AIDS Care (Chic) 2009; 8(1): 30-42.
[http://dx.doi.org/10.1177/1545109708330906] [PMID: 19211929]

[35] Emlet CA. An examination of the social networks and social isolation in older and younger adults living with HIV/AIDS. Health Soc Work 2006; 31(4): 299-308.
[http://dx.doi.org/10.1093/hsw/31.4.299] [PMID: 17176977]

[36] Fisher SD, Kanda BS, Miller TL, Lipshultz SE. Cardiovascular disease and therapeutic drug-related cardiovascular consequences in HIV-infected patients. Am J Cardiovasc Drugs 2011; 11(6): 383-94.
[http://dx.doi.org/10.2165/11594590-000000000-00000] [PMID: 22149317]

[37] Nutrition. 9th ed., AIDS Map 2011. Available at: http://www.nutrition.gov/.

[38] HIV/AIDS, TB and Nutrition Scientific inquiry into the nutritional influences on human immunity with special reference to HIV infection and active TB in South Africa 2011; 98(19): 10799-804.2007;
[PMID: 18000564]

Interaction of Behavior and Biomedical Prevention

Maryam Foroughi[1],* and **Pegah Valiollahi[2]**

[1] *Iranian Research Center for HIV/AIDS, Iranian Institute for Reduction of High Risk Behaviors, Tehran University of Medical Sciences, Tehran, Iran*

[2] *Department of Clinical and Experimental Medicine of Linköping University, Linköping, Sweden*

Abstract: Today we know that for new HIV infection prevention, there are some effective and feasible programs such as needle exchange, behavioral interventions and antiretroviral therapy (ART). The main component to maintaining behavioral changes is to find novel techniques and know how to stay motivated and also use combination of techniques and methods. This is what researcher and health providers call Biomedical and Behavioral interventions in prevention of HIV infection. Current evidence confirms the efficacy of behavioral interventions in lowering HIV acquisition versus standard care or no intervention. Biomedical intervention is another effective program for HIV prevention, where medical and clinical approaches are used to decrease HIV infection. As HIV infection rates are strongly influenced by human behavior, behavioral changes has long been understood as essential to curb the prevalence of infection. In all cases where a decrease in prevalence has been observed, broad-based changes in behavior were the key of success. Besides behavior change strategies, it is necessary to consider the accessibility to novel biomedical HIV prevention modalities such as vaccines and microbicides. The combination of behavioral changes and application of medical treatment (as ARV or Drug treatment such as Methadone and preventive treatments like microbicides) is regarded as the best effective intervention aganist HIV acquisition.

Keywords: ART, Bio Behaviors, Effective, HIV treatment, Interventions, Medical treatment, Methadone, Microbicides, Vaccines.

---

* **Correspondence to Maryam Foroughi:** Iranian Research Center for HIV/AIDS (IRCHA), Imam Khomeini Hospital, Keshavarz Blvd., Tehran, Iran; Tel/Fax: +98 (21) 66947984; E-mail: ma_foroughi@yahoo.com.

SeyedAhmad SeyedAlinaghi (Ed.)

1. INTRODUCTION

Human immunodeficiency virus (HIV) leads to acquired immune deficiency syndrome (AIDS) which is transmitted through contact with infected blood and bodily fluids.

Generally, HIV is associated with injection drug use and unprotected sexual contact. In other hand, although HIV infection is considered a sexual transmitted disease, there is also a strong influence of human behavior [1].

HIV leads to remarkable inflammation in the body. Some possible consequences of this inflammation are spinal cord and brain damages; dysfunction of nerve cells [1]. Neurological complications are the product of damage by the virus itself and do not usually set in, until advanced stages of HIV infection, characteristically in "AIDS" stage of infection. On the other hand, people with HIV or AIDS often develop anxiety disorders and depression. Hallucinations and remarkable changes in behavior can be experienced [1].

According to the route of transmission, several groups are at high risk for HIV acquisition, such as injection drug users (IDUs) by sharing needles and injecting equipments, non IDUs by impairment of judgment and also enhancement of sexual arousal which can lead to risky sexual behavior, commercial sex workers (CSW) by unprotected multi partner intercourse and their partners.

Drug use facilitates HIV infection progression by further compromising the immune system [2].

A reduction in the use of syringes and sexual risk behaviors of illicit drug users might have a great impact in the public health all around the world [3].

As supported by UNAIDS 2014 report on the global AIDS epidemic, the reduction in new HIV infections over the past 10 years is obviously accompanied with changes in behavior and social norms beside with increased awareness of HIV.

Today we know that for new HIV infection prevention, there are some effective and feasible programs such as needle exchange, behavioral interventions and antiretro viral therapy (ART).

2. BRAIN AND BEHAVIOR

The frontal lobe is an area in the brain, located at the front of each cerebral hemisphere. The frontal lobe covers most of the dopamine-sensitive neurons in the cerebral cortex. The dopamine system is associated with reward, attention, short-term memory tasks, planning, and motivation. The Frontal lobe is important for planning of movements, recent memory and some aspects of emotion as well as it is a component of the cerebral system, which supports goal directed behaviors and observed activity as a response to internal or external stimuli [4, 5].

When people wants to make changes such as lose weight, stop smoking, or accomplish another goal, there is no single solution that works for everyone. They have to try several different techniques, often through a process of trial-and-error, in order to achieve their goal. During the period of changing many people become discouraged and relinquish [5]. Therefore, changing behavior is difficult and the major practice to maintain behavioral changes is to seek new strategies and pave the ground to maintain motivations [5]. This is what researchers and health providers call biomedical and behavioral interventions in prevention of HIV infection.

3. BIOMEDICAL AND BEHAVIORAL INTERVENTIONS

In 2009, the Joint United Nations Program on HIV/AIDS (UNAIDS) reported that, the high rates of HIV infection among sex workers, as compared to most other population groups, has affected rates of heterosexual transmission of HIV particularly in low- and middle-income countries.

These trends have prompted the UNAIDS to call for an urgent redoubling of the effort in the fight against HIV/AIDS and many studies had been settled down for decrease the number of new HIV infection [6].

3.1. Behavioral Intervention

The underlying promise for the behavioral interventions is that human behaviors are mostly learned by interactions between an individual and the environment.

According to *McGahan, et al.* (2001), behavioral strategies can be divided into three periodic categories:

1. *Antecedent:* interventions that are implemented before a target behavior is likely to occur.
2. *Consequence:* interventions that are implemented following the occurrence of target behavior.
3. *Skill Development:* interventions or behavioral techniques that are designed to teach new skills and alternative, adaptive behaviors to reduce the frequency and severity of maladaptive behaviors [7].

The focus of behavioral HIV prevention programs can cover individuals, families, communities, entire societies, or (ideally) a combination of all these. Behavioral HIV prevention programs are strategies for decreasing HIV and sexually transmitted diseases. These interventions can be useful for both HIV positive and HIV negative population. Behavioral interventions aims at the expansion of targeted positive behaviors and lower or remove inappropriate or non-adaptive behaviors.

HIV tests and risk reduction counseling, condom use, HIV education, peer education and persuasion are some of examples of behavioral intervention in HIV prevention programs. According to the result of a meta-analysis study which was conducted in USA in 2006, interventions targeting People living with HIV/AIDS (PLWHA) are efficacious in lowering unprotected sex and acquisition of sexually transmitted diseases.

As a whole, interventions with the following characteristics remarkably lowered risky behaviors: based on behavioral theory, designed to change specifically HIV transmission risk behaviors, in an intensive manner; addressed a myriad of issues related to mental health, medication adherence, and HIV risk behavior [8, 9].

Crepaz and coworkers in 2006 using meta-analysis showed the reduction of unprotected sex and STIs among PLWHAs (OR: 0.57 and 0.20 respectively) [10].

In other study, held in 2006, Johnson confirm the increase of condom use (mean effect size –MES- = 0.16) by behavioral intervention in PLWHAs [11].

Also Herbst and coworkers in 2005 showed the reduce numbers of partners (OR, 0.85), and increase condom use during anal sex (OR, 1.61) as a result of behavioral intervention for men who have sex with men (MSM) [12].

The effectiveness of behavioral interventions is validated by international organization such as UNAIDS, WHO and CDC.

To obtain the best results, interventions must be enhanced to more significant purposes including a delay in the onset of the first intercourse, a reduction in number of sexual partners, an increase in condom use.

3.2. Biomedical Intervention

Another effective program in HIV prevention is biomedical intervention. Biomedical Interventions use medical and clinical approaches to reduce HIV infection.

Evidence of a direct relationship between HIV plasma viremia and HIV transmission events was first described by Quinn *et al.*, in Rakai, Uganda [13] through serodiscordant heterosexual couples. Today these findings have been confirmed by a study which showed a 96% decrease in HIV acquisition when the HIV-infected partner in the discordant couple was receiving ART [14].

Some examples of biomedical interventions in HIV prevention programs include drug treatment with opioid substitution therapy, needle and syringe provision, male circumcision, biomedical prophylaxis, ARTs in PMTCT services, post exposure prophylaxis, appropriate and accessible STD services, ART for prevention in sero-discordant couples.

As HIV infection is close related to human behavior, changes in behavior has long been understood as essential to curb the spread of infection. In all cases, where national epidemics have been reversed, broad-based behaviors changes were essential for success.

Besides behavior changes strategies, it is important to take the availability of new biomedical HIV prevention modalities, such as effective vaccines and microbicides when available should be considered [15].

Antimicrobial agents using discretely, either intra vaginally or intra rectally, are under development. Antiretroviral-based vaginal microbicides are in trials but they are also likely to be challenged by adherence requirements and drug resistance [16].

An example for microbicide intervention is Nonoxynal-9 (which kills HIV in the laboratory) as a vaginal microbicide but actually increased risk for HIV infection among female sex workers by damaging the mucosal barrier that forms part of the body's natural innate defense, against HIV [17]. In conclusion, Nonoxynal-9 is not recommended among the group for HIV prevention.

ART as a preventive program works by suppressing viral replication and reducing viral loads in blood, genitalia, and other tissues. Therefore, ART interventions are effective in potential risk reduction of HIV transmission. Also another success of ARTs is preventing mother-to-child transmission of HIV. By 2006, at least three million years of life have been saved in the United States as a direct result of Highly Active Antiretroviral Therapy (HAART) [18].

More recently, there has been an increased interest in the possible secondary effect of HAART in reducing HIV transmission [19]. Research on heterosexual HIV serodiscordant couples, for example, reported a reduction rate of HIV acquisition to more than 90%, [20]. Also reduction in community viral load as a result of HAART decreased incidence rate of HIV in injection drug users (IDUs) in Canada [21].

Combined biomedical and behavioral treatments have proved the effect on HIV risk behaviors and incidence rate of HIV acquisition. For example, recent research found that as a result of combinations of behavioral therapies with methadone treatment, approximately one-half of the participants who reported injection drug use at the beginning of the study, conveyed no longer use of intravenous drugs at the end of the study. Additionally, more than 90 percent of all participants confirmed no longer needle sharing [22].

In order to combine behavioral and biomedical prevention in HIV infected patients, three items should be considered [23].

Awareness: People who have high risk behaviors should be aware of these risky manners and also should be aware of biomedical preventive ways such as post-exposure (PEP) or pre-exposure prophylaxis (PrEP). Studies conducted around the world, have shown that awareness of PEP in MSMs is different among cities, 40% in California [24], 12% in New York [25], 50% in London [26] and 70% in Sydney [27].

Acceptability: It means that at risk population, should accept the use of ARTs or microbicides as recommended by the health system and organization, before or after risky behaviors.

Access: Although an individual may have knowledge of a certain preventive program and find it acceptable for use, they will only use them if they have access to them.

Intervention strategies on HIV prevention should be designed according to the needs of each society and based on population at risk, evidence based studies, cost effectiveness, *etc*.

The goal is deep-seated changes which are recommended by UNAIDS and it means that changes should be started from small focused studies of individuals on one area of HIV prevention to strategies that affected the whole community and groups of people.

As the final comment, individual behaviors and personal responsibilities, based on knowledge, will be the best protective strategy against AIDS and newly HIV infection. Behavioral changes have to be the social vaccine and this is the main goal in many preventive strategies, but like treatment, effective HIV prevention programs need a combination of different strategies.

The best weapon at this time especially in developing countries will be a combination of behavioral changes alongside with biomedical treatments and preventions.

CONFLICT OF INTEREST

The authors confirm that they have no conflict of interest to declare for this

publication.

ACKNOWLEDGEMENTS

Declared none.

REFERENCES

[1]   Harrison's Principles of Internal Medicine. 18 edition Part 8. Infectious diseases, section 14 infections due to human immunodeficiency virus and other human retroviruses. 2013. Available from: http://accessmedicine.mhmedical.com/book.aspx?bookId=331

[2]   Julio SG. Montaner, Expanded HAART coverage is associated with decreased population-level HIV-1-RNA and annual new HIV diagnoses in british columbia, canada. Lancet 2010; 376(9740): 532-9. [http://dx.doi.org/10.1016/S0140-6736(10)60936-1] [PMID: 20638713]

[3]   Meader N. Psychosocial interventions for reducing injection and sexual risk behavior for preventing HIV in drug users. The Cochrane Collaboration. Published by John Wiley & Sons, Ltd. 2010.

[4]   Giedd JN, Blumenthal J, Jeffries NO, *et al.* Brain development during childhood and adolescence: a longitudinal MRI study. Nat Neurosci 1999; 2(10): 861-3. [http://dx.doi.org/10.1038/13158] [PMID: 10491603]

[5]   Badre D, D'Esposito M. Is the rostro-caudal axis of the frontal lobe hierarchical? Nat Rev Neurosci 2009; 10(9): 659-69. [http://dx.doi.org/10.1038/nrn2667] [PMID: 19672274]

[6]   Sidibé M. UNAIDS. 2010. Available from:http://data.unaids.org/pub/BaseDocument/2010/20100216.

[7]   Deen Tisha L, Bridges Ana J, McGahan Tara C. Cognitive appraisals of specialty mental health services and their relation to mental health service utilization in the rural populationJ Rural Health. 2012; 28: pp. (2)142-51. [http://dx.doi.org/10.1111/j.1748-0361.2011.00375.x] [PMID: 22458315]

[8]   Kuchenbecker R. What is the benefit of the biomedical and behavioral interventions in preventing HIV transmission? Rev Bras Epidemiol 2015; 18 (1): 26-42. [http://dx.doi.org/10.1590/1809-4503201500050004] [PMID: 26630297]

[9]   Warik WM, Ota E, Mori R, *et al.* Behavioral interventions to reduce the transmission of HIV infection among sex workers and their clients in low- and middle-income 2 countries. Cochrane Database Syst Rev. JohnWiley & Sons, Ltd 2012.The Cochrane Collaboration [http://dx.doi.org/10.1002/14651858.CD005272] [PMID: 22336811]

[10]   Crepaz N, Lyles CM, Wolitski RJ, *et al.* HIV/AIDS Prevention Research Synthesis (PRS) Team. Do prevention interventions reduce HIV risk behaviours among people living with HIV? A meta-analytic review of controlled trials. AIDS 2006; 20(2): 143-57. [http://dx.doi.org/10.1097/01.aids.0000196166.48518.a0] [PMID: 16511407]

[11]   Johnson BT, Carey MP, Chaudoir SR, Reid AE. Risk reduction for persons living with human immunodeficiency virus: research synthesis of randomized controlled trials, 1993-2004. J Acquir Immune Defic Syndr 2006; 41(5): 642-50.

[http://dx.doi.org/10.1097/01.qai.0000194495.15309.47] [PMID: 16652039]

[12]   Herbst JH, Sherba RT, Crepaz N, *et al.* HIV/AIDS Prevention Research Synthesis Team. A meta-analytic review of HIV behavioral interventions for reducing sexual risk behavior of men who have sex with men. J Acquir Immune Defic Syndr 2005; 39(2): 228-41.
[PMID: 15905741]

[13]   Quinn TC, Wawer MJ, Sewankambo N, *et al.* Viral load and heterosexual transmission of human immunodeficiency virus type 1. N Engl J Med 2000; 342(13): 921-9.
[http://dx.doi.org/10.1056/NEJM200003303421303] [PMID: 10738050]

[14]   Cohen MS, Chen YQ, McCauley M, *et al.* HPTN 052 Study Team. Prevention of HIV-1 infection with early antiretroviral therapy. N Engl J Med 2011; 365(6): 493-505.
[http://dx.doi.org/10.1056/NEJMoa1105243] [PMID: 21767103]

[15]   Global HIV Prevention Working Group 2002. Available from:www.GlobalHIVPrevention.org

[16]   Wilson DP, Coplan PM, Wainberg MA, Blower SM. The paradoxical effects of using antiretroviral-based microbicides to control HIV epidemics. Proc Natl Acad Sci USA 2008; 105(28): 9835-40.
[http://dx.doi.org/10.1073/pnas.0711813105] [PMID: 18606986]

[17]   Hillier SL, Moench T, Shattock R, Black R, Reichelderfer P, Veronese F. *In vitro* and *in vivo*: the story of nonoxynol 9. J Acquir Immune Defic Syndr 2005; 39(1): 1-8.
[http://dx.doi.org/10.1097/01.qai.0000159671.25950.74] [PMID: 15851907]

[18]   Walensky RP, Paltiel AD, Losina E, *et al.* The survival benefits of AIDS treatment in the United States. J Infect Dis 2006; 194(1): 11-9.
[http://dx.doi.org/10.1086/505147] [PMID: 16741877]

[19]   Montaner JS, Hogg R, Wood E, *et al.* The case for expanding access to highly active antiretroviral therapy to curb the growth of the HIV epidemic. Lancet 2006; 368(9534): 531-6.
[http://dx.doi.org/10.1016/S0140-6736(06)69162-9] [PMID: 16890841]

[20]   Donnell D, Kiarie J, Thomas K. ART and risk of heterosexual HIV-1 transmission in HIV-1 serodiscordant African couples: A multinational prospective study 17th Conference on Retroviruses and Opportunistic Infections. San Francisco,CA. 2010; pp. 16-9.

[21]   Wood E, Kerr T, Marshall B, Li K. Longitudinal community plasma HIV-1 RNA concentrations and incidence of HIV-1 among injecting drug users: prospective cohort study. BMJ 2009; 338: b1649.
[http://dx.doi.org/10.1136/bmj.b1649]

[22]   Schroeder JR, Epstein DH, Umbricht A, Preston KL. Changes in HIV risk behaviors among patients receiving combined pharmacological and behavioral interventions for heroin and cocaine dependence. Addict Behav 2006; 31(5): 868-79.
[http://dx.doi.org/10.1016/j.addbeh.2005.07.009] [PMID: 16085366]

[23]   Socio-behavioral Issues of New Biomedical HIV Prevention Technologies. Canadian source for HIV HCV guideline 2011. Available frome:http://www.catie.ca/sites/default/files/pdf/NPT%20socio-behavioral_EN.pdf.

[24]   Liu AY, Kittredge PV, Vittinghoff E, *et al.* Limited knowledge and use of HIV post- and pre-exposure prophylaxis among gay and bisexual men. J Acquir Immune Defic Syndr 2008; 47(2): 241-7.
[http://dx.doi.org/10.1097/QAI.0b013e31815e4041] [PMID: 18340656]

[25] Daskalakis D, Bernstein KT, Hagerty R, *et al.* HIV pre- and post-exposure prophylaxis among bathhouse patrons [Abstract]. FL: Jacksonville 2006.

[26] de Silva S, Miller RF, Walsh J. Lack of awareness of HIV post-exposure prophylaxis among HIV-infected and uninfected men attending an inner London clinic. Int J STD AIDS 2006; 17(9): 629-30. [http://dx.doi.org/10.1258/095646206778113177] [PMID: 16942655]

[27] Poynten IM, Jin F, Mao L, *et al.* Nonoccupational postexposure prophylaxis, subsequent risk behaviour and HIV incidence in a cohort of Australian homosexual men. AIDS 2009; 23(9): 1119-26. [http://dx.doi.org/10.1097/QAD.0b013e32832c1776] [PMID: 19417578]

CHAPTER 17

Community Involvement in HIV Prevention

Lillian Mwanri* and Banafsheh Moradmand Badie

Discipline of Public Health, School of Health Sciences, Faulty of Medicine, Nursing and Health Sciences, Flinders University, South Australia

Abstract: The Human Immunodeficiency Virus and AIDS (HIV/AIDS) pandemic remains a public health challenge and a significant obstacle to socioeconomic development especially in developing countries. HIV/AIDS is a serious disease and has claimed millions of lives across the world in recent years. Many Individuals, families and communities including adults and children from across the world, particularly in low-and middle-income countries have been affected by this scourge. To address this problem, community involvement in HIV/AIDS prevention has been recognized, particularly because HIV/AIDS acquisition and transmission occur through community interactions and via complex social networks. Recognition of factors contributing to susceptibility and the spread of HIV/AIDS within countries, societies, communities and populations groups is necessary in order to halt this pandemic. Recognising these factors will inform the development of strategies to address the epidemic within general communities and within specific key population groups. Networks of individuals such as sexual partners, community members and societies need to be recognised as important in HIV transmission and prevention and understanding of communities dynamics including within families, friends and acquaintances should be the first entry point for HIV/AIDS management strategies. Involvement of communities will include developing and implementing community-based approaches to HIV counseling, testing, treatment and prevention. Effective linkages of these approaches with health facility-based services and eradicating the barriers that key populations face in accessing these services are necessary measures. Improving policies and interventions including providing effective education to various key populations and subgroups will facilitate effective life-saving choices.

---

* **Correspondence to Lillian Mwanri:** Discipline of Public Health, School of Health Sciences, Faulty of Medicine, Nursing and Health Sciences, Flinders University, South Australia. GPO Box 2100, Adelaide 5001; Tel: (618) 72218417; Fax: 08 (+618) 72218424; E-mail: lillian.mwanri@flinders.edu.au.

SeyedAhmad SeyedAlinaghi (Ed.)

Keywords: A global challenge, AIDS, Communities, Community involvement, HIV, Key populations, Public health threat, Social networks.

1. INTRODUCTION

Since its initial reporting over three decades ago, the HIV/AIDS contagion has remained a deadly disease without cure, and a significant cause of impairment in public health and development among families, communities and nations across the world. Globally, HIV/AIDS has affected individuals, families and communities with millions of lives lost. Importantly, developing nations and middle income countries are the most affected [1, 2]. Further reports on HIV/AIDS have revealed that more than 30 million people have become victims of this scourge globally, including children [3 - 6]. However, the reported HIV/AIDS prevalence across the globe is variable, with good and not so good stories. For example, it has been reported that HIV/AIDS rates in some countries such as Malawi and Kenya have been declining [3, 6 - 8], while in other countries such as Thailand and in other South East Asian countries, the HIV/AIDS rates are increasing despite earlier reports of declining trends [9]. Additionally, in some countries including the Middle East, the Pacific region, China and India, HIV/AIDS prevalence are reported to be increasing [1, 3, 10]. It has also been noted that, the determinants of susceptibility and acquisition of HIV infection include behaviors of people who have one or more commonalities and interests [10]. In recent years, the importance of community involvement in disease prevention including HIV/AIDS prevention has been recognised [11]. As such, because HIV acquisition and transmission occur between people who interact in one way or another [12], it is necessary to address HIV/AIDS issues through sociocultural networks and community groups. Recognition of the multiplicity of factors contributing to people's susceptibility and the spread of HIV infection within countries, societies, communities and groups of population is critically important to prevent and halt the transmission of this pandemic. It is therefore necessary to recognise dynamics in the society of individuals, community members and social networks in order to develop necessary strategies for prevention of HIV and protection of communities [13]. Communities including families, friends and acquaintances are the first entry point to preventing HIV transmission. Prevention can be done by providing education and reinforcing HIV risk evading behaviors among members of such networks. The family for example, plays a key role in taking care and educating its members who are infected by HIV/AIDS [14]. Because of the advancement of HIV treatment, HIV and related opportunistic infections have become more of chronic health conditions rather than a death sentence and when many individuals are affected within a community, it is necessary to involve the whole community in addressing many complex issues of HIV prevention, including treatment options [15].

2. COMMUNITIES

Medical and public health specialists and practitioners, sociologists, anthropologies, demographers, social workers and other relevant professionals in sectors dealing with HIV pandemic hold varying perspective of what the community is [16]. However, one definition and that will be used in this chapter stands up highly and defines the community as a group of people sharing a common value system, having common needs and sharing interests and have similar or shared experiences [17]. It has also been described that, next to the families, the community is the most important framework in which an individual learns to grow and develop socially and is the center of activities which contribute significantly to the development of human values [18], including those related to HIV transmission. The community provides a space whereby its members develop a sense of attachment with each other through interaction in a variety of social groupings [18 - 20]. Many characteristics of the community structure and interaction have been identified as complex, but overall, members of the community socialise and communicate with each other to share thoughts, feelings, experiences, skills and knowledge [15, 17, 21]. These interactions offer a sense of togetherness among people and are developed in different ways in different communities [12, 21]. Societal member interactions range from simple actions including individual lovers or communities groups' interactions [13]. Communities interact when community members and groups are connected for a common goal including the sharing of resources [16, 17, 22].

Multiple and complex community factors including socio-cultural, economic and structural are involved in the interplay of HIV/AIDS matrix of infection acquisition and transmission [13, 23]. As such, in order to combat the HIV/AIDS complex issues including its prevention, it is crucially important that the community itself is involved for effective outcomes and sustainability.

3. THE ROLE OF THE COMMUNITY IN SUSCEPTIBILITY, TRANSMISSION AND PREVENTION OF HIV INFECTION

The concept of susceptibility often acknowledges the risk factors or circumstance which create the opportunity for community members to acquire HIV infection, and risky behaviors that one does or is forced to engage in, and to become vulnerable and susceptible to this scourge [24, 25]. In terms of HIV/AIDS acquisition and vulnerability, this can be further explained by the following descriptions:

i. increased exposure to the HIV infection is associated with risky environment and social status, and
ii. the potential of acquiring infection due to individual's behaviors.

These facts indicate that there are several factors contributing to the susceptibility of people to HIV infection. These factors include a wide range of individual patterns of behaviors and circumstances such as:

- engaging in multiple sex partners and unsafe sex [26 - 30];
- individuals being involved in drug usage [29, 30];
- economic and social aspects including poverty, unemployment, low-paid that are compounded by high responsibility for family needs or living expenses [31 - 33];
- a wide range of socio-cultural and environmental determinants such as the HIV prevalence in the population, beliefs, literacy and basic knowledge of HIV/AIDS, limited access to HIV/AIDS-related health services, migration and gender inequality [28, 34, 35, 31, 36];
- physiological factors such as differences between men and women's body compositions that lead to enhanced likelihood of women than men being susceptible to HIV/AIDS infection [35, 37].

These factors denote that susceptibility could occur at different levels such as at individual, household and subgroups in the community [38]. In addition, this susceptibility could also occur at a broader context that enhances the transmission of infection in the community. All these indicate that multitude of factors within the community support the susceptibility and the spread of HIV among community members. These factors together, have been described as economic and socio- environmental determinants of HIV/AIDS, *i.e.* factors that could increase or decrease the risk of epidemic and HIV/AIDS transmission in the community [39] (Table **1**). Acknowledgement and understanding of these factors are necessary if the community were to be involved in the prevention of HIV [40].

Table 1. Determinants of HIV/AIDS (Adapted from Barnett and Whiteside, 2006).

Distal determinants →			Proximal determinants
Macro Environment	Micro Environment	Behavior	Biology
Wealth	Mobility and migration	Rate of partner change	Virus sub type
Income Distribution	Urbanization	Prevalence of concurrent partner	Stage of Infection and vial load
Cultural and social norms	Access to Health Care	Sexual interactions	Presence of other sexually transmissible infections (STIs)
Religion	Level of Violence	Condom Use	Sex
Governance	Women's rights and Status		Circumcision
Unemployment	Literary level	Breast Feeding	
Civil unrest	The Prevalence of HIV	Multiple sexual partners	
	Availability of treatment	Peer Pressures	

4. COMMUNITY GROUPS AND HIV PREVENTION

It is a common knowledge that in any community, there is no single group or individuals who are completely protected from HIV/AIDS susceptibility. However, HIV infections impact some community groups more than others; therefore, identifying the risk groups (key populations) is of paramount importance for the success in community-based prevention and other interventions. Economic, social, cultural and structural factors have direct or indirect effects on heightening the rates of HIV infection among subgroups in the community. Identification of groups and tailoring prevention activities across them is necessary. The following community groups have been identified as 'at high risk' or 'key populations' in many communities [41]:

4.1. Female Sex Workers

Female Sex Workers (FSWs) are a group of people (women) who provide sexual services in return for payment [42]. Although there has been improved diagnosis, access to the treatment with antiretroviral therapy (ART) [43], and increased condom use [44], HIV prevalence among FSWs has consistently been higher when compared to other groups in some countries [45 - 47]. For example, in Cambodia, HIV/AIDS prevalence among 'direct' FSWs (brothel based) was 14% in 2006 and over 25% in more recent data from 'indirect' FSWs [47]. This has been reported to be significantly higher rates compared to the prevalence in the general population in Cambodia [47]. Male clients were reported to be drivers of FSWs having unprotected sex because men have more economical power when compared to females [48]. Economic disempowerment has been attributed to driving FSWs to engage in a multiplicity of high-risk activities in order to survive and to meet their needs or wants. The link between economic status and the susceptibility to HIV infection based on the view of economic need (poverty) *versus* economic want (the desire for the material goods) have been described as the main pull and push factors that can drive women's behaviors or render them participate in sex work. To understand these dynamics, it is necessary to involve communities themselves (*i.e.* FSWs) in order to effectively prevent HIV in such groups [32]. In addition, evidence supports the notion that the control of the transmissible diseases including HIV in sex workers, and their clientele is a valuable and cost effective intervention to contain the spread of HIV [42].

4.2. Drug Users

The intravenous drug abuse, addiction and associated behaviors have been linked with HIV since the beginning of the HIV/AIDS epidemic. This link is also associated with a heightened risk for both contracting and transmitting HIV/AIDS and of worsening its consequences [49]. Several studies have found that HIV rates are higher in Injecting Drug Users (IDUs) than non-IDUs [50, 51]. A wide range of studies [47, 52, 53] have demonstrated the link between the use of Amphetamine Type Stimulants (ATS) and the risk of HIV in FSWs. This link may be a direct result of the limited economic opportunities available to particular demographic groups, thus driving vulnerable individuals to engage in harmful economic activity. It has been stated that the use of ATS provides a simultaneous sense of happiness and forgetfulness [47]. These effects have been recognised to impair judgment and can influence poor decision-making during negotiation of the sexual act [54]. Overall, FSWs who use ATS are known to have higher sexual social capital and far reaching sexual networks when compared to non-ATS users. It has also been reported that the use of ATS leads to forgetfulness in condom use with a resultant increase in the risk of HIV transmission and acquisition [54]. It has been recognised that, ATS is commonly used by male clients as a means to delay ejaculation, resulting in prolonged sexual activity [47]. Prolonged and unprotected sexual intercourse has been linked to enhanced HIV/AIDS risk due to damaged tissues due to friction that occurs [47, 52]. Female sex workers also report that ATS using clients are more likely to either encourage the use of ATS or actively seek out ATS using FSWs [52]. Male customers who prefer unprotected sex may also want FSWs who are drug users and often they offer drugs in exchange for unsafe sex [48]. The ATS using FSWs may also accept unprotected sexual intercourse to substitute funding of their own ATS addition [55]. The dynamics between drug use, sex work and HIV risky behaviours are complex and are driven by complex economic and socio-cultural determinants.The FSWs research suggests ATS are often used for occupational reasons such as increasing sociability and lowering inhibitions as a way of dealing with sex work and to increase energy or productivity. The use of ATS has also been reported to have other negative features including impairment of decision-making ability leading to forgetfulness and poor condom use. Female sex workers generally have limited formal education and thus are left with few choices for sustainable income generation [47]. For many FSWs, ATS use is common in the sex work settings and is expected as a necessity for their work [47]. By understanding many of the external factors associated with the ATS use; such as poverty, and how these exacerbate HIV/AIDS, prevention initiatives can be tailored to have much greater impact. This can only be achieved through involving FSWs, gauge their collaboration and for them to be participants in the entire process. Sex workers involvement is very important and is supported by the

Ottawa Charter of Health Promotion which recognises the community involvement as a necessity in any interventions that are required to impact community health's outcomes [40].

4.3. Men Who have Sex with Men

It is recognised that the magnitude of HIV/AIDS scourge differs greatly from setting to setting including within and between countries and from community to community. Globally, men who have sex with men (MSM) engage in anal sex and at times without condom for their own protection from HIV. This practice carries a highly significant risk of HIV transmission when compared to vaginal sex [56]. It is known that HIV was first recognised among young homosexual men in the United State of America (USA) and in other developed countries; and that the global prevalence of HIV is higher among MSM communities in many developed settings [57]. It is thus necessary to understand group dynamics in the community if one wants to address HIV prevalence and its determinants. For example, in America, young African American MSM are more affected by HIV compared to other groups in the same settings even though they are a minority group in the nation [57]. Of importance to note in this group is that in many developed nations, MSM have a disproportionately higher risk of HIV/AIDS due to unprotected anal sex [57, 58]. For example, in Australia 80% of HIV diagnoses are MSM even though they form the minority of the population [58]. In developed countries, cities with bigger communities of MSM have relatively higher HIV infection rates [58]. The high HIV prevalence documented among MSM highlights the necessity to plan and develop special interventions to protect key and vulnerable MSM groups in many countries. Consistently, understanding behaviors and dynamics in MSM groups, intervention targeting them can be effective in the HIV prevention in the community.

4.4. Gender and the Risk of HIV

Women particularly in developing countries have a disproportionately high risk of contracting HIV/AIDS [59 - 62]. It is well acknowledged that women are physiologically more susceptible to HIV than men, and are more likely to be infected with HIV when they have sex with HIV positive men than *vice versa*

[63]. Young women in particular are more vulnerable because their vaginal mucosa is still immature and exposes the inoculums of infected seminal fluid on a large surface area that may be susceptible to trauma during sexual activity, leading to a heighten risk of HIV infection [64]. Cultural and social determinants in some cultures dictate *"gender norms that make it difficult for young women to negotiate safe sex with male partners"* [60, 63]. It is also recognised that women from across the globe are particularly vulnerable when it comes to HIV transmission because of their inability to protect themselves. Many factors including physical, economic, cultural and socio-environmental contribute to their vulnerability [65 - 67]. Furthermore, inequities including in education and in decision making have often heightened women's vulnerability to HIV infection in many communities [7, 9, 68]. In addition, women vulnerability increases directly or indirectly due to violence including sexual or physical violence which they often suffer [65, 69 - 71], often from their closest community members including from past or recent intimate sexual partners [65, 72, 73]. Some studies have reported that group level and cultural empowerment intervention programs for communities who practice polygamous marriages are necessary. Some programs have been instrumental in empowering women at both individual level and as a group. Such programs incorporate interventions that have cultural relevance and help linking individuals to relevant communities [73 - 75]. It is necessary to consider group perspectives especially gender issues in addressing HIV transmission in the future and this should be applicable globally. In circumstances when violence against women is accepted, factors such as the lack of power by women may lead to failure of using protective equipment such as condom. In this context, the interventions that encourage the use of condoms may not be very effective [67], thus effecting other measures may deem necessary. It is imperative to involve the community to enhance the understanding of prohibitive factors to HIV prevention. In addition, the understanding of these factors is necessary in designing HIV prevention interventions in communities.

4.5. Mobile and/or Migrant Groups

The ability to migrate in the past few decades has been considered an important cause of the spread of HIV infection across groups, communities and countries. The International Organisation for Migration (IOM) reported a significant increase in the number of migration and population mobility worldwide [76]. For example, in the inception of the twenty first century one out of every thirty five persons is an international migrant and such condition has vastly contributed to the wider spread of HIV across the world [77]. Globalisation factors including communication technology, financial transfer and ability to travel have led to increased interdependence and movement of people across continents. These factors have also influenced changes in the epidemiology of many diseases including facilitating the transmission of HIV to many geographical and cultural boundaries. Mobility and migration, therefore, are identified as a risk factor for HIV/AIDS within country and across countries [2]. As such, mobility and migration capabilities have implications in many communities and they also challenge the prevention and management of HIV in aforementioned groups, communities and countries across the globe [78 - 80]. Migrants and mobile groups migrate from one place to another due to multiple and complex reasons. Examples include to escape civil unrests in their home environment and/or to search for better opportunities temporarily, seasonally or permanently [78, 81]. The mobility itself does not pose problems, but the environment in which people move to or in, may contribute to their susceptibility to contracting and spreading HIV infection [82, 83]. Some studies have demonstrated the ways through which migration and mobility play pivotal role for the transmission of HIV infection within and across countries. For example, migrant workers have faced significant and complex environmental changes such as being away from their social network of friends, families and communities. This has led to the disruption of social networks which further weakens supervision and sanction against non-normative behaviors. Consequently, they experience changes in culture restraints, live anonymously and they can be socially isolated and lonely. In addition, most migrant groups have poor access to health care due to a myriad of complex factors such as poverty, language barriers and unfamiliarity with the environment and different health and social systems. Under these circumstances they are exposed and succumb to a wide range of pressure and may engage in high-risk behaviors which predispose them to HIV infection. Due to poverty and economic pressure, which forced them to migrate in the first instance, vulnerability to HIV infection increases [78, 83 - 85]. For example, migrant workers have been reported to be disproportionately involved in injecting drugs use, having multiple sex partners and unprotected sex including with Commercial Sex Workers (CSWs). Many have also been reported to have multiple sex partners, which make them more susceptible to HIV infection [77 - 80, 84, 86, 87]. Gazi and colleagues studied behaviors of a specific mobile group of Bangladesh boatmen working across the border with Myanmar and reported that members of this particular group were susceptible to HIV epidemic not only because of the engagement in sexual activities with CSWs but also due to engagement in unprotected sex with other men and in group sex that comprised several people at a time [88]. In addition, several studies inquiring about susceptibility factors to HIV infection among female migrant workers point out that owing to low income and economic pressure the female migrants are engaged in high-risk sexual practices including selling unsafe sex for goods, services and cash, or taking part-time job as CSWs to earn some income for their own survival and to support their families back home [9, 14, 77, 78, 85]. The susceptibility of migrant workers to the epidemic is also exacerbated by exploitation, sexual harassment, sexual violence including rapes and the lack of social protection in their work places [76, 78, 85]. In their study at the Mexico- USA border, Maxwell and colleagues investigated the use of drugs and risk of HIV. Their findings revealed that migrant workers were at risk of contracting HIV due to risky sexual behaviors (engaging in unprotected sex with other males and CSWs, being under the influence of alcohol or drugs when engaging in sexual activities) [89]. Additionally, the lack of knowledge of issues of HIV transmission and prevention has also been cited as one of the risk factors for HIV transmission [89]. In the same study, it was demonstrated that migrants observed low or inconsistent condom use, and share needles and/or injection equipment [89]. In addition, the lack of access to services including the HIV information contributed to increased susceptibility to acquiring HIV infection [77, 86]. UNAIDS has pointed out that migrant workers should be recognised as one of the key populations at increased risk of HIV infection [78]. Additional factors that hinder migrant workers from accessing services and information about HIV include socio-cultural, linguistic, legal and behavioral barriers faced by these groups in the host communities or countries [78, 82, 85]. Other mobile groups who have been reported to be as high-risk for HIV infection are bus drivers, truck drivers and their assistants, sex workers, construction personnel and their sex partners, boatmen and military and/or people in the navy [34, 90, 91]. In order to effectively prevent HIV in these communities, and in accordance with Ottawa Charter and Health Promotion, it is imperative that they are involved and supported in the implementation of activities that may facilitate the prevention of this scourge [40]. Re-orientation of resources and the development of infrastructure that supports the community involvement are all crucial factors [40].

CONCLUSION

This chapter has demonstrated that some groups are more vulnerable to HIV/AIDS than others in many communities. Several factors including financial, human, environmental and social disadvantages place these groups in a more vulnerable position to transmitting and acquiring HIV/AIDS. Un understand of the dynamics and deep issues among these subgroups is required in order to develop targeted programs and interventions for prevention of HIV in their communities [21, 22, 40]. Having identified these groups, it is necessary to tailor prevention messages that reflect the group specific needs and to deliver services and information using pathways and mechanisms including networks that are appropriate for a particular group [40]. Understanding dynamics and networks of specific groups would lead to the development of effective strategies to halt the HIV/AIDS scourge in the community [92, 93]. As communities provide rules and values within which individuals and subgroups operate, it is imperative to identify, consult and involve groups and communities when developing interventions for prevention of HIV. Recognition of multiple and complex factors contributing to the susceptibility and the spread of HIV infection within groups of population, societies, communities and countries is critically important to prevent and restrain the transmission of HIV pandemic. Successful implementation of community health programs and prevention interventions depend in large part on the accurate analysis and understanding of many community and social factors. Community profiling will be required and will need a comprehensive assessment of many complex factors that play role in HIV transmission, resources and potential avenues for prevention.

CONFLICT OF INTEREST

The authors confirm that they have no conflict of interest to declare for this publication.

ACKNOWLEDGEMENTS

Declared none.

REFERENCES

[1]   World Health Organisation.. HIV/AIDS 2012. Available from: http://www.who.int/mediacentre/ factsheets/fs360/en/index.html.

[2]   ADB. Roads and HIV/AIDS, A Resource Book for the Transport Sector. Philippines: Asian Development Bank 2008.

[3]   UNAIDS. HIV/AIDS Epidemic Update Geneva; UNAIDS 2009.

[4]   Cornia GA. UNICEF Innocenti Research Centre. Overview of the impact and best practice response in favour of children in a world affected by HIV/AIDS. AIDS, pub policy and child well-being. Florence: UNESDOC 2006. Available at: http://www.eldis.org/go/home#&id=14526& type=Document#.Vt0Q2kDRpkg

[5]   Save the Children (UK). Children, HIV/AIDS and the Law: A Legal Resource. Pretoria: Save the Children 2001. Available at: http://www.savethechildren.org.uk/

[6]   Phiri S, Webb D. The Impact of HIV/AIDS on Orphans and Program and Policy Responses. In: Cornia GA, Ed. AIDS, Public Policy and Child Well-Being. Florence: UNICEF, Eastern and Southern Africa Regional Office 2002. Available at: http://www.unicef-irc.org/publications/476.

[7]   UNAIDS. Report on the Global HIV/AIDS Epidemic. Geneva: UNAIDS 2004.

[8]   Sweat M, Gregorich S, Sangiwa G, *et al.* Cost-effectiveness of voluntary HIV-1 counselling and testing in reducing sexual transmission of HIV-1 in Kenya and Tanzania. Lancet 2000; 356(9224): 113-21.
[http://dx.doi.org/10.1016/S0140-6736(00)02447-8] [PMID: 10963247]

[9]   UNAIDS. Gender and HIV/AIDS: taking stock of research and programmes. Geneva: UNAIDS 1999.

[10]   WHO. World Health Statistics. Geneva: World Health Organisation 2011.

[11]   Bundara N, Mwanri L, Masika J. Addressing Childhood undernutrition in Tanzania: Challenges and Opportunities. African J Food, Agricul Nutr Develop 2013; 13(1): 7288-306.

[12]   Smith KP, Christakis NA. Social networks and health. Annu Rev Sociol 2008; 34: 405-29.
[http://dx.doi.org/10.1146/annurev.soc.34.040507.134601]

[13]   Towle M, Lende DH. Community approaches to preventing mother-to-child HIV transmission: perspectives from rural Lesotho. Afr J AIDS Res 2008; 7(2): 219-28.
[http://dx.doi.org/10.2989/AJAR.2008.7.2.7.524] [PMID: 25864398]

[14]   Makoae MG, Mokoman Z. 'Examining Women's Vulnerability to HIV Transmission and the Impact of AIDS: The Role of Peer Education/Peer Support in Lesotho's Garment Industry'Final Report to CARE Lesotho-South Africa Country Office Cape Town. Queensland, Australia: Human Science Research Council 2008.

[15]   Crystal S, Kersting RC. Stress, social support, and distress in a statewide population of persons with AIDS in New Jersey. Soc Work Health Care 1998; 28(1): 41-60.
[http://dx.doi.org/10.1300/J010v28n01_03] [PMID: 9711685]

[16]   Bracht N. Health Promotion at the Community Level: New Advances. 2nd ed., Calfornia: SAGE Publications, Inc 1999.

[17]   Hillery J. definition of community: Areas of agreement. Rural Sociol 1955; 20(2): 118-27.

[18]   Feaster D, Robbins M, Szapocznik J. Using individual level data in family assessment: hierarchical linear modeling with African American HIV+ mothers and their families. Miami, FL: University of Miami, Center for Family Studies 2000.

[19]   UNICEF. The Situation of Families and Children affected by HIV/AIDS in Vietnam. Vietnam: UNICEF 2004.

[20]   Ishikawa N, Pridmore P, Carr-Hill R, Chaimuangdee K. The attitudes of primary schoolchildren in Northern Thailand towards their peers who are affected by HIV and AIDS. AIDS Care 2011; 23(2): 237-44.
[http://dx.doi.org/10.1080/09540121.2010.507737] [PMID: 21259137]

[21]   Mwanri L, Hiruy K, Masika J. Empowerment as a tool for a healthy resettlement: a case of new African settlers in South Australia. Int J Migr Health Soc Care 2012; 8(2): 86-98.
[http://dx.doi.org/10.1108/17479891211250021]

[22]   Hiruy K, Mwanri L. End-of-life experiences and expectations of Africans in Australia: Cultural implications for palliative and hospice care Nursing Ethics , 2013 [Last date access: 03-12-2014]; Availabe at: http://nej.sagepub.com/ content/early/2013/03/04/0969733012475252

[23]   Latkin CA, Knowlton AR. Micro-social structural approaches to HIV prevention: a social ecological perspective. AIDS Care 2005; 17 (Suppl. 1): S102-13.
[http://dx.doi.org/10.1080/09540120500121185] [PMID: 16096122]

[24]   Masanjala W. The poverty-HIV/AIDS nexus in Africa: a livelihood approach. Soc Sci Med 2007; 64(5): 1032-41.
[http://dx.doi.org/10.1016/j.socscimed.2006.10.009] [PMID: 17126972]

[25]   Morton J. Conceptualizing the Links between HIV/AIDS and Pastoralist Livelihoods, inThe. Eur J Dev Res 2006; 18(2): 235-54.
[http://dx.doi.org/10.1080/09578810600708247]

[26]   Loevinsohn M, Gillespie S. HIV/AIDS, Food Security and Rural Livelihoods: Understanding and Responding, International Food Policy Research Institute. Washington, D.C., USA: IFPRI 2003.

[27]   Müller TR. HIV/AIDS and Human Development in sub-Saharan Africa. The Netherlands: Wageningen Academic Publishers 2005.
[http://dx.doi.org/10.3920/978-90-8686-560-4]

[28]   De Santis JP. HIV infection risk factors among male-to-female transgender persons: a review of the literature. J Assoc Nurses AIDS Care 2009; 20(5): 362-72.
[http://dx.doi.org/10.1016/j.jana.2009.06.005] [PMID: 19732695]

[29]   Peretti-Watel P, Spire B, Schiltz MA, *et al*. VESPA Group. Vulnerability, unsafe sex and non-adherence to HAART: evidence from a large sample of French HIV/AIDS outpatients. Soc Sci Med 2006; 62(10): 2420-33.
[http://dx.doi.org/10.1016/j.socscimed.2005.10.020] [PMID: 16289743]

[30]   Nemoto T, Operario D, Keatley J, Han L, Soma T. HIV risk behaviors among male-to-female transgender persons of color in San Francisco. Am J Public Health 2004; 94(7): 1193-9.
[http://dx.doi.org/10.2105/AJPH.94.7.1193] [PMID: 15226142]

[31]   Paudel V, Baral KP. Women living with HIV/AIDS (WLHA), battling stigma, discrimination and denial and the role of support groups as a coping strategy: a review of literature. Reprod Health 2015; 12: 53.
[http://dx.doi.org/10.1186/s12978-015-0032-9] [PMID: 26032304]

[32]   Byron E, Gillespie S, Hamazakaza P. Local Perceptions of HIV Risk and Prevention in Southern Zambia, International Food Policy Research Institute. Zambia: IFPRI 2006.

[33]   Chapoto A. The impact of AIDS-related prime-age mortality on rural farm households: Panel survey evidence from Zambia, Ph.D. dissertation, Michigan State University, East Lansing, Michigan. 2006.

[34]   Fauk KN. Factors Contributing to the Susceptibility to HIV Infection: A Case of Ojek Community in Belu District, East Nusa Tenggara, Indonesia, Master Thesis, Van Hall Larenstein University, Wageningen, The Netherlands 2010.

[35]   Karim A Q, Sibeko S, Baxter C. Preventing HIV infection in women: a global healthimperative. Clin Infect Dis 2010; 50 (4): 122-9.

[36]   Durban. Using rights and law to reduce women's vulnerability to HIV. Can HIV AIDS Policy Law Rev 2000; 5(4): 1-12.
[PMID: 11833150]

[37]   Higgins JA, Hoffman S, Dworkin SL. Rethinking gender, heterosexual men, and women's vulnerability to HIV/AIDS. Am J Public Health 2010; 100(3): 435-45.
[http://dx.doi.org/10.2105/AJPH.2009.159723] [PMID: 20075321]

[38]   ITDG. Impact of HIV/AIDS among Pastoral Communities in Kenya. Nairobi, Kenya: International Technology Development Group 2005.

[39]   Barnett T, Whiteside A. AIDS in the Twenty-First Century. London: Palgrave Macmillan 2006.

[40]   World Health Organisation. The Ottawa Charter for Health Promotion. Geneva: WHO 1986.

[41]   Zinberg N. Drugs, Set and Setting: The Basis for Controlled Intoxicant Use. New Haven: Yale University Press 1984.

[42]   Laga M, Alary M, Nzila N, *et al*. Condom promotion, sexually transmitted diseases treatment, and declining incidence of HIV-1 infection in female Zairian sex workers. Lancet 1994; 344(8917): 246-8.
[http://dx.doi.org/10.1016/S0140-6736(94)93005-8] [PMID: 7913164]

[43]   Charles M. HIV epidemic in Cambodia, one of the poorest countries in Southeast Asia: a success

story. Expert Rev Anti Infect Ther 2006; 4(1): 1-4.
[http://dx.doi.org/10.1586/14787210.4.1.1] [PMID: 16441203]

[44] Saphonn V, Parekh BS, Dobbs T, *et al.* Trends of HIV-1 seroincidence among HIV-1 sentinel surveillance groups in Cambodia, 1999-2002. J Acquir Immune Defic Syndr 2005; 39(5): 587-92.
[PMID: 16044012]

[45] Sopheab H, Morineau G, Neal JJ, Saphonn V, Fylkesnes K. Sustained high prevalence of sexually transmitted infections among female sex workers in Cambodia: high turnover seriously challenges the 100% Condom Use Programme. BMC Infect Dis 2008; 8: 167.
[http://dx.doi.org/10.1186/1471-2334-8-167] [PMID: 19077261]

[46] NCHADS. Ministry of Health National Center for HIV, AIDS, Dermatology and STDs: Annual Report National Centre for HIV/AIDS, Dermatology and STDs , 2006 [Accessed 19th September 2012]; Available at: http://www.nchads.org/report.php

[47] Maher L, Phlong P, Mooney-Somers J, *et al.* Amphetamine-type stimulant use and HIV/STI risk behaviour among young female sex workers in Phnom Penh, Cambodia. Int J Drug Policy 2011; 22(3): 203-9.
[http://dx.doi.org/10.1016/j.drugpo.2011.01.003] [PMID: 21316935]

[48] Johnston CL, Callon C, Li K, Wood E, Kerr T. Offer of financial incentives for unprotected sex in the context of sex work. Drug Alcohol Rev 2010; 29(2): 144-9.
[http://dx.doi.org/10.1111/j.1465-3362.2009.00091.x] [PMID: 20447221]

[49] WHO. Assessment of compulsory treatment of people who use drugs in Cambodia, China, Malaysia and Viet Nam: An application of selected human rights principles, World Health Organisation , 2009 [Accessed 19th February 2013]; Available at: http://www.wpro.who.int/publications/docs/FINALforWeb_Mar17_Compulsory_Treatment.pdf

[50] Bassols AM, Santos RA, Rohde LA, Pechansky F. Exposure to HIV in Brazilian adolescents: the impact of psychiatric symptomatology. Eur Child Adolesc Psychiatry 2007; 16(4): 236-42.
[http://dx.doi.org/10.1007/s00787-006-0595-7] [PMID: 17200792]

[51] Rhodes T, Singer M, Bourgois P, Friedman SR, Strathdee SA. The social structural production of HIV risk among injecting drug users. Soc Sci Med 2005; 61(5): 1026-44.
[http://dx.doi.org/10.1016/j.socscimed.2004.12.024] [PMID: 15955404]

[52] Couture M, Neth S, Vonthanak S, *et al.* Correlates of amphetamine-type stimulant use and associations with HIV-related risks among young women engaged in sex work in Phnom Penh, Cambodia. Drug Alcohol Depend 2012; 120(1-3): 119-26.
[http://dx.doi.org/10.1016/j.drugalcdep.2011.07.005] [PMID: 23186171]

[53] Kab V, Evans J, Sansothy N, *et al.* Young Women's Study Collaborative. Testing for amphetamine-type stimulant (ATS) use to ascertain validity of self-reported ATS use among young female sex workers in Cambodia. Addict Sci Clin Pract 2012; 7: 11.
[http://dx.doi.org/10.1186/1940-0640-7-11] [PMID: 23186171]

[54] Halkitis PN, Jerome RC. A comparative analysis of methamphetamine use: black gay and bisexual men in relation to men of other races. Addict Behav 2008; 33(1): 83-93.
[http://dx.doi.org/10.1016/j.addbeh.2007.07.015] [PMID: 17825996]

[55]   Needle R, Kroeger K, Belani H, Achrekar A, Parry CD, Dewing S. Sex, drugs, and HIV: rapid assessment of HIV risk behaviors among street-based drug using sex workers in Durban, South Africa. Soc Sci Med 2008; 67(9): 1447-55.
[http://dx.doi.org/10.1016/j.socscimed.2008.06.031] [PMID: 18678437]

[56]   Grant RM, Lama JR, Anderson PL, *et al.* iPrEx Study Team. Preexposure chemoprophylaxis for HIV prevention in men who have sex with men. N Engl J Med 2010; 363(27): 2587-99.
[http://dx.doi.org/10.1056/NEJMoa1011205] [PMID: 21091279]

[57]   Koblin B, Chesney M, Coates T, *et al.* EXPLORE Study Team. Effects of a behavioural intervention to reduce acquisition of HIV infection among men who have sex with men: the EXPLORE randomised controlled study. Lancet 2004; 364(9428): 41-50.
[http://dx.doi.org/10.1016/S0140-6736(04)16588-4] [PMID: 15234855]

[58]   Victorian AIDS Council. Gay Men's Health Centre fact Sheet , 2013 [Accessed 24/04/2013]; Available at: http://www.vicaids.asn.au/

[59]   Van Loggerenberg F, Dieter AA, Sobieszczyk ME, Werner L, Grobler A, Mlisana K. CAPRISA 002 Acute Infection Study Team. HIV prevention in high-risk women in South Africa: condom use and the need for change. PLoS One 2012; 7(2): e30669.
[http://dx.doi.org/10.1371/journal.pone.0030669] [PMID: 22363467]

[60]   Mantell JE, Harrison A, Hoffman S, Smit JA, Stein ZA, Exner TM. The Mpondombili Project: preventing HIV/AIDS and unintended pregnancy among rural South African school-going adolescents. Reprod Health Matters 2006; 14(28): 113-22.
[http://dx.doi.org/10.1016/S0968-8080(06)28269-7] [PMID: 17101429]

[61]   Jewkes RK, Levin JB, Penn-Kekana LA. Gender inequalities, intimate partner violence and HIV preventive practices: findings of a South African cross-sectional study. Soc Sci Med 2003; 56(1): 125-34.
[http://dx.doi.org/10.1016/S0277-9536(02)00012-6] [PMID: 12435556]

[62]   Eaton L, Flisher AJ, Aarø LE. Unsafe sexual behaviour in South African youth. Soc Sci Med 2003; 56(1): 149-65.
[http://dx.doi.org/10.1016/S0277-9536(02)00017-5] [PMID: 12435558]

[63]   Fourie P. The Political Management of HIV and AIDS in South Africa: One Burden Too Many. New York: Palgrave Macmillan 2006.
[http://dx.doi.org/10.1057/9780230627222]

[64]   Leclerc-Madlala S. Age-disparate and intergenerational sex in southern Africa: the dynamics of hypervulnerability. AIDS 2008; 22(4) (Suppl. 4): S17-25.
[http://dx.doi.org/10.1097/01.aids.0000341774.86500.53] [PMID: 19033752]

[65]   Amaro H. Love, sex, and power. Considering women's realities in HIV prevention. Am Psychol 1995; 50(6): 437-47.
[http://dx.doi.org/10.1037/0003-066X.50.6.437] [PMID: 7598292]

[66]   Ehrhardt AA, Sawires S, McGovern T, Peacock D, Weston M. Gender, empowerment, and health: what is it? How does it work? J Acquir Immune Defic Syndr 2009; 51 (Suppl. 3): S96-S105.
[http://dx.doi.org/10.1097/QAI.0b013e3181aafd54] [PMID: 19553784]

[67]   Wingood GM, Scd , DiClemente RJ. Application of the theory of gender and power to examine HIV-related exposures, risk factors, and effective interventions for women. Health Educ Behav 2000; 27(5): 539-65.
[http://dx.doi.org/10.1177/109019810002700502] [PMID: 11009126]

[68]   Padian NS, Shiboski SC, Jewell NP. Female-to-male transmission of human immunodeficiency virus. JAMA 1991; 266(12): 1664-7.
[http://dx.doi.org/10.1001/jama.1991.03470120066034] [PMID: 1886189]

[69]   Huda S. Sex trafficking in South Asia. Int J Gynaecol Obstet 2006; 94(3): 374-81.
[http://dx.doi.org/10.1016/j.ijgo.2006.04.027] [PMID: 16846602]

[70]   Upchurch DM, Kusunoki Y. Associations between forced sex, sexual and protective practices, and sexually transmitted diseases among a national sample of adolescent girls. Womens Health Issues 2004; 14(3): 75-84.
[http://dx.doi.org/10.1016/j.whi.2004.03.006] [PMID: 15193635]

[71]   Wyatt GE, Myers HF, Loeb TB. Women, Trauma, and HIV: an overview. AIDS Behav 2004; 8(4): 401-3.
[http://dx.doi.org/10.1007/s10461-004-7324-3] [PMID: 15690113]

[72]   Hunter M. The changing political economy of sex in South Africa: the significance of unemployment and inequalities to the scale of the AIDS pandemic. Soc Sci Med 2007; 64(3): 689-700.
[http://dx.doi.org/10.1016/j.socscimed.2006.09.015] [PMID: 17097204]

[73]   Epstein H. The invisible cure: Africa, the west, and the fight against AIDS. New York: Farrar Straus & Giroux 2007.

[74]   DiClemente RJ, Wingood GM, Blank MB, Metzger DS. Future directions for HIV prevention research: charting a prevention science research agenda. J Acquir Immune Defic Syndr 2008; 47 (Suppl. 1): S47-8.
[http://dx.doi.org/10.1097/QAI.0b013e3181605e5d] [PMID: 18301134]

[75]   Wingood GM, DiClemente RJ. The ADAPT-ITT model: a novel method of adapting evidence-based HIV Interventions. J Acquir Immune Defic Syndr 2008; 47 (Suppl. 1): S40-6.
[http://dx.doi.org/10.1097/QAI.0b013e3181605df1] [PMID: 18301133]

[76]   IOM. Population, Mobility and HIV/AIDS. Geneva, Switzerland: International Organization for Migration 2003.

[77]   Ahn ND, Hung NL, Tra BT, Quynh VH. Mobility and HIV Vulnerability in Viet Nam: A review of published and unpublished data and implications for HIV prevention programmes, Canada South East Asia Regional HIV/AIDS Programme (CSEARHAP); Canada 2008.

[78]   Population Mobility and AIDS. UNAIDS: Geneva, Switzerland 2001.

[79]   Saggurti N, Mahapatra B, Swain N S, Jain K N. Male maigration and risky sexual behavior in Rural India: is the place of origin critical for HIV prevention programs? BMC Public Health 2011; 11 (1): 1-13.

[80]   Halli SS, Buzdugan R, Saggurti N, *et al.* Migration/Mobility and Vulnerability to HIV among Male Migrant Workers. Karnataka, India: Population Council 2008.

[81]   Butt L, Numbery G, Morin J. Preventing AIDS in Papua. Papua: Kotaraja 2002.

[82]   JUNIWA. The Threat Posed by the Economic Crisis to Universal Access to HIV Services For Migrants. Bangkok: Joint United Nations Initiative on Mobility and HIV/AIDS 2009.

[83]   Anh ND. The HIV/AIDS Vulnerability of Labour Out-Migrants and its Consequences on the Left-behind at the Household Level. Hanoi, Viet Nam: Institute of Sociology 2009.

[84]   Greif MJ, Nii-Amoo Dodoo F. Internal migration to Nairobi's slums: linking migrant streams to sexual risk behavior. Health Place 2011; 17(1): 86-93.
        [http://dx.doi.org/10.1016/j.healthplace.2010.08.019] [PMID: 20884274]

[85]   IOM. HIV and Bangladeshi Women Migrant Workers: An Assessment of Vulnerabilities and Gaps in Services. Geneva, Switzerland: International Organization for Migration 2012.

[86]   Pandey H, Shukla KK. The probability model for risk of vulnerability to STDs/or HIV infection among pre-marital female migrants in Urban India. J Appl Quant Methods 2010; 5(1): 145-51.

[87]   Yang H, Li X, Stanton B, *et al.* Workplace and HIV-related sexual behaviours and perceptions among female migrant workers. AIDS Care 2005; 17(7): 819-33.
        [http://dx.doi.org/10.1080/09540120500099902] [PMID: 16120499]

[88]   Gazi R, Mercer A, Wansom T, Kabir H, Saha NC, Azim T. An assessment of vulnerability to HIV infection of boatmen in Teknaf, Bangladesh. Confl Health 2008; 2(5): 5.
        [http://dx.doi.org/10.1186/1752-1505-2-5] [PMID: 18341696]

[89]   Maxwell C J, Cravioto P, Galvan F. Drug use and risk of HIV/AIDS on the Mexico-UAS border: a comparison of treatment admissions in both countries. Drug Alcohol Depend 2006; 82 (5): 85-93.

[90]   Jabbari H. Lack of HIV infection among truck drivers in Iran by rapid HIV test. J Rese Med Sci 2010; 15(5): 287-9.

[91]   Jabbari H, Aghamollaie S. Frequency of HIV infection among sailors in south of Iran by rapid HIV Test. AIDS Res Treat 2011; 2011: 612475.
        [http://dx.doi.org/ 10.1155/2011/612475] [PMID: 612475]

[92]   Browning CR, Leventhal T, Brooks-Gunn J. Neighborhood context and racial differences in early adolescent sexual activity. Demography 2004; 41(4): 697-720.
        [http://dx.doi.org/10.1353/dem.2004.0029] [PMID: 15622950]

[93]   Cohen S, Janicki-Deverts D. Can we improve our physical health by altering our social networks? Perspect Psychol Sci 2009; 4(4): 375-8.
        [http://dx.doi.org/10.1111/j.1745-6924.2009.01141.x] [PMID: 20161087]

CHAPTER 18

Positive Prevention

Seyed Ramin Radfar[*]

University of California, Los Angeles, Integrated Substance Abuse Programs, Los Angeles, USA

Abstract: In order to control HIV epidemic, people should avoid high-risk behaviors related to the transmission of HIV regardless of their HIV status. The practice of best known strategies for avoiding HIV infection is both true for People Living with HIV (PLHIVs) and the sero-negative people. However, HIV may be transmitted via two scenarios: the first is that the HIV-positive person is unaware of his/her sero-status, and the second is that the HIV-positive person ignores his/her sero-positivity.

Positive Health, Dignity and Prevention (PHDP) covers a broad spectrum of policies and activities not only for PLHIVs but also for all of the members of a community, hence we all have responsibilities in the control of HIV epidemic.

Positive Health, Dignity and Prevention is not just a new name for the concept of HIV prevention for and by people living with HIV, formerly known as 'positive prevention'. Implementation of PHDP would not be similar in different settings (*i.e.* available resources, stages of the epidemic, *etc.*); but in all communities, eight major components have been introduced as the framework of PHDP activities, that are: advocacy, building evidence, coverage scale up, increase in access to services, serodiscordant couples protection, influence the responsibilities of PLHIVs, stigma and discrimination reduction and scaling up and supporting the social capital

Keywords: Advocacy, Evidence based, Dignity, Health, HIV transmission, Human Rights, Most at risk populations, Positive Prevention, Prevention, Quality of life, Research, Sero discordant couples.

[*] **Correspondence to Seyed Ramin Radfar:** UCLA Integrated Substance Abuse Programs, University of California, 11075 Santa Monica Blvd., Suite 200, Los Angeles, CA 90025, USA; Tel: +3102675399; Fax: +3103120538; E-mail: raminradfar@yahoo.com.

SeyedAhmad SeyedAlinaghi (Ed.)

1. INTRODUCTION

In order to control HIV epidemic, people should avoid high-risk behaviors related to the transmission of HIV regardless of their HIV status. The practice of best known strategies for avoiding HIV infection is both true for People Living with HIV (PLHIVs) and the sero-negative people. However, HIV may be transmitted *via* two scenarios: the first is that the HIV-positive person is unaware of his/her sero-status, and the second is that the HIV-positive person ignores his/her sero-positivity. Subsequently, unsafe sexual contacts and/or needle sharing practices are the main routes of transmission which occur after the first two states.

Tailoring appropriate and effective interventions for PLHIVs is one of the most important strategies for the control of epidemic. It means that for having a nationally effective response to epidemic, we need to get PLHIVs participation in different levels of interventions from policy making to field work [1]. HIV transmission in almost all of the cases is highly related to human behaviors. Unfortunately, changing high-risk behaviors to safe behaviors is not usually simple, and the desirable change in marginalized and most at risk populations is considerably harder compared to the other sections of a community. Moreover, anti-retroviral therapy increases the lifespan of PLHIVs and decreases their morbidity. Accordingly, a larger population of PLHIV should control their risky behaviors for halting the spread of the infection. For example, practicing safer sex for PLHIVs is probably hard in the long term [2]. In this regard, some studies found that different factors such as self-efficacy, responsibility, drug use, mental health and the context of the community that the PLHIVs are living should be considered as factors that can promote or demote positive prevention activities among PLHIVs [3].

2. POSITIVE HEALTH, DIGNITY AND PREVENTION

Positive prevention may be considered as an approach [4] or strategy [4, 5] or simply as a package of activities; but all of such definitions are similar in the fact that they focus on PLHIVs. According to the current literature, there was a misconception about the continuum and definition of positive prevention until 2008 [6]. In 2011, UNAIDS introduced a new framework for what we called

Positive Prevention as well as the Global Network of People Living with HIV [7]. The new term contains not only the concept of positive prevention, but also health and dignity and is "Positive Health, Dignity and Prevention". Positive Health, Dignity and Prevention (PHDP) covers a broader spectrum of policies and activities not only for PLHIVs but also for all of the members of a community, hence we all have responsibilities in the control HIV epidemic.

"Positive Health, Dignity and Prevention is not just a new name for the concept of HIV prevention for and by people living with HIV, formerly known as 'positive prevention'. Rather, Positive Health, Dignity and Prevention is built on a broader basis that includes improving and maintaining the dignity of the individual living with HIV, to support and enhance that individual's physical, mental, emotional and sexual health, and which, in turn, among other benefits, creates an enabling environment that will reduce the likelihood of new HIV infections".

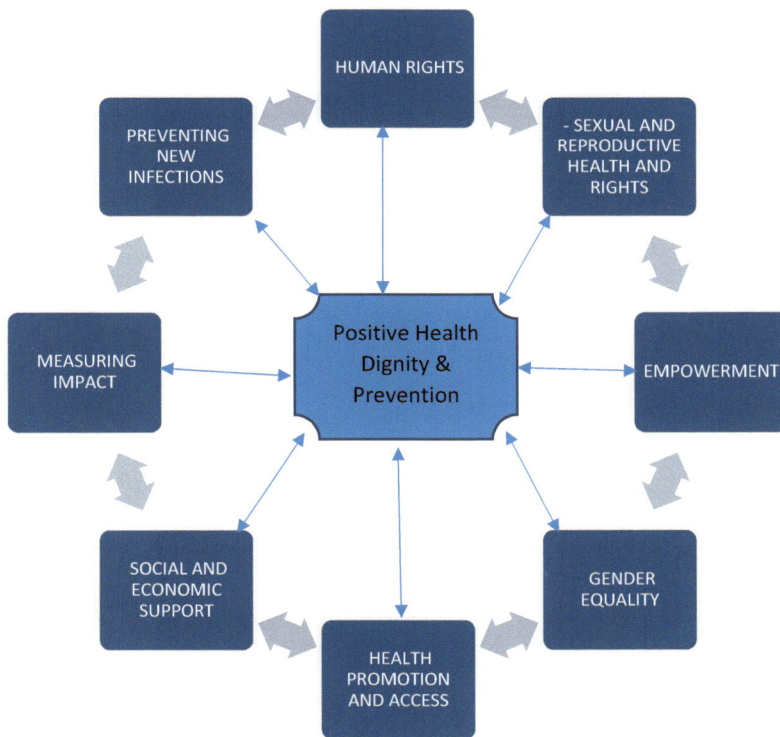

Fig. (1). Major components of Positive Health, Dignity and Prevention (PHDP).

Implementation of PHDP would not be similar in different settings (*i.e.* available resources, stages of the epidemic, *etc.*); but in all communities, eight major components have been introduced as the framework of PHDP activities [7]. (Fig. **1**) shows these components.

According to this framework, nine groups of activities should be considered prior to implementation of interventional programs at the community level [7]:

1. Advocacy: for having a meaningful and broad-based mobilization of PLHIVs in HIV prevention, not only at individual level but also at organizational level such as NGOs and CBOs from local to international levels.
2. Building Evidence: The discovery of HIV and its related interventions goes back to less than 40 years ago; accordingly, more evidence is needed to better judge the health concerns.

The other activities include dissemination, policy dialogue, planning, implementation, integration, monitoring and evaluation and finally adaptation and improvement (For more study please see Positive Health, Dignity and Prevention: A Policy Framework. Amsterdam, GNP+).

1. Researchers have to address the following questions in the field of positive prevention: How to increase and scale up coverage of the evidence-based interventions in different settings and different target groups that usually have dynamic changes?
2. How to increase the access and use interventions that have been designed for increasing the quality of life of PLHIVs?
3. How to protect serodiscordant couples? How we can promote safer sex practices among the couples?
4. Which factors influence the responsibilities of PLHIVs regarding their health and the health conditions of other people?
5. How we can eliminate or at least decrease the stigma and discrimination toward PLHIVs in different levels of a community?
6. How we can scale up and support the social capital programs that focus on community-driven, sustainable responses to HIV?

CONFLICT OF INTEREST

The author confirms that author has no conflict of interest to declare for this publication.

ACKNOWLEDGEMENTS

Declared none.

REFERENCES

[1]   Practical Guidelines for Intensifying HIV Prevention; towards universal access 2007.Geneva: Joint United Nations Programme on HIV/AIDS (UNAIDS), Switzerland. Available from: http://www.stopaidsnow.org/practical-guidelines-intensifying-hiv-prevention-towards-universal-access

[2]   Gordon CM, Stall R, Cheever LW. Prevention interventions with persons living with HIV/AIDS: challenges, progress, and research priorities. J Acquir Immune Defic Syndr 2004; 37 (Suppl. 2): S53-7. [http://dx.doi.org/10.1097/01.qai.0000142321.27136.8b] [PMID: 15385900]

[3]   Wolitski RJ, Parsons JT, Gómez CA. SUMS Study Team, SUMIT Study Team. Prevention with HIV-seropositive men who have sex with men: lessons from the Seropositive Urban Men's Study (SUMS) and the Seropositive Urban Men's Intervention Trial (SUMIT). J Acquir Immune Defic Syndr 2004; 37 (Suppl. 2): S101-9.
[http://dx.doi.org/10.1097/01.qai.0000140608.36393.37] [PMID: 15385906]

[4]   Positive Prevention Prevention Strategies for People with HIV/AIDS. International HIV/AIDS Alliance 2003. Available from: http://www.cdc.gov/hiv/topics/prev_prog/AHP/resources/other/pdf/Positive_Prevention_IHA_Marked.pdf

[5]   Kennedy CE, Medley AM, Sweat MD, O'Reilly KR. Behavioural interventions for HIV positive prevention in developing countries: a systematic review and meta-analysis. Bull World Health Organ 2010; 88(8): 615-23.
[http://dx.doi.org/10.2471/BLT.09.068213] [PMID: 20680127]

[6]   Positive Prevention; towards a Pan-Canadian Framework; A discussion paper. Canadian AIDS Society 2012. Available from: www.cdnaids.ca/Positive_Prevention.

[7]   Mallouris Christoforos. Positive Health, Dignity and Prevention: A Policy Framework. UNAIDS, Switzerland 2011; pp.2-47. Available from: http://www.unaids.org/sites/default/files/media_asset/20110701_PHDP_0.pdf

Management Model of Positive Clubs

SeyedAhmad SeyedAlinaghi[1,2], May Sudhinaraset[3], Hamid Emadi Koochak[1], Koosha Paydary[1,4,*], Sahra Emamzadeh-Fard[5], Sepideh Khodaei[1] and Sara Sardashti[1]

[1] *Iranian Research Center for HIV/AIDS, Iranian Institute for Reduction of High Risk Behaviors, Tehran University of Medical Sciences, Tehran, Iran*

[2] *Tehran Positive Club, Tehran, Iran*

[3] *Global Health Sciences, University of California San Francisco, CA, USA*

[4] *Students' Scientific Research Center (SSRC), Tehran University of Medical Sciences (TUMS), Tehran, Iran*

[5] *Department of Radiology, Division of Interventional Radiology, Memorial Sloan-Kettering Cancer Center, New York, USA*

Abstract: Aiming the positive prevention, psychosocial support and reduction of stigma and discrimination, positive clubs have been established in Iran since 2006. We created a systematic management procedure using the Logical Framework Approach (LFA) and Work Breakdown Structure (WBS). Based on this model, a central council including trained people living with HIV (PLHIV) provides the management for positive clubs. Subsequently, under the supervision of this council, different practical committees are formed. These committees are in close interaction with each other and by participation of HIV positive and negative volunteers, we may anticipate the empowerment of people living with HIV as well as reduction of stigma and discrimination at the community level. The objective of this chapter is to discuss a conceptual model based on LFA and WBS in order to identify appropriate management and increase participation and empowerment of PLHIV in positive clubs. Challenges and recommendations of implementing this type of model for prevention efforts are also discussed.

*** Correspondence to Koosha Paydary:** Iranian Research Center for HIV/AIDS (IRCHA), Imam Khomeini Hospital, Keshavarz Blvd., Tehran, Iran; Tel/Fax: +98 (21) 66947984; E-mail: paydarykoosha@gmail.com.

Keywords: Committees, Council, Discrimination, Logical framework approach, Model, People living with HIV, Positive club, Positive prevention, Psychosocial support, Stigma, Work breakdown structure.

1. INTRODUCTION

It would certainly be impossible to develop a successful national program to control HIV/AIDS without participation of People Living with HIV (PLHIV). Organizations of PLHIV are significant in the response to the global HIV/AIDS epidemic where by sufficient support, PLHIV may play a key role in the delivery of AIDS programs in their communities [1, 2]. The active participation of PLHIV empowers and urges the AIDS efforts further encouraging other people into action [1, 2]. Also, the Greater Involvement of People Living with AIDS (GIPA) in principle aims to enhance the quality and effectiveness of the AIDS response at the community and social level. Public involvement of PLHIV may break down the fear and prejudice and demonstrate that they may be productive members of the society [1, 3].

One of the most remarkable achievements in Iran is the establishment of positive clubs in 2006 under the supervision of relevant medical universities. Such clubs were designed to use community resources (non-governmental organizations) and the specialist, technical assistance of medical universities [2]. Objectives of positive clubs are positive prevention, psychosocial support with the aim of empowering and developing the capacities of PLHIV for the management and improvement of life skills as well as reduction of stigma and discrimination [4, 5]. The positive prevention is a collection of strategies which help PLHIV for adhering to healthier and longer lives. Thus, positive prevention is about maintaining the reproductive health, preventing sexually transmitted infections (STIs) and HIV infection progress in addition to increasing PLHIV responsibilities for prevention of HIV/AIDS [6]. Also, this approach strengthens the national response by mobilizing peer groups to promote the personal health of PLHIV, comply with treatment and prevention, fight stigma and social discrimination, and provide them with psychosocial support [6].

The objective of this chapter is to discuss a conceptual model based on Logical

Framework Approach (LFA) and Work Breakdown Structure (WBS) in order to identify appropriate management and increase participation and empowerment of PLHIV in positive clubs.

2. THE MODEL

We designed a unique method to address the issue of management of positive clubs including who should manage the positive clubs and the processes of implementing a positive club, outlined in Table **1**, Figs. (**1a** and **1b**). Supervisory tools are also outlined in Table **1**.

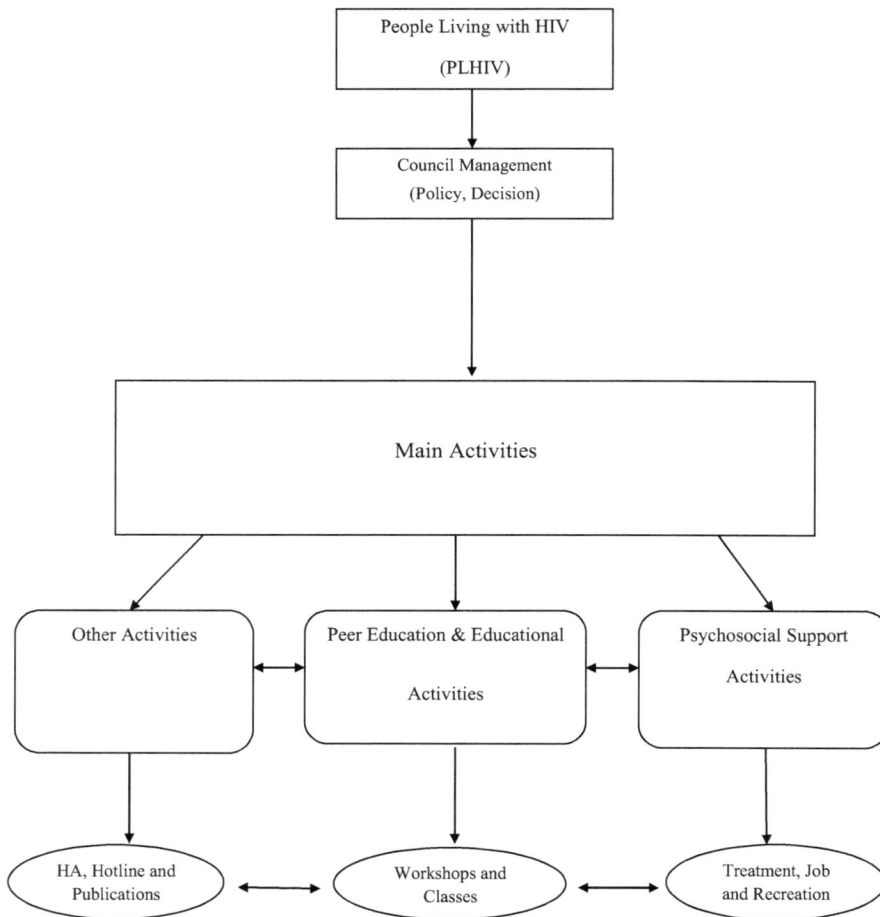

Fig. 1(a). Work Breakdown Structure (WBS) based on tasks.

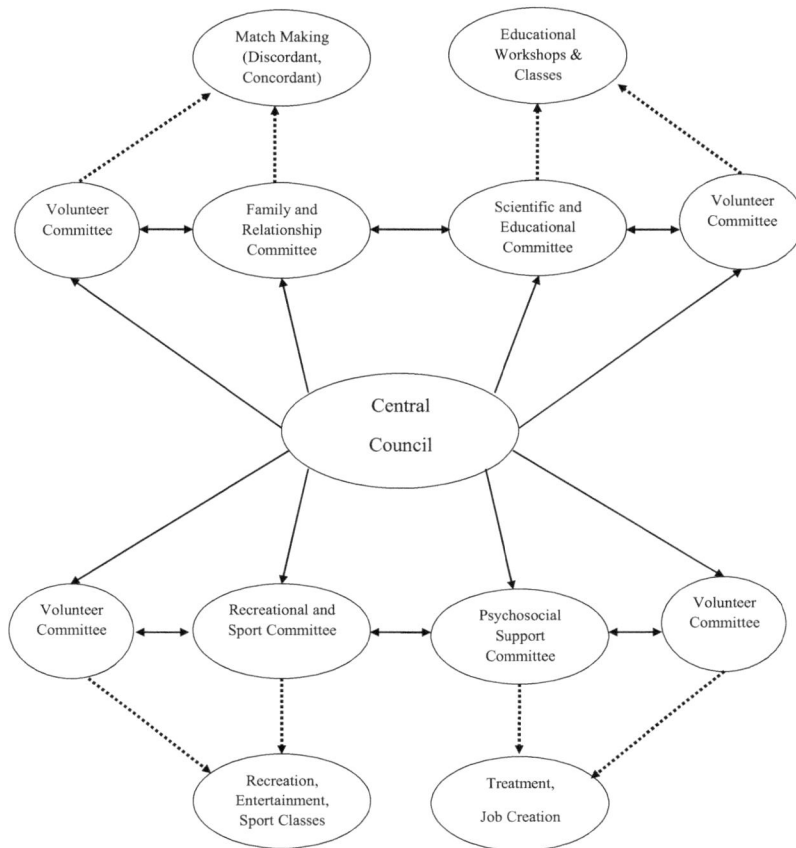

Fig. 1(b). The final model based on both the organization and tasks. The committees do the activities in close interaction with each other. The filled (→), spot (⋯→) and bilateral (↔) arrows show the committees, the tasks and interaction between various committees, respectively.

Table 1. Logical Framework Approach (LFA) for the model at positive clubs.

Components	Indicators	Supervision Tools
Impact •Reduction of HIV incidence in society	HIV incidence in society	•Report of CDC •Report of WHO •Report of UNAIDS
Outcome •Positive Prevention •Psychosocial Support •Reduction of Stigma and Discrimination	•Number of PLHIV who are member of PCs divided to all PLHIV	•Using checklists •Results of studies

(Table 1) contd.....

Components	Indicators	Supervision Tools
Output •Increasing participation of PLHIV •Empowerment of PLHIV	•Number of PLHIV who attend in the activities divided to total PLHIV of PCs	•PCs visits (regular and periodic) •Written reports •Using checklists
Process •Quantity of the activities (start and finish time, duration, location, number of staff, trainers and trainees, materials) •Quality of the activities (content, location, materials, educational level of trainers and trainees)	-	•PCs visits (regular and periodic) •Written reports •Using checklists
Input • Recreational activities • Registering PLHIV at centers related to the Technical and Vocational Training Organization • Providing sessions of psychiatrist visits, counseling and medication for PLHIV or affected by HIV • Holding training sessions on life skills • Holding sessions of peer education for key populations at higher risk of HIV exposure • Organizing sport activities • Holding birthday gathering for members • Holding group therapy • Holding refreshing sessions for peer educators to keep their information updated • Holding educational sessions such as Nutrition and HIV, how to refer people with high risk behaviors to VCT centers, adherence to treatment for PLHIV who receive ART, Prevention of Mother to Child Transmission (PMTCT) for women living with HIV • Referring the new cases of HIV from VCT centers to the PCs in collaboration of psychologists of VCT centers • Entertainments: movies and music • Meditation and Yoga classes • Books and pamphlets regarding the issue of HIV/AIDS • Hotline counseling • HIV Anonymous (HA) sessions	•Number of implemented activities divided to all activities	•PCs Visits (regular and periodic) •Written Reports

PLHIV: people living with HIV, VCT: Voluntary Counseling and Testing, PCs: Positive Clubs, ART: Anti-Retroviral Therapy, CDC: Centers for Disease Control and Prevention, WHO: World Health Organization, UNAIDS: Joint United Nations Programme on HIV/AIDS

2.1. Management Model of Positive Clubs

Based on this model, management of a club is performed by a central council including five PLHIV who are elected by the club members. Under the supervision of this council, five sub-committees are formed including:1) Recreational and Sport committee, 2) Scientific and Educational committee, 3) Psychosocial Support committee, 4) Family and Relationship (Positive Match Making) committee, and 5) Volunteers committee. Such committees interact closely with each other and employ volunteers specifically PLHIV as well as other members of the society (see Fig. **1b**).

2.2. Increasing Participation and Empowerment of PLHIV

To reduce societal stigma associated with HIV, the central council plans and organizes common activities to raise awareness about HIV and increase the status of PLHIV by providing activities where infected individuals may interact with the general public. In this regard, we specifically encourage those who are not living with HIV to participate and to get involved with activities of HIV positive members in various committees. This approach, however, should be implemented considering two important issues: first, the equal participation of volunteers who are not living with HIV in the committees is of utmost importance and secondly, to increase the involvement of HIV negative volunteers with family and friends in the HIV community. The participation of HIV negative volunteers is beneficial not just for those infected, but also the community in general because it increases knowledge, lowers social stigma [5], and promotes greater understanding for all.

Subcommittees target specific needs of PLHIV and are set up to promote collaboration in the community. There are practical and service oriented committees according to the needs of the members in the mentioned model. Additionally, these committees function as a monitoring and evaluating system to transfer the concerns of PLHIV to the main council at the higher level (Fig. **1b**). Subsequently, the council can establish appropriate decisions and policies which may serve the club more efficiently (Fig. **1a**).

The committees with their branches provide related services when demanded by members. The main activities (see Fig. **1a**) in the committees include:

Peer Education and Educational Activities:

- Educational workshops such as teaching life skills, nutrition and HIV, HIV transmission and prevention, clinical manifestations, how to refer people with high risk behaviors to Voluntary Counseling and Testing (VCT) centers, adherence to treatment for PLHIV who receive Antiretroviral (ARV) therapy, Prevention of Mother to Child Transmission (PMTCT) for women living with HIV, treatment and care, side effects of antiretroviral medications, co-infections (*i.e.* hepatitis B and C) and pregnancy hygiene.
- Trainings and workshops on the issue of HIV/AIDS transmission and prevention for peer educators at the clubs, in order to provide trainings at Narcotics Anonymous (NA) camps followed by referring of people with high risk behaviors to VCT centers.

Psychosocial Support Activities

- Treatment Activities:

-Group therapy with a psychologist for PLHIV or affected people.

-Meditation and Yoga classes.

-Psychiatrists visits of PLHIV and affected people for medical treatment.

- Job Creation Activities:

In the job creation section, the club can send PLHIV to the Technical and Vocational Training School in order to participate at workshops regarding vocational and professional skills. The PLHIV may sell their products in different exhibitions and social events. In addition, the members act as instructor to teach vocational and professional skills which they already have learned in the training centers outside of the club to new members.

- Recreational Activities:

-Sport classes such as: ping pong, football, volleyball, swimming, chess, mountain climbing and camping.

-Birthday gatherings, traditional festivals and religious celebrations.

-Entertainments: movies and music.

Other Activities:

- HIV Anonymous (HA) sessions: During these sessions, PLHIV get to talk about their feelings and personal, familial, financial, and social problems.
- Hotline counseling: Providing counseling services by educated PLHIV.
- Publications: Books and pamphlets regarding the issue of HIV/AIDS.

After introducing the basics, it is noteworthy that this model is unique considering its core value and inner practical system (see Fig. **1b**). In order to foresee convincing results, certain issues should be systematically appraised in terms of the model's fundamental elements. For example, one of such fundamental elements is the people who substantially get involved in the ongoing development of positive clubs (*i.e.* professionals, instructors, volunteers who want to help and cooperate with PLHIV). By closely inter-relating the PLHIV and other members of the society, we can anticipate an automatic decrease in stigma and discrimination in addition to producing better results at work. The proposed model is a multipurpose concept and can be used for other types of health outcomes with the objective of incorporating positive clubs in prevention and intervention efforts.

3. DISCUSSION

This chapter outlines a proposed model based on existing framework in order to explore how positive clubs can be organized and managed, and how to promote the participation of PLHIV and those in the general communities for HIV prevention efforts. In order to more efficiently manage positive clubs applying such model, two important issues should be addressed as the main challenges: First, the recruitment of staff among those who are not living with HIV is a significant challenge. Meanwhile, we presume that providing an environment for PLHIV in order to confidently work alongside those who are not living with HIV may effectively decrease stigma and further empower PLHIV. Strategies to engage individuals not living with HIV need to be further developed, including the recruitment by infected individuals of peers and family. Besides, psychosocial support is crucial to offer professional capacities for dealing with the real life conditions in the working environment. The second is that working with PLHIV may be sometimes quite challenging. In fact, the interesting concept of responsibility and its role in the life of PLHIV is an important and broad topic; since in reality, getting PLHIV to effectively work and systematically participate in the long or even short term activities would not be an easy task. There are a number of reasons why involving PLHIV as managers remains difficult. This fact mainly roots in type of PLHIV personality towards other members of the society, and might be quite frequently observed in the actions. Since the establishment of the clubs, we have been noticing a wide gap between the seropositive and seronegative groups. Such gap is more obviously observed among the new seropositive members who recently joined the club but it is also observed in those who joined the club long before them. This could be in part attributed to the fact that new members may feel inconvenient to get involved in any activity alongside HIV negative members considering the fear of facing stigma and discrimination. However, this case is less of a problem among PLHIV with longer membership durations and therefore strategies to improve continuing membership should remain a priority. In addition, the unwillingness to work with or even refusing to cooperate with HIV negative members is a challenge and needs to be addressed. Correspondingly, we have acknowledged and addressed the need to seek for a fundamental approach to deal with this issue; however, there will always be certain challenges in the day to day life of PLHIV regarding their interactions with negative people.

It is true that lives of many PLHIV are inevitably changed after that they are diagnosed with HIV infection. Many of them experience adverse life events such as divorce or death of their spouse and have to suffer from loneliness due to stigma and discrimination. It should be mentioned that in the clubs, this model works efficiently just by checking the activity of committee called positive match making. This idea came to the surface after reviewing the result of a study done in Tehran Positive Club in 2010 [7]. The study showed that one of the main challenges of PLHIV was the issue of life partnership which is believed to have a root in the existing stigma [8]. The study showed that marriage is one of the most socio-cultural problems for PLHIV in the society [7]. Therefore, we decided to provide an opportunity for people in the clubs to have a chance to meet right person so that they would be able to engage in a positive, healthy and hopeful relationship. Subsequently, on one day both single and married seropositive and seronegative members may gather and then the married people talk about their shared life experiences so that they would encourage the singles for marriage.

CONCLUSION

The model presented here in shows that we can thoroughly expand our activities as a club to the whole community. This model explores how HIV positive and negative people can work together to increase participation and empowerment of not only PLHIV, but also their families and reduce stigma and discrimination. Thus, this management model of positive clubs can be applied as a prototype and a successful model, in order to more efficiently decrease stigma and increase the quality of life of PLHIV in the community.

CONFLICT OF INTEREST

The authors confirm that they have no conflict of interest to declare for this publication.

ACKNOWLEDGEMENTS

Declared none.

REFERENCES

[1]   UNAIDS. From Principle to Practice: Greater Involvement of People Living with or Affected by HIV/AIDS (GIPA). Best Practice Key Material 1999. Available at: http://www.unaids.org/en/ resources/presscentre/featurestories/2007/march/20070330gipapolicybrief

[2]   Positive Clubs: Psychosocial support to people living with HIV in the Islamic Republic of Iran Joint United Nations Programme on HIV/AIDS (UNAIDS) 2010. Available at: http://www.un.org/ youthenvoy/2013/08/unaids-joint-united-nations-programme-on-hivaids/

[3]   International HIV/AIDS Alliance and Horizons. The Involvement of People Living with HIV/AIDS in Community-based Prevention, Care and Support Programs in Developing Countries Washington D.C: Horizons 2003.

[4]   Positive Clubs: Psychosocial support to people living with HIV in the Islamic Republic of Iran" Joint United Nations Programme on HIV/AIDS (UNAIDS) 2011. Available at: http://www.unaids.org/

en/resources/presscentre/featurestories/2010/october/20101013fsiran

[5]   SeyedAlinaghi SA, Daraei RB, Mohraz M. A new social modeling approach for reduction of HIV related stigma and discrimination. Glob Adv Res J Soci Sci 2012; 1(1): 9-11.

[6]   Joint United Nations Programme on HIV/AIDS (UNAIDS). Guidelines of Positive clubs in Iran 2011. Available at: www.ijhpm.com/pdf_2958_17ec072d51fb77857e51716aa3f7915f.html

[7]   Mohraz M, SeyedAlinaghi SA. [Prevalence of psychosocial problems in HIV positive patients]. Tehran Univ Med J 2010; 8: 311-3.

[8]   SeyedAlinaghi SA, Paydary K, Afsar Kazerooni P, *et al.* Evaluation of stigma index among people living with HIV/AIDS (PLWHA) in six cities in Iran. Thrita 2013; 2(4): 69-75. Available at: http://thritajournal.com/11801.fulltext
[http://dx.doi.org/10.5812/thrita.11801]

CHAPTER 20

Integration of HIV Services into Primary Health Care (PHC) System

SeyedAhmad SeyedAlinaghi[1], Hossein Malekafzali Ardakani[2], Hamid Emadi Koochak[1], Mona Mohammadi Firouzeh[1], Ghobad Moradi[3] and Minoo Mohraz[1,*]

[1] *Iranian Research Center for HIV/AIDS (IRCHA), Iranian Institute for Reduction of High-Risk Behaviors, Tehran University of Medical Sciences, Tehran, Iran*

[2] *Department of Epidemiology and Biostatistics, School of Public Health, Tehran University of Medical Sciences, Tehran, Iran*

[3] *Social Determinants of Health Research Center, Kurdistan University of Medical Sciences, Sanandaj, Iran*

Abstract: Various factors should be considered when deciding whether integration of HIV/AIDS services into Primary Health Care (PHC) would be beneficial or not. Many studies have stated the necessity of integrating HIV/AIDS programs and Sexually Transmitted Infections (STIs) in PHC and the positive impacts of this integration on a number of PHC goals; however, lack of a monitoring and evaluation (M&E) system makes it difficult to assess the efficiency of the integration into PHC. Considering the scale-up of care and treatment for HIV/AIDS in developing countries, there is increased debate that intensified attention to HIV programs may lead to declines in delivery of other PHC services.

Overall most evidences establish that integrated services can exert a positive effect on client satisfaction, leading to improved access to component services, and reduced HIV stigma, and also these are cost-effective. Key aspects of integration programs include: co-location of services, provision of effective substance use treatment, cross-training of care providers, and provision of enhanced monitoring of drug-drug interactions. Key components in implementing this agenda will be fostering the political tendency to

* **Correspondence to Minoo Mohraz:** Iranian Research Center for HIV/AIDS (IRCHA), Imam Khomeini Hospital, Keshavarz Blvd., Tehran, Iran; Tel/Fax: +98 (21) 66947984; E-mail: minoomohraz@ams.ac.ir.

fund infrastructure and service delivery, expanding street-level outreach services to injection drug users, and training community health workers able to cost effectively delivering these services.

Keywords: AIDS, Decentralization, HIV, Integration, Prevention, Primary Health Care (PHC), Service delivery, Stigma, Substance use, Treatment and Care.

1. INTRODUCTION

More than three decades ago, the world's Ministries of Health declared Primary Health Care (PHC), the delivery of basic preventive and curative services as "Health for all" a top priority at Alma-Ata. Since then, the world's poorest countries have not met most PHC goals [1]. Factors have included insufficient political prioritization of health, structural adjustment policies, poor governance, population growth, inadequate health systems, and scarce research and assessment on PHC [2].

Although HIV is one of the most important infectious cause of adult mortality in many countries of the world, AIDS prevention and care are not clearly ranking priorities for PHC, yet arguments occur among international health policy makers [1]. Therefore, inclusive strategies are required for effective delivery of preventive, diagnostic and curative services to these complex patient populations [3].

In this chapter, we discuss the integration of HIV/AIDS services into PHC, the benefits and pitfalls, and the world experiences.

2. BENEFITS OF INTEGRATION OF HIV/AIDS SERVICES IN PHC

Recently, the concern of integrating HIV services finds an increasingly high priority on public health agendas [1, 3]. HIV/AIDS has shifted to a chronic disorder and despite of disease causes, an integrated approach to the management of chronic diseases is needed in the PHC [4, 5]. The integration of HIV/AIDS programs into PHC has taken place in some countries around the world either partially or completely (Table **1**). However, the success of its implementation varies from country to country. Numerous factors come into play when deciding whether the integration of HIV/AIDS programs would be beneficial or not to a region. Factors such as the careful monitoring of the government, community involvement, and skilled personnel have to a strong impact on the success of such programs [6]. An analytical approach is necessary to discover the potential barriers, adopt effective strategies for dealing with these barriers and to facilitate the integration. Generally speaking, the integration of such programs is a challenging topic that needs both appropriate funding and staff. Planning for HIV-related services depends on HIV prevalence in each country and the level of services differ from country to country and even differ between the different districts of a country. Countries, and even districts with a higher prevalence of HIV, should be provided with more services as well as more clinics than those with a lower prevalence. It is believed that the need for the integration is higher in developing countries because it has been shown that in such countries, HIV as well as Sexually Transmitted Infections (STIs) prevalence is higher than in developed countries [4, 5].

Table 1. An overview of different countries' status in providing the most important services regarding HIV/AIDS in Primary Health Care (PHC) System worldwide.

Country	Integration in PHC	Important services regarding HIV/AIDS	Centers providing services regarding HIV/AIDS	Consequences
Iran	Is not applied.	-Narcotics Anonymous (NA) -Providing programs for harm reduction (syringe and needle exchange, methadone therapy, condom distribution) -Providing HIV testing	-Voluntary counseling & Testing (VCT) centers -Positive clubs -Drop-in center (DIC)	-Increasing access to HIV testing -Become slow progression of the epidemic among injection drug users. -Control of HIV transmission through blood and its products were successful. -HIV Prevalence is low among the general population in the country.

(Table 1) contd.....

Country	Integration in PHC	Important services regarding HIV/AIDS	Centers providing services regarding HIV/AIDS	Consequences
Thailand	Has been applied.	-HIV/AIDS prevention and cares -Providing STIs treatment -Providing women's health services	-PHC centers -VCT centers -Positive clubs	-Each region understands and resolves its own health care needs. -Health care instructions are transferred from one to another.
South Africa	Reliable information is not available.	-HIV/AIDS prevention and Cares -Diagnosis of Tuberculosis -Providing STIs treatment -Providing women's health services	-Non governmental sectors -Sanatoriums -STIs clinics	-Private institutions have filled the gaps that existed in PHC. -Training the nurses in the field of antiretroviral therapy resulted in increased adherence to treatment.
Brazil	Has been applied.	-Syringe and needle exchange -Creating public participation by holding meetings, seminars and working groups in schools and public places -Providing mother to child transmission prevention services with establishment of the networks (PHC, reference centers, clinics and women's wards) -Providing services regarding prevention in the workplace -Organizing a network of testing and follow-up -Developing reward system for voluntary testing -Providing access to rapid tests	-HIV and STIs clinics	-Increasing adherence to treatments -Increasing family and social support -Raising awareness of ways to prevent HIV/AIDS infection

(Table 1) contd.....

Country	Integration in PHC	Important services regarding HIV/AIDS	Centers providing services regarding HIV/AIDS	Consequences
China	Has been applied.	-Syringe and needle exchange -Providing alternative treatment with Opioid	-PHC centers	-Transferring doctors from hospitals to PHC centers -Inadequate coverage of antiretroviral treatments -New cases are not effectively controlled.
India	Reliable information is not available.	-Providing home care services -Establishing centers for voluntary counseling and testing -Providing services to prevent infection transmission from mother to child -Providing services regarding STIs and condom distribution -Providing antiretroviral treatment and syringe and needle exchange -Providing alternative treatment with Opioid	-Centers providing ART -Community based health centers	-Increasing of awareness in the society -Shortage of medicines, equipment and personnel -Having coverage problems specially in rural areas
Malaysia	Has been applied.	-Syringe and needle exchange -Providing alternative treatment with Opioid -Having plans of preventing infection transmission from mother to child in antenatal clinics -Implementing HIV/AIDS programs in health centers, polyclinics and home visits -Having educational programs, particularly for young people	-PHC centers -Polyclinics	-Increasing of awareness in the society -Careful following-ups are done by patients.

(Table 1) contd.....

Country	Integration in PHC	Important services regarding HIV/AIDS	Centers providing services regarding HIV/AIDS	Consequences
Indonesia	Has been applied.	-Having programs for expanding the use of condom -Prevention of HIV/AIDS through STIs treatment -Prevention of HIV infection among injection drug users -Providing services regarding VCT -Providing services regarding HIV treatment and care -Providing services to prevent infection transmission from mother to child -Providing services regarding HIV/AIDS in the work place -Providing services regarding HIV/AIDS in non-governmental organizations -Prevention of HIV infection among the youth -Having harm reduction programs (syringe and condom distribution, methadone therapy as an alternative treatment) -Providing legal services specially publishing regional policies regarding HIV/AIDS	-Health care centers -Health care clinics	-The lack of government accurate supervision specially on the NGO's -Limited places for providing services -Limited number of skilled personnel in the field of HIV/AIDS services -Unfair distribution of services as well as inappropriate behavior of service providers with patients

(Table 1) contd.....

Country	Integration in PHC	Important services regarding HIV/AIDS	Centers providing services regarding HIV/AIDS	Consequences
SriLanka	Has been applied.	-Giving free education specially to the illiterate population -Having training programs specially for vulnerable people and ones with high-risk behaviors and having HIV/AIDS programs with the title of Health Promotion -Providing health services for the youth	-STIs clinics	-Raising awareness -Providing access to HIV test -Providing access to STIs screening services -Providing access to antiretroviral medications -Prevention of Mother to Child Transmission
Morocco	Has been applied.	-Having social communication campaign against AIDS -Having prevention programs for youth, women and populations at risk -Having harm reduction programs (syringe and condom distribution, methadone therapy as an alternative treatment) specially for injection drug users -Providing access to VCT particularly by the NGO's -National testing days programs -Providing access to antiretroviral treatment for all patients -Development of prevention programs in schools -Instructing people by outreach team	-STI clinics	-Lack of sufficient services for the whole community

(Table 1) contd.....

Country	Integration in PHC	Important services regarding HIV/AIDS	Centers providing services regarding HIV/AIDS	Consequences
Oman	Has been applied.	-They are based on network creation between Primary Health Centers -They focus on high-risk groups and prisoners -Prevention programs in workplaces -Harm reduction programs	-New PHC centers -Developed health centers -Local hospitals -Provincial hospitals -Regional hospitals	-Has been successful.
Uganda	Has been applied.	-HIV/AIDS prevention and Cares -Diagnosis of Tuberculosis -STIs treatment	-PHC clinics	-Increasing psychological and social support specially in the rural community
Spain	Has been applied.	-Syringe and needle exchange programs provided by non-governmental sectors and centers of drug abuse prevention -Social services provided by non-governmental sectors -Safer sex practices	-Polyclinics	-
Turkey	Reliable information is not available.	-Programs are not known exactly. -Using the help of family doctors regarding HIV/AIDS programs particularly with prevention -Instructing HIV/AIDS prevention in the workplace	-VCT centers	-Has recently started. -It is still not clear.

(Table 1) contd.....

Country	Integration in PHC	Important services regarding HIV/AIDS	Centers providing services regarding HIV/AIDS	Consequences
Canada	Has been applied.	-All public and private sectors are involved, such as: Urban society, Public health divisions, People who live with HIV/AIDS or are exposed to it, Non-governmental sections, and Nurses -Setting up telephone counseling lines by the private sectors -Prevention programs in prisons performed by peer training -Doing research in HIV/AIDS with intersectional collaboration	-PHC centers	-Health Promotion
Haiti	Has been applied.	-Providing AIDS-related care like DOT-HAART and HIV/AIDS prevention and Cares -Diagnosis of Tuberculosis -Providing STIs treatment -Providing women's health services	-PHC centers	-Increasing community awareness about transmission and prevention of HIV -Spreading the prevention of transmission from mother to child -Increasing demands for VCT -Reducing the stigma associated with HIV -Increasing the quality of other services related to PHC

Primary Health Care (PHC), Sexually Transmitted Infections (STIs), Men who have Sex with Men (MSM), Directly Observed Therapy (DOT), Highly Active Anti-Retroviral Therapy (HAART).

Many studies reported the importance and the necessity of integrating HIV/AIDS programs and STIs in PHC. The integration of HIV/AIDS programs into PHC has shown to be the most effective strategy to control and prevent HIV infection [1, 5, 6].

The integration of HIV and STIs care and treatment into family planning services can have a positive effect on patient satisfaction, make access to services more convenient, and can reduce HIV related stigma in clinics. A study in Uganda

(2002) showed that offering a comprehensive package which included: Voluntary Counseling and Testing (VCT), family planning, care and support services for illnesses such as Tuberculosis (TB), STIs and HIV/AIDS can help make a patient feel more comfortable to talk to their physician about HIV, reduce stigma and also increase pre-test counseling of HIV [1, 4, 7].

It was found that the integration of AIDS prevention and care, consisting of the application of antiretroviral agents, is beneficial in resource-poor settings. These activities show favorable and measurable effects on various PHC goals, like vaccination, family planning, tuberculosis case finding and cure, and health promotion. Other collateral benefits, though less readily measured, include improved staff morale and enhanced confidence in public health and medicine [1, 8]. Therefore, HIV VCT is an effective tactic to protect against the HIV transmission in developing countries [9].

3. PITFALLS OF INTEGRATION OF HIV/AIDS SERVICES IN PHC

A variety of pitfalls are described that may occur with the push to rapidly expand access to antiretroviral therapy (ART) in sub-Saharan Africa. Undesirable opportunity costs, the fragmentation of health systems, worsening health care inequities as well as poor and relenting treatment outcomes are also involved [10]. The integration approach allows the public sector of the PHC system to assess more subjects for HIV, place patients on ART in a more fast and effective manner, reduce loss-to-follow-up, and obtain higher geographic HIV care coverage. Through the integration process, HIV resources have been applied to rehabilitate PHC infrastructure including laboratories and pharmacies, strengthen supervision, fill workforce gaps, and improve patient flow between services and facilities in ways that can benefit all programs. PHC systems can be strengthened with aid resources used for integrating and better linking HIV care with existing services [11].

To integrate care services, HIV primary care is combined with mental health and substance abuse services as to offer a single coordinated treatment program, rather than fragmented and often hard to navigate system. It addresses the various clinical complexities-whether mental health, substance abuse, and/or HIV care -

associated with having various needs and conditions in a holistic, easily accessed manner [12]. Integrated HIV management with health centers and polyclinics-in order to decentralize the management of HIV patients from a hospital based setting to the primary care level-would help to promote and upgrade the best care for HIV patients. The Malaysian Ministry of Health is currently maintains an integrated management of HIV patients into health centers and polyclinics. This program consists of several stages. Now, more than 160 clinics are offering services like risk assessment, HIV testing, counseling, medical examination, treatment, follow-up, case notification, contact tracing, referral, and home visits by trained clinical personnel [13]. Without an integration system to monitor and evaluate (M&E), it is difficult to investigate the efficiency of HIV and family planning (FP) service integration. Since 2007, Nigeria has been integrating FP and HIV M&E systems. A pre-post survey conducted a comparative analysis for the availability and use of FP-HIV integration M&E tools six months before the integration and 12-months after the integration in 71 health facilities, supported by the Global HIV/AIDS Initiative Nigeria (GHAIN). Pre-integration, four facilities (6%) had national FP registers, 32 (45%) had monthly aggregated FP data and 33 (46%) reported data up to national level. Post-integration, all (100%) facilities used national FP register with FP-HIV integration indicators, and reported data up to national level. Sixty six facilities (93%) had at least one monthly supervisory visit. The average count of FP clients per facility pointed for HIV testing enhanced from five in the first months to 15 by month 12 post-integration. Improving resources of HIV programs led to enhanced monitoring of FP-HIV services integration [14].

With the intensive scale-up of care and HIV/AIDS therapy in developing countries, some people think that a distribution of financial resources focused on HIV programs may overcome health care systems and result in reductions in delivery of other PHC services. There is a little data confirming the negative or positive synergies on health care provision obtained from HIV-dedicated programs [8]. An increasing debate rises about the role of scaled-up investments in HIV/AIDS programs on nourishing or exhausting the fragile health systems of many developing countries. Considerably increased resources have been brought into countries for HIV/AIDS programs by major Global Health Initiatives. An increase in awareness and priority for public health from governments are exemplified some positive effects. Furthermore, delivery of services to people living with HIV/AIDS (PLWHA) has been increased significantly. In many countries, infrastructure and laboratories have been strengthened, and in some cases PHC services have been improved. The impact of AIDS on the health work force has been lowered according to various parameters including the provision of ART to HIV-infected health care workers, training, and task-shifting. However, many reports are of concerns, among them a temporal relationship between increasing AIDS funding and inactive reproductive health funding, and accusations that scarce personnel are siphoned off from other health care services by offers of better-paying jobs in HIV/AIDS programs. Since delivery of AIDS services has not yet obtained a conceivable level "as close to Universal Access as possible", countries and development partners must maintain the momentum of investment in HIV/AIDS programs. At the same time, it should be found that global action for health is even more underfunded than the response to the HIV epidemic. Therefore, the real issue is not whether to fund AIDS or health systems, but how to enhance funding for both [9, 11, 15].

4. THE WORLD EXPERIENCES

Table **1** shows the integration status of HIV programs into PHC in different countries.

In developing countries where the integration of HIV/AIDS programs has taken place, such as Thailand, Uganda, and Haiti, it is believed that the use of volunteers in these programs is very beneficial. Volunteers are trained extensively and then sent out to communities and homes around the country to raise awareness and if necessary, refer those who engage in high risk behaviors to come into the clinic. In such communities, educational services can be more easily accessible to hard-to-reach populations and the work of volunteers can increase the quality of such services. Volunteers also play a key role in reducing the stigma of HIV and AIDS. South Africa's health system is based on home care and peer education through the use of volunteers. In this system, people who engage in high risk behaviors are referred to the PHC clinics by the volunteers [1, 10, 11, 13, 15].

The health systems in countries such as Brazil, India, Malaysia and Indonesia are based on decentralization. The government distributes clinics all over the country as opposed to just one central area. STIs clinics and related health care services in different areas also provide HIV/AIDS related services. In Lusikisiki, a rural area of South Africa with a population of 150,000 persons serviced by one hospital and 12 clinics, MÉdecins Sans FrontiÈres has been supporting a program to deliver HIV services through decentralization to PHC clinics, task shifting (including nurse-initiated as opposed to physician-initiated treatment), and community support. This approach has allowed for a rapid scale-up of treatment with satisfactory outcomes. Although the general approach in South Africa is to provide ART through hospitals which seriously limits access for many people, if not the most people one year outcomes in Lusikisiki are comparable in the clinics and hospital. The greater proximity and acceptability of services at the clinic level has led to a faster enrollment of people into treatment and better retention of patients in treatment (2% *vs.* 19% lost to follow-up). In all, 2200 people were receiving ART in Lusikisiki in 2006, which represents 95% coverage [13, 16].

Among countries in the Middle East, the PHC system of Oman (like Iran) includes the primary and developed health centers and local, velayati and regional hospitals. If it is necessary, patients will be referred from their PHC centers to the regional hospital in Oman. It seems that HIV-related care and prevention has been integrated in this system, but the magnitude and amount of integration is unknown. In 2004, Iran's Ministry of Health integrated substance use treatment and HIV prevention into the rural PHC system. Four hundred seventy eight active opium or heroin users were enrolled in a rural clinic. Participants received counseling for abstinence from substances, or daily needle exchange and condoms. Participants receiving daily needle exchange/condoms stayed in the program longer than those not. This project indicates that HIV risks persist in rural Iran, demonstrating the innovative application of Iran's rural health care system to develop prevention and treatment services to the populations [5, 15, 17].

The feasibility, the demand, and the effect of integrating on-site primary care services into VCT were examined at a stand-alone VCT center in Port au Prince, Haiti. Through a retrospective review of patient records, it was described the integration of primary care services at the Groupe Haitien d'Etude du Sarcome de

Kaposi et des Infections Opportunistes (GHESKIO) VCT center between 1985 and 2000. Between 1985 and 1999, services for HIV care, tuberculosis care, treatment of STIs, and reproductive health were succinctly integrated into HIV VCT at GHESKIO. The counts of new individuals trying VCT at GHESKIO enhanced from 142 in 1985 to 8175 in 1999, with an increasing percentage of women, adolescents, symptom-free clients, and self-referred clients. Of new adults seeking VCT in 1999, the center has the capacity to offer AIDS care to 17%, tuberculosis treatment to 6%, STIs management to 18%, and family planning to 19%. HIV transmission between discordant couples was 0 infections/100 follow-up years; vertical transmission from mother to child was 11 infections/100 live births; these rates are remarkably less than expected rates of transmission in Haiti. This report indicated the feasibility, demand, and effective synergy of integrating on-site primary care services into HIV VCT in Haiti [9].

In collaboration with the Zambian Ministry of Health, TB-HIV integration activities started in December 2005 and extended to seven health centers by March 2007. Principal activities consisted of developing staff capability to manage co-infected patients, conducting HIV tests within TB departments and generating referral systems between departments. Through a provider-initiated approach, 2053 TB patients were provided HIV tests. Seventy-seven percent agreed to be tested; 69% of those tested were HIV-infected. Of these, 59% were enrolled in HIV care. The proportion of ART program enrollees who were TB-HIV co-infected increased by 38% after program implementation [18].

In Brazil, access to free HIV testing concentrates in the Counseling and Testing Referral Centers. PHC units can greatly expand the access to HIV testing and counseling and reaching out for people at risk who would never go to the referral centers. The project was launched in December 1st, 2001. Curitiba has 1.6 million populations, with 93 PHC units. Professionals from all 93 PHC units were trained on counseling. On the overall, from December 1st to the 28th, 4551 people were tested, with a seropositivity of 0.99%, which is higher than the Ministry of Health estimates [19].

Offering HIV testing in PHC units is feasible. It can advance disease control in the micro-environment, focusing in people with higher risks. Notions that people would not seek the PHC unit to test because it is close to their homes were not a major obstacle. Some health units tended to organize counseling with some limiting access: large groups, fixed schedule, *etc*. This was opposed by the Municipal Health Secretary. It is understood that those who seek the unit should be received with individual counseling and immediate testing. PHC teams or family doctors can, if properly trained, assist HIV positive asymptomatic patients in their health units, facilitating treatment adherence as well as family and community support centers resulted in detection [6].

CONCLUSIONS AND RECOMMENDATIONS

A variety of evidence shows the positive impact of integrated services on client satisfaction, improved access to component services, and lowered clinic-based HIV-related stigma. These services are cost-effective. Integrating HIV testing and referral services into urban primary care centers resulted in detection of co-infected patients and remarkably enhanced the proportion of TB patients among people accessing HIV care. Continued challenges cover to maximize the counts of patients accepting HIV tests and removing barriers to enrollment into HIV care. As proposed, through continuing scale-up access to antiretroviral medications for drug users, developing co-located integrated care delivery systems must concentrate on national programs. Current data indicates that such programs can extend disease-specific services; enhance detection of TB and HIV; increase medication adherence; improve entry into substance use treatment; lower the possibility of adverse drug events; and enhance the efficiency of prevention interventions. Major dimensions of integration programs are: co-location of services convenient to the patient; provision of effective substance use treatment, including pharmacotherapies; cross-training of generalist and specialist care providers; and provision of enhanced monitoring of drug-drug interactions and adverse side effects. Key components to implement this agenda is to strengthen the political intent to fund infrastructure and service delivery, extend street-level outreach services to injection drug users, and train community health workers capable of cost effectively delivering these services [20].

Most importantly, in developing countries the best route to provide HIV prevention programs is through the use of trained volunteers. In this model, health personnel train volunteers and then these volunteers take their education and training to educate members of the community. This not only reduces HIV stigma, but also leads to a rise in awareness as well as knowledge about the disease. Developed countries are based on making polyclinics, providing HIV related services in these polyclinics, using more non-governmental organizations (NGOs) and networks between the different parts of health system [20].

CONFLICT OF INTEREST

The authors confirm that they have no conflict of interest to declare for this publication.

ACKNOWLEDGEMENTS

Declared none.

REFERENCES

[1]   Walton DA, Farmer PE, Lambert W, Leandre F, Koenig SP, Mukherjee JS. Integrated HIV prevention and care strengthens primary health care: lessons from rural Haiti. J Pub health policy 2004; 25(2): 137-58.   Available   from: http://www.chwcentral.org/sites/default/files/Integrated%20HIV%20prevention%20and%20care%20strengthens%20primary%20health%20care_Lessons%20from%20rural%20Haiti_0.pdf
        [PMID: 1525538]

[2]   Walley J, Lawn JE, Tinker A, *et al.* Lancet Alma-Ata Working Group. Primary health care: making Alma-Ata a reality. Lancet 2008; 372(9642): 1001-7.
        [http://dx.doi.org/10.1016/S0140-6736(08)61409-9] [PMID: 18790322]

[3]   Sylla L, Bruce RD, Kamarulzaman A, Altice FL. Integration and co-location of HIV/AIDS, tuberculosis and drug treatment services. Int J Drug Policy 2007; 18(4): 306-12.
        [http://dx.doi.org/10.1016/j.drugpo.2007.03.001] [PMID: 17689379]

[4]   Mayhew S. Integrating MCH/FP and STD/HIV services: current debates and future directions. Health Policy Plan 1996; 11(4): 339-53.
        [http://dx.doi.org/10.1093/heapol/11.4.339] [PMID: 10164192]

[5]   Beaglehole R, Epping-Jordan J, Patel V, *et al.* Improving the prevention and management of chronic disease in low-income and middle-income countries: a priority for primary health care. Lancet 2008; 372(9642): 940-9.
        [http://dx.doi.org/10.1016/S0140-6736(08)61404-X] [PMID: 18790317]

[6]   PHC community based health services delivery framework. "A model on delivering PHC services within communities" 2009. Draft 25th January

[7]   Nuwaha F, Kabatesi D, Muganwa M, Whalen CC. Factors influencing acceptability of voluntary

counselling and testing for HIV in Bushenyi district of Uganda. East Afr Med J 2002; 79(12): 626-32.
[http://dx.doi.org/10.4314/eamj.v79i12.8669] [PMID: 12678445]

[8]   Price JE, Leslie JA, Welsh M, Binagwaho A. Integrating HIV clinical services into primary health care in Rwanda: a measure of quantitative effects. AIDS Care 2009; 21(5): 608-14.
[http://dx.doi.org/10.1080/09540120802310957] [PMID: 19444669]

[9]   Peck R, Fitzgerald DW, Liautaud B, *et al.* The feasibility, demand, and effect of integrating primary care services with HIV voluntary counseling and testing: evaluation of a 15-year experience in Haiti, 1985-2000. J Int Assoc Provid AIDS Care 2003; 33(4): 470-5.
[PMID: 12869835]

[10]   McCoy D, Chopra M, Loewenson R, *et al.* Expanding access to antiretroviral therapy in sub-saharan Africa: avoiding the pitfalls and dangers, capitalizing on the opportunities. Am J Public Health 2005; 95(1): 18-22.
[http://dx.doi.org/10.2105/AJPH.2004.040121] [PMID: 15623853]

[11]   Pfeiffer J, Montoya P, Baptista AJ, *et al.* Integration of HIV/AIDS services into African primary health care: lessons learned for health system strengthening in Mozambique - a case study. J Int AIDS Soc 2010; 13(1): 3.
[http://dx.doi.org/10.1186/1758-2652-13-3] [PMID: 20180975]

[12]   Hoffman HL, Castro-Donlan CA, Johnson VM, Church DR. The Massachusetts HIV, hepatitis, addiction services integration (HHASI) experience: responding to the comprehensive needs of individuals with co-occurring risks and conditions. Public Health Rep 2004; 119(1): 25-31.
[PMID: 15147646]

[13]   Talib Rozaidah. Malaysia: Fighting a Rising Tide: The Response to AIDS in East Asia (eds Tadashi Yamamoto and Satoko Itoh). Tokyo: Japan Centre for International Exchange 2006; pp. 195-206.

[14]   Chukwujekwu O, Chabikuli NO, Merrigan M, Awi D, Hamelmann C. Integrating reproductive health and HIV indicators into the Nigerian health system--building an evidence base for action. Afr J Reprod Health 2010; 14(1): 109-16.
[PMID: 20695143]

[15]   Yu D, Souteyrand Y, Banda MA, Kaufman J, Perriëns JH. Investment in HIV/AIDS programs: does it help strengthen health systems in developing countries? Global Health 2008; 4(1): 8.
[http://dx.doi.org/10.1186/1744-8603-4-8] [PMID: 18796148]

[16]   Bedelu M, Ford N, Hilderbrand K, Reuter H. Implementing antiretroviral therapy in rural communities: the Lusikisiki model of decentralized HIV/AIDS care. J Infect Dis 2007; 196 (Suppl. 3): S464-8.
[http://dx.doi.org/10.1086/521114] [PMID: 18181695]

[17]   Mojtahedzadeh V, Razani N, Malekinejad M, *et al.* Injection drug use in Rural Iran: integrating HIV prevention into Iran's rural primary health care system. AIDS Behav 2008; 12(4) (Suppl.): S7-S12.
[http://dx.doi.org/10.1007/s10461-008-9408-y] [PMID: 18521737]

[18]   Harris JB, Hatwiinda SM, Randels KM, *et al.* Early lessons from the integration of tuberculosis and HIV services in primary care centers in Lusaka, Zambia. Int J Tuberc Lung Dis 2008; 12(7): 773-9.
[PMID: 18544203]

[19]   Simao MBG, Cubas RF, Battaglin C, Luhm KR. Early HIV detection in primary health care units in Curitiba, Brazil. Poster Exhibition: The XIV International AIDS Conference: Abstract no. ThPeF8039.

[20]   Mohraz M, Malekafzali H, Gooya MM, *et al.* [Recommended Model for Integration of HIV/AIDS in Primary Health Network]. Project Report, October 2011.

CHAPTER 21

Community Involvement: New HIV Monitoring Strategies

Donald J. Hamel[*]

Department of Immunology and Infectious Diseases, Harvard School of Public Health, 651 Huntington Avenue, Boston MA 02115 USA

Abstract: HIV testing strategies should be carefully tailored to specific settings and populations. Screening algorithms typically include rapid test, ELISA and Western blot testing cascades. Over the counter consumer tests for oral fluids are expanding in developed countries, and early infant diagnosis screening programs such as Dried Blood Spot (DBS) testing are expanding in developing countries with high HIV prevalence. Advanced nucleic and PCR based testing platforms continue to be simplified as Point of Care (POC) equipment by numerous manufacturers. Psychosocial support and counseling are critical components of effective HIV testing programs in any community, and serve as a bridge between testing activities and early uptake to treatment regimens.

Keywords: DBS, EID, ELISA, Harm reduction, HIV testing, Oral fluid tests, Point of Care, Psychosocial support, Rapid tests, Serology, Western blot.

1. INTRODUCTION

Monitoring strategies for HIV are complex and require consideration of purpose, population, setting, technology, budgets as well as other factors. Groups for evaluation may range from patients, adolescents, infants, the general public, blood donors, sex workers, Injection Drug Users (IDU) to Sexually Transmitted Infections (STI) clinic attendees. The populations might have very specific

[*] **Correspondence to Donald J. Hamel:** Department of Immunology and Infectious Diseases, Harvard School of Public Health, 651 Huntington Avenue, Boston MA 02115, USA; Tel: 617-432-3413; Fax: 617-432-3575; E-mail: dhamel@hsph.harvard.edu

SeyedAhmad SeyedAlinaghi (Ed.)

characteristics, such as strict religious beliefs or varied educational backgrounds [1]. Settings for monitoring could be a hospital, a Voluntary Counseling and Testing (VCT) clinic, private homes in a door-to-door outreachservice, blood banks, urban settings, or very rural locations [2 - 4]. Technology and cost of screening tests continue to evolve and improve over time and require periodic reevaluations [5]. Studies may be undertaken to screen large numbers of patient samples, to confirm patients who previously were tested HIV positive, to monitor ART treatment, or to conduct an epidemiological survey. Monitoring may be driven by individual study as well, to assess viral loads or the emergence of drug resistance mutations. For any such endeavor, one needs to pay thoughtful attention to these, and other diverse issues. Even human subjects review committees and political factors can influence design of an appropriate HIV monitoring strategy [6 - 11].

2. TESTS FOR HIV INFECTION AND POINT OF CARE

Broadlyspeaking, HIV screening technologies typically are serologic tests, which detect antibodies specific to HIV, as well as more sophisticated Nucleic Acid Tests (NATs), which detect genetic particles of the HIV genome directly. More specifically, serologic assays may target antibodies in whole blood, plasma, dried blood spots, saliva or urine [12]. Detuned assays, which deliberately raise the detection limit of certain types of assays, can estimate the time of infection to examine HIV incidence [13]. NATs can provide qualitative infection information, or quantitative measurement of a patient's viral burden. Viral culture can characterize viral tropism and DNA sequencing can provide the HIV subtype information for patients.

Historically, first generation Enzyme Linked Immunosorbent Assays (ELISAs, viral lysate with IgG detection) emerged in the mid-1980s and was targeted toward high-risk populations. Improvements were driven by the need to reduce false positives as well as to screen for additional viral variants (various HIV-1 subtypes, HIV-2). Hemagglutination assays were followed by second (recombinant antigen) and third generation (IgG and IgM detection) ELISAs. The current fourth generation ELISA detects both HIV-1 and HIV-2 antibodies as well as p24 antigen. As with all HIV testing and screening, initial positive results by a screening assay absolutely need to be confirmed by a second test before any result is reported to a patient [14]. Western blot confirmatory assays have largely been replaced by standardized NAT confirmatory testing in developed countries, and with secondary ELISA rapid test confirmation predominating in developing countries. Screening assays should be of high sensitivity, and the confirmatory test must have equal or higher specificity [5].

A milestone in HIV monitoring was passed with the US FDA approval of the over-the-counter OraQuick test kit in 2012 [15]. Designed for personal home use by the public, for a price under US$30 and the result in less thanone hour, the test can detect antibodies to HIV-1 and HIV-2 from a saliva sample. The manufacturer provides 24 hours telephone support in the US for technical assistance, and also can refer callers to social support networks. While the impact of this widespread testing capacity is still pending, enthusiasm runs high that this can expand early HIV screening and increase a much earlier access to care, particularly in marginalized populations less likely to see a physician on a regular basis [16]. However, testing in a medical setting still provides the best quality of care, and efforts to expand this capacity must be strengthened [17].

Routine oral fluid screening at dental office during exams is another new field of research [18]. The greatest burden of responsibility is perhaps the dental professional communicating sensitive information and acting in a counseling role. Blood bank screening remains an extremely important function at the community level, and the monitoring has evolved in this setting with technology such as gene chip arrays. In 1995 antibody testing of blood was expanded to include p24 antigen testing as well [19, 20]. Many countries worldwide now screen with fourth generation ELISA to reduce the number and cost of tests performed. The US FDA has recommended NAT testing of collected blood products and pooled screening is the current standard protocol of screening in this setting [21, 22].

With broad applications for developing countries and rural settings, point of care platforms for screening and testing have been expanding greatly in the past five years [23, 24]. CD4 testing platforms (Pointcare, PartecMiniPOC) are now available and viral load platforms continue to move toward improved versions [25]. Dried Blood Spot (DBS) collection and screening has become part of national early infant diagnosis programs in many large developing countries, such as Nigeria [26]. DBS allows both detection of infection by DNA PCR assay, and also provides the possibility of viral load determination. Large corporations including bioMeriux, Roche, Abbott and Siemens continue to develop and refine their HIV viral load platforms for wider use, particularly in developing countries [27].

3. THE ROLE OF PSYCHOSOCIAL SUPPORT

Psychosocial support is also an important community contribution to HIV screening, monitoring and comprehensive care. Anxiety and depression are to be expected when considering HIV testing and a possible HIV positive outcome. This is the case with not only individuals from marginalized groups, but also those with strong family and social support networks. With any HIV screening endeavor that includes patient reporting, it is ideal to have support groups in place, with people of similar background who have worked their own way through the difficult process of self acceptance. Understanding 'where the person is coming from' and having peer groups and health counselors available and reaching out can greatly assist in navigating the first stages of accepting life with HIV [28]. Psychosocial support networks also provide linkage to proper medical care, as well as fostering healthy and responsible attitudes for persons living with HIV [29]. These connections may also leverage other interventions on acommunity widebasis, such as harm reduction counseling, topical microbicide use, PrEP, male circumcision, needle exchange, *etc.* [30].

Returning to the social context of HIV screening, the use of social networks has recently been shown to have a place in prevention, being shown to help engage at risk communities. Secret, or hidden Facebook groups allow private forums for frank discussions and they have been shown to improve the frequency of HIV testing requests by engaging persons who are not exposed to traditional medical settings [31].

CONFLICT OF INTEREST

The author confirms that author has no conflict of interest to declare for this publication.

ACKNOWLEDGEMENTS

Declared none.

REFERENCES

[1]   Bayer R. Ethical and social policy issues raised by HIV screening: the epidemic evolves and so do the challenges. AIDS 1989; 3(3): 119-24.
[http://dx.doi.org/10.1097/00002030-198903000-00001] [PMID: 2496728]

[2]   Christopoulos KA, Zetola NM, Klausner JD, *et al.* Leveraging a rapid, round-the-clock HIV testing system to screen for acute HIV infection in a large urban public medical center. J Acquir Immune Defic Syndr 2013; 62(2): e30-8.
[http://dx.doi.org/10.1097/QAI.0b013e31827a0b0d] [PMID: 23117503]

[3]   Kroeger K, Taylor AW, Marlow HM, Fleming DT, Beyleveld V, Alwano MG. Perceptions of door-t--door HIV counselling and testing in Botswana. SAHARA J: journal of Social Aspects of HIV/AIDS Research Alliance / SAHARA. Human Sci Res Council 2011; 8(4): 171-8.

[4]   Evolution in testing technology enables some urban EDs to implement HIV screening at relatively low cost. ED Manag 2011; 23(10): 109-12.
[PMID: 21972754]

[5]   WHO World Health Organization Report: HIV antigen/antibody assays : operational characteristics : report 16 rapid assays 2009. Available from: http://www.who.int/diagnostics_laboratory/evaluations/hiv/en/

[6]   Carballo-Diéguez A, Frasca T, Balan I, Ibitoye M, Dolezal C. Use of a rapid HIV home test prevents HIV exposure in a high risk sample of men who have sex with men. AIDS Behav 2012; 16(7): 1753-60.
[http://dx.doi.org/10.1007/s10461-012-0274-2] [PMID: 22893194]

[7]   Cherutich P, Bunnell R, Mermin J. HIV testing: current practice and future directions. Curr HIV/AIDS Rep 2013; 10(2): 134-41.
[http://dx.doi.org/10.1007/s11904-013-0158-8] [PMID: 23526423]

[8]   Kasedde S, Luo C, McClure C, Chandan U. Reducing HIV and AIDS in adolescents: opportunities and challenges. Curr HIV/AIDS Rep 2013; 10(2): 159-68.
[http://dx.doi.org/10.1007/s11904-013-0159-7] [PMID: 23563990]

[9]   Strain MC, Richman DD. New assays for monitoring residual HIV burden in effectively treated individuals. Curr Opin HIV AIDS 2013; 8(2): 106-10.
[http://dx.doi.org/10.1097/COH.0b013e32835d811b] [PMID: 23314907]

[10]   Becker M, Ramanaik S, Halli S, *et al.* The Intersection between sex work and reproductive health in northern karnataka, India: Identifying gaps and opportunities in the context of HIV prevention. Aids Res Treat 2012; 2012(12): 842576.
[PMID: 23346390]

[11]   Chou R, Selph S, Dana T, *et al.* Screening for HIV: Systematic Review to Update the U.S. Preventive Services Task Force Recommendation. Rockville MD 2012.

[http://dx.doi.org/10.7326/0003-4819-157-10-201211200-00007] [PMID: 23165662]

[12]   Lawn SD, Kerkhoff AD, Vogt M, Wood R. Diagnostic accuracy of a low-cost, urine antigen, point-o-
       -care screening assay for HIV-associated pulmonary tuberculosis before antiretroviral therapy: a
       descriptive study. Lancet Infect Dis 2012; 12(3): 201-9.
       [http://dx.doi.org/10.1016/S1473-3099(11)70251-1] [PMID: 22015305]

[13]   Bärnighausen T, McWalter TA, Rosner Z, Newell ML, Welte A. HIV incidence estimation using the
       BED capture enzyme immunoassay: systematic review and sensitivity analysis. Epidemiology 2010;
       21(5): 685-97.
       [http://dx.doi.org/10.1097/EDE.0b013e3181e9e978] [PMID: 20699682]

[14]   Constantine NT, Kabat W, Zhao RY. Update on the laboratory diagnosis and monitoring of HIV
       infection. Cell Res 2005; 15(11-12): 870-6.
       [http://dx.doi.org/10.1038/sj.cr.7290361] [PMID: 16354562]

[15]   Ng OT, Chow AL, Lee VJ, et al. Accuracy and user-acceptability of HIV self-testing using an oral
       fluid-based HIV rapid test. PLoS One 2012; 7(9): e45168.
       [http://dx.doi.org/10.1371/journal.pone.0045168] [PMID: 23028822]

[16]   Pant Pai N, Sharma J, Shivkumar S, et al. Supervised and unsupervised self-testing for HIV in high-
       and low-risk populations: a systematic review. PLoS Med 2013; 10(4): e1001414.
       [http://dx.doi.org/10.1371/journal.pmed.1001414] [PMID: 23565066]

[17]   Paltiel AD, Walensky RP. Home HIV testing: good news but not a game changer. Ann Intern Med
       2012; 157(10): 744-6.
       [http://dx.doi.org/10.7326/0003-4819-157-10-201211200-00545] [PMID: 23044643]

[18]   Hutchinson MK, VanDevanter N, Phelan J, et al. Feasibility of implementing rapid oral fluid HIV
       testing in an urban University Dental Clinic: a qualitative study. BMC Oral Health 2012; 12: 11.
       [http://dx.doi.org/10.1186/1472-6831-12-11] [PMID: 22571324]

[19]   Takizawa K, Nakashima T, Mizukami T, et al. Degenerate polymerase chain reaction strategy with
       DNA microarray for detection of multiple and various subtypes of virus during blood screening.
       Transfusion 2013; 53(10 Pt 2): 2545-55.
       [http://dx.doi.org/10.1111/trf.12193] [PMID: 23590180]

[20]   Saksena NK, Conceicao V, Perera SS, Wu J. Gene array data relevant to immunological and
       virological monitoring of human immunodeficiency virus type 1 infection. Curr Opin HIV AIDS
       2013; 8(2): 132-9.
       [http://dx.doi.org/10.1097/COH.0b013e32835ccae1] [PMID: 23380654]

[21]   O'Brien SF, Zou S, Laperche S, Brant LJ, Seed CR, Kleinman SH. Surveillance of transfusion-
       transmissible infections comparison of systems in five developed countries. Transfus Med Rev 2012;
       26(1): 38-57.
       [http://dx.doi.org/10.1016/j.tmrv.2011.07.001] [PMID: 21944935]

[22]   Constantine NT, Callahan JT, Watts DM. Retroviral testing: Essentials for quality control and
       laboratory diagnosis. Boca Raton, FL: CRC Press 1992; p. 228.

[23]   Lehe JD, Sitoe NE, Tobaiwa O, et al. Evaluating operational specifications of point-of-care diagnostic
       tests: a standardized scorecard. PLoS One 2012; 7(10): e47459.

[http://dx.doi.org/10.1371/journal.pone.0047459] [PMID: 23118871]

[24]   Faraoni S, Rocchetti A, Gotta F, *et al*. Evaluation of a rapid antigen and antibody combination test in acute HIV infection. J Clin Virol 2013; 57(1): 84-7.
[http://dx.doi.org/10.1016/j.jcv.2013.01.007]

[25]   Bergeron M, Daneau G, Ding T, *et al*. Performance of the PointCare NOW system for CD4 counting in HIV patients based on five independent evaluations. PLoS One 2012; 7(8): e41166.
[http://dx.doi.org/10.1371/journal.pone.0041166] [PMID: 22912668]

[26]   Jordan JA, Ibe CO, Moore MS, Host C, Simon GL. Evaluation of a manual DNA extraction protocol and an isothermal amplification assay for detecting HIV-1 DNA from dried blood spots for use in resource-limited settings. J Clin Virol 2012; 54(1): 11-4.

[27]   Mendoza Cd. Soriano, Vincent. Update on HIV viral-load assays: New technologies and testing in resource-limited settings. Future Virol 2009; 4(5): 423-30.
[http://dx.doi.org/10.2217/fvl.09.24]

[28]   Bucharski D, Reutter LI, Ogilvie LD. "You need to know where we're coming from": Canadian Aboriginal women's perspectives on culturally appropriate HIV counseling and testing. Health Care Women Int 2006; 27(8): 723-47.
[http://dx.doi.org/10.1080/07399330600817808] [PMID: 16893808]

[29]   MacPherson P, MacPherson EE, Mwale D, *et al*. Barriers and facilitators to linkage to ART in primary care: a qualitative study of patients and providers in Blantyre, Malawi. J Int AIDS Soc 2012; 15(2): 18020.
[http://dx.doi.org/10.7448/IAS.15.2.18020] [PMID: 23336700]

[30]   Long EF, Stavert RR. Portfolios of biomedical HIV interventions in South Africa: a cost-effectiveness analysis. J Gen Intern Med 2013; 28(10): 1294-301.
[http://dx.doi.org/10.1007/s11606-013-2417-1] [PMID: 23588668]

[31]   Young SD, Jaganath D. Online social networking for HIV education and prevention: a mixed-methods analysis. Sex Transm Dis 2013; 40(2): 162-7.
[http://dx.doi.org/10.1097/OLQ.0b013e318278bd12] [PMID: 23324979]

CHAPTER 22

Monitoring and Evaluation of HIV/AIDS Interventions

Omid Zamani*

HIV/STI Surveillance Research Center, and WHO Collaborating Center for HIV Surveillance, Institute for Futures Studies in Health, Kerman University of Medical Sciences, Kerman, Iran

Abstract: Monitoring and evaluation is necessary for any program management endeavor however it has been a challenge for application to HIV/AIDS projects globally because of the multidisciplinary and multidimensional aspects of the epidemic. Results-based management has been the main driver behind monitoring and evaluation efforts with various methodologies and indicators used for different stages of the results chain. Complexity of the HIV/AIDS epidemic necessitates the use of triangulation approach and complexity science related methods in studying various HIV aspects from biology to social dynamics and policy-making. Participatory methods have also been utilized for enhancing trust, ownership and empowerment within affected communities. Some frameworks are introduced to help planning and implementing national monitoring and evaluation systems. The future of monitoring and evaluation could be more promising for ensuring accountability and scientific rigor.

Keywords: Accountability, Assessment, Effectiveness, Efficiency, Evaluation, Indicator, Monitoring, Participatory, Planning, Results, Triangulation.

1. INTRODUCTION

HIV/AIDS emerged as a public health concern in a world where evaluation science and practice was also developing rapidly. In fact, the complexity of biopsychosocial factors involved in HIV/AIDS epidemic was helpful in

---

* **Correspondence to Omid Zamani:** HIV/STI Surveillance Research Center, and WHO Collaborating Center for HIV Surveillance, Institute for Futures Studies in Health, Kerman University of Medical Sciences, Kerman, Iran; Tel:+98 (912) 3757353; Fax: +98 (21) 22632159 ; E-mail: omid.zamani@gmail.com

SeyedAhmad SeyedAlinaghi (Ed.)

developing novel approaches for monitoring and evaluation of HIV/AIDS projects around the world."Increases in scrutiny, fierce competitions for decreased funding levels, strong demand for results, and great emphasis on accountability yielded higher pressure on non-profits and government organizations for providing the results, being accountable, demonstrating great performance, and acting like business users" [1].

HIV/AIDS program management and interventions dealing with the quality of life assessment in the target population and People Living with HIV (PLHIV), in particular, have generally faced the challenge for monitoring and evaluation (M&E) of projects and programs. The answers to the questions such as how certain practices would be proved to make different outcomes, whether a change is needed in programs, or whether there is an essential need for a new intervention, with some other questions in relation to accomplishment, effectiveness and accountability are provided through this process. When a state, for example, aims to make harm reduction policies, the M & E process will explain the pre-determined implementation of various components and services, like needle and syringe exchange, increasing used of condom, voluntary counseling and testing, and sentinel sites; and determine the levels of success in the strategies, individually and collectively, as the entire package.

The M&E is regarded as an applied research. The M&E seeks to improve decision-making process, develop knowledge with actions and problem-solving in health and social settings. According to The OECD, "Monitoring is defined as a continuous performance, applying systematic data collections on given indicators as to inform management and main stakeholders about ongoing projects with progress towards achievements, and utilization of allocated funds" [2]. Also, "Evaluation refers to a systematic and targeted evaluation of projects, programs, or strategies, in progress and completed, together with design, implementation, and outcome. The purpose is to demonstrate the extent of relevance and fulfillment of goals, efficiency, effectiveness, influence, and sustainability. Any evaluation should bring valid and useful knowledge, which allows the utilization of lessons learned for making decisions, whether of recipients or donors" [2].

On the other hand, the Results-Based Management (RBM) has changed the traditional approach to M&E from measuring performance and outputs to assessment of outcomes and impact of health interventions. In RBM approach, a results chain or model is regarded as a manifestation of a program, defining how to achieve development goals (an aspect of the quality of human life). The approach covers causal associations and key assumptions for any level of results. This will be elaborated in details below.

Some experts prefer to integrate M&E in an inclusive frame to stress on a lifecycle approach in programming. Table **1** shows a framework with monitoring as a "process evaluation".

Table 1. Comprehensive evaluation framework.

Types of Evaluation	Broad Purpose	Main Questions Answered by it
Baseline Analysis / Formative Evaluation Research	Determines Concept and Design	Where are we now? Is an intervention needed? Who needs the intervention? How should the intervention be carried out?
Monitoring / Process Evaluation	Monitors Inputs and Outputs, Assesses Service Quality	How are we doing? To what extent are planned activities actually realized? How well are the services provided?
Effectiveness Evaluation	Assesses Outcome and Impact	How did we do? What outcomes are observed? What do the outcomes mean? Does the program make a difference?
Future plans / Cost-Effectiveness Analysis	Assesses Value-for-Resources Committed Including Sustainability Issues	Should program priorities be changed or expanded? To what extent should resources be reallocated? What are the next steps and needed resources?

2. INDICATORS FOR THE M&E FRAMEWORK

An indicator refers to a measure used to examine a condition, progress in a procedure, or results of an activity or project. There are a wide range of M&E indicators:

- **Direct indicators** match exactly the results at any level. For example, viral load is a good indicator for HIV replication.
- **Indirect** or **"proxy" indicators** provide changes or results when direct measures are impossible. The spread of *Neisseria Gonorrhea*, is an indirect gauge of high risk behaviors, or the number of positive public speeches for HIV&AIDS is a proxy indicator of increased knowledge around HIV/AIDS among the policy-makers.
- **Quantitative measures** are usually expressed as numbers, percentages or shares, such as a rate or a ratio (for example, percentage of PLWHA needing antiretroviral drugs during the treatment).
- **Qualitative observations** involved, for example, the individuals' practices within an organization in pursuit of engagement in training workshops.
- **Aggregate measures** bring data from individuals together, and summarized at the country- or region- levels (*e.g.*, rates of IDU or HIV) [3].
- **Environmental indicators** represent physical or social features of the place where people live. These determine factors external to an individual, such as drug quality, or the number of neighborhood associations. These indicators have analogues at the individual level [4].
- **Global indicators** lack clear analogue for the individual level. Contextual indicators are good examples, including the presence of healthy public policies, anti-discrimination acts, or equity in access to care, social cohesion, *etc.*[4].

An M&E indicator refers to a gauge which provides results compared to what was previously planned during different levels of a "results chain". Table **2** shows some examples. While some people may argue that the level of indicators may vary based on the definition of program and/or project and the scales – *i.e.* national, regional or local-; experts from the United Nations suggest a Human Rights Based Approach to Programming (HRBAP) where the fulfillment of different human rights for every human being is considered at impact (top) level.

Many intergovernmental organizations including UNAIDS, United Nations Children's Fund, the Global Fund and WHO have encouraged the countries for development of a mutually accepted action framework for HIV/AIDS which could offer the underlying principle for the integration of activities of all partners; a coordinating leadership for AIDS at the national level, with a broad multi-sector governing body, and a totally accepted system for national monitoring and evaluation process [3], known as Three-Ones principles and they annually aggregate and report reconciliation of nationally reported data, usually in a joint reporting form. "Through fundamental collaborations of the World Bank, global agencies pledged to a general HIV M&E framework, called the "12 Components Framework". This covered the definition of M&E systems with the underlying base for assessments, and capacity development of M&E systems" [4].

Table 2. Classified M&E indicators *[adapted and revised from monitoring and evaluation toolkit, the global fund].*

Level	Characteristic	Examples
Impact	Measure the quality and quantity of long-term results (widespread improvements in a society) generated by program outputs.	• *reduction in morbidity and mortality of HIV&AIDS* • *Percentage of most-at-risk populations who are infected with HIV* • *Incidence of HIV among 15 to 24 year old young individuals (male and female)*
Outcome	Measure the intermediate results generated by program outputs. They often correspond to any change in people's behavior as a result of the program.	• *proportion of target population who meet prescribed standards of behavior (e.g. continuous condom use)* • *number of people whose behavior changes* • *percentage of young people who have had sex before the age of 15* • *percentage of Injecting Drug Users (IDUs) who practice safer injecting and sexual activity*
Output	Measure the quantity, quality and timeliness of the products — goods or services — that are the result of an activity/project/program.	• *number of people whose opinions/attitudes change (e.g. accept a colleague living with HIV)* • *Adults' support in educating condom use to prevent HIV/AIDS among young people* • *number of people who learn the facts (e.g. can cite 3 routes of HIV transmission)* • *Number or percentage of target population covered by intervention (e.g. ART, harm reduction or care)* • *number of active peer/community educators* • *number of counseling provided at Voluntary Confidential Counseling and Testing (VCCT) centers*

(Table 2) contd.....

Level	Characteristic	Examples
Process	Measure the progress of activities in a program/project and the way such activities are carried out.	• *number of people who receive/read the communication materials* • *Number of providers trained according to national standards for an intervention (e.g. VCCT)* • *Number of students received participatory life-skills based HIV&AIDS education in schools*
Input	Measure the quantity, quality and timeliness of resources provided for an activity/project/program.	• *amount of communication materials (posters, pamphlets,...) produced/distributed* • *Number of VCCT centers established* • *Policy and guidelines are in place at national level* • *Percentage of national expenditure for HIV&AIDS programs*

"The 12 components should not be regarded as implementation steps. There is no requirement to implement in a sequential consistency. Rather, these components should all be present with acceptable standards in order to enhance the effectiveness of the national HIV M&E system" [5].

An equity-focused evaluation [6] approach has also been introduced to look at the equity dimensions of development interventions and to take process and contextual analysis into consideration, rather than just ensuring achievement of results. Similarly a gender-responsive approach tries to address realization of inclusion, participation and fair power relations as principles of gender equality throughout the process and results of evaluation plans [7]. Both are recommending the use of multiple methods and mixed methods for evaluation.

3. TRIANGULATION

Compared to a more limited approach, any method of evaluation which uses several quantitative and qualitative techniques is probably intended to investigate various requirements of evaluation. To survey a problem from different angles by using different methods is called triangulation which aims to enhance the reliability of results. According to Denzin [8] four basic forms are introduced for triangulation: data triangulation (with time, space, and person); investigator triangulation (involving the use of different observers); theory triangulation (the use of more than one theoretical scheme for explanation of a phenomenon); and methodological triangulation (involving more than one method, including within-method or between-method strategies). However, the 5th form could be multiple triangulations (*i.e.* combining some of them in the same investigation). Triangulation has the advantage of enhanced reliability of findings. Also, it can be used in quantitative (validation) and qualitative (inquiry) research.

4. COMPLEXITY SCIENCE APPROACH

Complexity of causal network of HIV control at national level requires more sophisticated approach to planning, monitoring and evaluation, especially when considering the demand for scaling up the HIV prevention, care and treatment. Complexity theory provides some insight to understand such issues and to help shaping new approaches to evaluation. Complexity theory tries to consider nonlinear, adaptive and self-regulated nature of individual and social change in an inter-dependent environment. This is completely different from the usual practice of monitoring and evaluation where simplifying assumptions just yield a tunneled-vision of the reality. Complexity-science- related quantitative techniques such as time-series analysis, machine learning, data mining, nonlinear dynamics, network modeling and agent-based modeling [9] together with some qualitative methods such as participatory action research [10] and Qualitative Comparative Analysis (QCA) [11] provide opportunities for evaluating change in a complex realm such as HIV/AIDS. These methods have been used in studying various HIV aspects from biology to social dynamics and policy-making [12 - 14].

5. PARTICIPATORY MONITORING AND EVALUATION

In general, typical M&E uses a quantitative and non-participatory research design which is developed by some external evaluators, remained uninvolved in the program or project. However, we can consider people as agents rather than objects of M&E; with the capability to analyze their situations and obtain specific solutions. This approach has been increasingly adopted recently, because it not only satisfies the interests groups, including funding organizations and policymakers, but also provides opportunities for all who were involved to express their own views and decisions. "What maybe discriminate "Participatory

M&E" from conventional techniques is the fact that this focuses on the engagement of a broad range of interest parties in the M&E process. Trust, ownership and empowerment are the basic values of Participatory M&E" [13].

Further, participatory M&E uses groundbreaking indicators, like pictures and stories, instead of those applied by conventional M&E. Various participatory evaluation approaches can be taken into account and even introduced within national M&E systems; for example, Participatory Rural Appraisal (PRA), Most Significant Change (MSC), Participatory Learning and Action (PLA), Beneficiary Assessment (BA) and Forum Theatre.

6. PLANNING M&E SYSTEMS

Development of an M&E plan prior to implementation of any project/program is a prerequisite for robust and rigorous assessment of its results. In addition to defining scope and conceptual outline of the M&E, methodological approach including the choice of indicators, designs, protocols and tools for evaluation studies, implementation plan and dissemination choices should be determined in this plan. A Community Randomized Controlled Trial (C-RCT) is considered as theoretical gold standard for impact assessment in large scale interventions however usually they are not financially, logistically or ethically feasible when applied to HIV/AIDS settings. An alternative, suggested by Boily *et al.*, includes "an integrated mathematical framework to merge empirical, biological, and behavioral information from various subpopulations in areas of intervention, by an application of tailor-made models for transmission dynamics which are introduced in the Bayesian framework" [14]. Some strategies for more effective M&E in settings with limited resource are suggested by Nash *et al.* [15]:

1. Web-specific applications with decentralized data entry and actual accessibility of summary reporting.
2. Timely feedback to site and district employees.
3. Integration of indicators of traditionally siloed program areas at the site level.
4. Longitudinal survey of program and site features.
5. Geographic information systems, and
6. Application of routinely collected aggregate data for epidemiologic and

operational studies.

The following could be recommended as best practices for M&E systems:

- M&E funding should be developed with appropriate resources (preferably, about 10 percent of the program budgeting) [16].
- M&E should cover all levels of results in a logical sequence with comprehensive indicators relevant to context.
- Incorporating mixed methods and triangulation in M&E systems may ensure validity and reliability of data and may assist in holistics conclusions.
- To minimize cost burden in limited resource settings, M&E interventions should be harmonized, effectively organized and integrated with current systems.
- Maximum participation of key stakeholders including the program participants is needed to increase the utilization of evaluation results, having a communication and utilization plan is a prerequisite as well.
- There should be mechanisms in place for revision and improving the M&E systems.

7. FUTURE OF M&E

The field of M&E has significantly evolved. Michael Quinn Patton has suggested the followings as the future trends in evaluation [17]:

1. Enhanced evaluation at the international and cross-cultural levels with increased globalization and variety,
2. Improvement in knowledge and value of the profession and trans-discipline of evaluation,
3. Growing political interests to promote accountability, performance indicators, and transparency,
4. Increased focus on building capacity and developing skills of evaluation,
5. Persistent debates around the nature of methodological rigor, and
6. Applying systems-thinking and complexity science as the evaluation process frameworks.

CONFLICT OF INTEREST

The author confirms that author has no conflict of interest to declare for this

publication.

ACKNOWLEDGEMENTS

Declared none.

REFERENCES

[1]   Calidoni-Lundberg F. Evaluation: definitions, methods and models. ITPS: Swedish Institute for Growth Policy Studies 2006. Available from: http://www.tillvaxtanalys.se/download /18.1af15a1f152a3475a818975/1454505626167/Evaluation+definitions+methods+and+models-06.pdf

[2]   OECD-DAC Working Party on Aid Evaluation. Glossary of Key terms in Evaluation and Results-based Management and Evaluation 2002; p17-21. Available from: http://www.oecd.org/dataoecd/29/21/2754804.pdf

[3]   UNAIDS. "Three Ones" key principles; "Coordination of National Responses to HIV/AIDS" Guiding principles for national authorities and their partners UNAIDS 2004. Available at: http://data.unaids.org/una-docs/three-ones_keyprinciples_en.pdf

[4]   Porter LE, Bouey PD, Curtis S, *et al.* Beyond indicators: advances in global HIV monitoring and evaluation during the PEPFAR era. J Acquir Immune Defic Syndr 2012; 60 (Suppl. 3): S120-6. [http://dx.doi.org/10.1097/QAI.0b013e31825cf345] [PMID: 22797733]

[5]   UNAIDS Monitoring and Evaluation Reference Group (MERG) 12 Components Monitoring & Evaluation System Assessment. New York: UNAIDS 2010; pp. 4-32. Available from: http://www.unaids.org/sites/default/files/sub_landing/files/1_MERG_Assessment_12_Components_ME_System.pdf

[6]   Bamberger M, Segone M. How to design and manage Equity-focused evaluations. UNICEF 2011. Available from: http://mymande.org/sites/default/files/EWP5_Equity_focused_evaluations.pdf

[7]   Integrating Human Rights and Gender Equality in Evaluation: Towards UNEG Guidance. UNEG 2011. Available from: http://www.uneval.org/document/detail/980

[8]   Denzin NK. Sociological Methods: A Sourcebook. Aldine Transaction 2006.

[9]   Chalizi CR. Methods and techniques of complex systems science: An overview chapter 1 , complex systems science in biomedicine. New York:Springer 2006; pp. 33-114.

[10]   Panos London. How can complexity theory contribute to more effective development and aid evaluation?. London: Panos London 2009. Available from: http://panos.org.uk/wp-content /files/2011/03/Panos_London_Complexity_and_Evaluation_dialogueCK5gVc.pdf

[11]   Schensul JJ, Chandran D, Singh SK, Berg M, Singh S, Gupta K. The use of qualitative comparative analysis for critical event research in Alcohol and HIV in Mumbai, India. AIDS Behav 2010; 14 (Suppl. 1): S113-25. [http://dx.doi.org/10.1007/s10461-010-9736-6] [PMID: 20563636]

[12]   Lanham HJ, *et al.* How complexity science can inform scale-up and spread in health care: Understanding the role of self-organization in variation across local contexts. Social Science & Medicine 2012.

[http://dx.doi.org/http://dx.doi.org/10.1016/j.socscimed.2012.05.040] [PMID: 21516198]

[13]   Parks Will, Gray-Felder Denise, Hunt Jim, Byrne Ailish. Who measures change, an introduction to participatory monitoring and evaluation of communication for social change. Communication For Social Change Consortium 2005.

[14]   Boily MC, Lowndes CM, Vickerman P, *et al.* CHARME-India team. Evaluating large-scale HIV prevention interventions: study design for an integrated mathematical modelling approach. Sex Transm Infect 2007; 83(7): 582-9.
[http://dx.doi.org/10.1136/sti.2007.027516] [PMID: 17942574]

[15]   Nash D, Elul B, Rabkin M, *et al.* Strategies for more effective monitoring and evaluation systems in HIV programmatic scale-up in resource-limited settings: Implications for health systems strengthening. J Acquir Immune Defic Syndr 2009; 52 (Suppl. 1): S58-62.
[http://dx.doi.org/10.1097/QAI.0b013e3181bbcc45] [PMID: 19858942]

[16]   Cooper D , Cahn P , Lewin S , *et al.* The Sydney Declaration: a call to scale-up research (Letter). Lancet 2007; 370(9581): 7-8. Available from: http://www.stopaidsnow.org/sites/stopaidsnow.org /files/General_SydneyDeclaration.pdf

[17]   Patton MQ. Future trends in evaluation. In: Segone M, Ed. From policies to results. America: UNICEF in partnership with DevInfo, IDEAS, ILO, IOCE, the World Bank, UNDP, UNIFEM and WFP 2010. Available from: http://www.mymande.org/elearning-unit/start-unit/3/22/story_content/external_files/ readingmaterial_unit3.1.pdf

CHAPTER 23

Sampling Methods for Hidden Populations

Omid Zamani[*]

HIV/STI Surveillance Research Center, and WHO Collaborating Center for HIV Surveillance, Institute for Futures Studies in Health, Kerman University of Medical Sciences, Kerman, Iran

Abstract: In many countries access to some populations most at risk of contracting HIV is limited. Thus conventional sampling methods cannot be utilized for studying various aspects of the epidemic among those populations. Respondent-Driven Sampling (RDS) and Time-Location Sampling (TLS) methods are developed during the recent years to allow having more accurate and more generalizable estimates on the characteristics of the participants. RDS uses the links in the social network of participants for recruitment of new ones and TLS uses the places where the potential participants usually gather. Both methods have assumptions and limitations which should be considered when applying them to different groups and situations. Prior formative research may provide invaluable information on some factors which may influence the researchers' choice for using these methods including cost, time, feasibility and coverage of target population. This may also help in guiding development of public health interventions to mitigate the risks. Some statistical software is available for analysing data gathered from samples together with some modifications and tricks to decrease bias.

Keywords: Bias, Epidemic, HIV, Location, Population, Respondent, Risk, Sampling, Selection, Snowball.

1. INTRODUCTION

HIV/AIDS is associated with some high risk behaviours such as Injection Drug Use (IDU) and unprotected sex which in many societies impose stigma and discrimination to those committing them. The most at risk populations (MARPs)

[*] **Correspondence to Omid Zamani:** HIV/STI Surveillance Research Center, and WHO Collaborating Center for HIV Surveillance, Institute for Futures Studies in Health, Kerman University of Medical Sciences, Kerman, Iran; Tel:+98 (912) 3757353; Fax: +98 (21) 22632159 ; E-mail: omid.zamani@gmail.com

SeyedAhmad SeyedAlinaghi (Ed.)

are usually hidden populations who are hard reached by health workers and researchers. Conducting a conventional survey with random sampling is not feasible through these groups because usually there is not a sampling frame available for them and they are usually a very small part of the general population, facing with stigma and discrimination. So simply doing a household survey cannot catch enough target participants. In the past decades, some efforts were deployed to find innovative approaches to overcome the problem of not having a representative sample. Two general strategies were used in this regard; using the links in the social network of participants and going to places where and when they are concentrated [1].

One of the earliest solutions was using snowball sampling in which a few selected participants function as seeds to invite other participants from their own social network. This process is replicated with the new participants until the desired sample size is achieved. In this way, convenient reaching of the sample size is achieved, however there are still some concerns which remain about non-random sample *e.g.* selection bias toward those who have a larger social network and might be at higher risk of HIV, but leaving the isolated individuals out of the sample. "Non-probability sampling methods such as snowball sampling are useful in formative research and in problem definition, but they are not suitable for producing data that can be confidently generalized to larger populations, although they are sometimes–incorrectly-used in this manner" [1].

2. RESPONDENT-DRIVEN SAMPLING

Respondent-driven sampling (RDS) was introduced in late 90's to minimize the bias in snowball sampling through a mathematical model which puts greater weight on the information received from "isolated" participants compared to those who have more connections [2]. In RDS the researchers select 5-10 seeds (or index cases) among target group who are well-connected to others and can recruit 2-4 other participants each. The recruitment is done through a fixed predetermined number of coupons or tickets which will be given to seeds and the new recruits. The cascade of new recruitment waves will continue until researches reach to the desired sample size or the stability of results among waves which is called "equilibrium". One of the main issues in RDS is following the chain of coupons through coupon manager software. Also special softwares exist for statistical analysis of results.

There are three assumptions for an RDS study; 1) respondents know one another as members of the target population, 2) respondents' networks are linked and form a single network and 3) sample size is small relative to size of the target population. Lansky *et al.*, have proposed quantitative measures to evaluate, post-hoc, the extent to which the three assumptions were met [3].

An RDS sample is self-weighting only when two conditions are encountered: (1) network sizes for groups of analytic interest (*e.g.*, gender, race) are equivalent, and (2) efficacy of recruit are equal between groups. Unfortunately these two conditions are not met usually, so post-stratification weights are required to yield population estimates that control for these sources of bias [4].

Goel and Sharad have argued that having a greater sample size in RDS does not necessarily lead to more accurate estimates and suggested reduction of recruitment coupons for each participant [5]. They also showed that bottlenecks, anywhere in the network, impact the quality of RDS estimates [5].

"Two main estimation methods are generally used. The RDS-1 estimator, currently in wide use, can be implemented with the standard respondent-driven sampling analysis software. RDS-1 accounts for patterns of recruitment between subgroups and the average number of other members of the target group who the recruiters know (the "network size") in each subgroup. RDS-2 is a more recently developed estimator that relates respondent-driven sampling estimation to widely used survey estimation through the use of a generalized Horvitz–Thompson estimator. RDS-2 accounts for network size only. Initial theoretical analysis has asserted that the RDS-2 estimator is asymptotically unbiased as long as six key assumptions are met, including that respondents accurately report the size of their "network" (the number of other members of the target group they know), that respondents randomly recruit from their network, and that respondents have reciprocal relationships with members of the target population" [6]. RDS data are usually analysed with RDSAT software which generates appropriately weighted estimated proportions with confidence intervals. However RDSAT software is not capable to calculate bivariate or multivariate statistics, for which researchers transfer data to other softwares. Thus, recently an implementation in R and another in Stata were introduced [7].

Salganik presented a bootstrap method for constructing confidence intervals around respondent-driven sampling estimates and demonstrated in simulations that it outperforms the usual method [8]. Wylie and Jolly showed that using self-presenting seeds may improve access to hidden populations [9].

Xin Lu *et al.*, developed an estimator which is based on prior information about the average indegrees of estimated variables. "When the indegree is known, such as for RDS studies over internet social networks, the estimator can greatly reduce estimate error and bias as compared with current methods; when the indegree is not known, which is most common for interview-based RDS studies, the estimator can, through sensitivity analysis, be used as a tool to account for uncertainties of network directedness and error in self-reported degree data" [10].

RDS conducted among injecting drug users generally have faster recruitment compared with studies among sex workers [11]. Malekinejad *et al.*, found that RDS has been somewhat more successful in IDU studies in terms of recruitment efficiency, as measured by the number of new participants referred per seed for week and that RDS studies took nine weeks to complete on average [11]. Johnston *et al.*, (2008) have investigated some challenges in the implementation of RDS including those of appropriately defining eligibility criteria, structuring social network size questions, selecting design effects and conducting statistical analysis [12].

Since the design effect can be relative to the length of recruitment chains, Johnston *et al.*, (2013) recommended that a design effect of three or four for RDS studies might be more appropriate [13]. They also observed that design effect generally appeared to increase with increased homophily, but it did not appear to be related to mean network size [13].

A recent study suggested more distant contacts were less likely to be reported, and therefore recruited, but if reported, more distant contacts were as likely as closer contacts to be recruited and people living closer to an interview site were more likely to be recruited [14]. So researchers should be careful in choosing the network size question and interview site location(s). Jeness *et al.*, showed while the spatial structure of RDS recruitment may be biased in heterogeneous urban settings, the impact of this bias on estimates of outcome measures appears minimal [15].

The utility of RDS can be extended beyond surveillance into intervention research through participatory methods as Tiffany elaborated [16]. RDS can also be combined with population size estimation methods such as capture-recapture to estimate the size of most at risk populations in a given area [17]. More recently Wejnert has used RDS to do a social network analysis [18].

RDS studies have a lot of ethical considerations that Semaan *et al.*, suggested to be reported, including "data on variables related to the process of participant-driven recruitment and to the options for informing participants of their discordant partnerships" [19]. Ethical issues involved in research implementing respondent-driven sampling of at-risk populations in developing countries, should be more explicit because ethical review mechanisms may be weak and special circumstances with regard to security and services may exist, for example sending mobile interviewers out instead of inviting participants to a 'marked' location [20].

Finally some public health professionals may feel that RDS as an intervention may affect the participants, however it seems there is no association between RDS recruitment and changes in network composition or HIV risk behaviours [21].

3. TIME LOCATION SAMPLING

Time Location Sampling (TLS) [also called Time Space Sampling (TSS)] is the approach for finding participants where and when they gather. This technique was utilized in 1990's for studies among MSM [22]. TLS is a modified cluster sampling in which the researcher considers the list of different time slots at various venues (locations) where target group gathers as a clustering frame and selects a random number of those clusters for recruiting participants. In the other word, VDT (Venue, Day and Time) units form the sampling frame. For example if we have three clubs with four time slots for each we will have 12 clusters. In practice the researchers need a mapping before TLS for identifying available venues and time slots to be able to develop the sampling frame.

Sampling should be preferably done with a probability proportional to the number of the eligible persons at each VDT. It is better to sample entrances of VDTs in proportion to frequency of use as well [4]. Staff members should count the venue attendants, screen prospective participants, invite eligible participants, use random or systematic sampling to choose potential respondents, conduct the surveys, and collect relevant data on those who refuse to participate in the survey or on those who withdraw from the survey [4]. With regard to potentially changing conditions that may have an influence on the sampling process (*e.g.* changes in attendance patterns caused by seasonal weather variations or by social, economic, or legal forces), it is recommended regularly (*i.e.* monthly) identifying new VDTs and to evaluate the effective output of VDTs already listed in the sampling frame [4].

TLS permits researchers to get a large, diverse sample of the target population and to generalize the findings to the target population. TLS also allows for identifying locations where the target population can receive services, if this is a goal of the project. TLS has two important limitations; the first is when VDTs that were not easily identifiable or approachable were excluded from the sampling frame and the second is when the target populations in the included VDTs differ from those that could have been selected at the excluded VDTs on important variables associated with the outcomes of interest [4].

Since members of the target population who do not attend public venues are excluded from the sampling frame and venue regulars have many more chances of being interviewed than occasional patrons, TLS is criticized to have bias in favour of frequent venue attendees [23]. To tackle this issue Karon and Wejnert propose that TLS data be analysed as a two-stage sample survey using a simple weighting procedure based on the inverse of the approximate probability that a person was sampled and using sample survey analysis software to estimate the standard errors of estimates to account for the effects of clustering within locations and variation in the weights [24].

TLS and RDS have been used in many different countries and for a variety of target populations. In some countries they are used for periodic bio-behavioural surveillance among most at risk populations which provides HIV and risky behaviour trend data after 2-3 rounds.

The choice between TLS and RDS should consider ease of implementation, time needed to complete the study, cost of the study, coverage of the population of interest, assumptions required for the analysis to be valid, data required for the analysis, difficulty in doing the analysis, and feasibility in doing the analysis [24]. TLS generally takes a longer period of time and is more expensive than RDS and might be more appropriate for some mobile populations such as truck drivers [25]. RDS may have advantages in reaching higher risk individuals who are most hidden from intervention research and service delivery [26, 27]. The importance of conducting detailed formative research to properly plan TLS or RDS surveys is vital. Qualitative data are critical to well-designed sampling procedures, *e.g.*, venue selection for TLS or seed selection for RDS, the required spectrum of indicators, the correct phrasing of questions, determine appropriate types of incentives; to assess the economic value of goods in each setting; and to understand the larger population and the accessible population [28].

CONFLICT OF INTEREST

The author confirms that author has no conflict of interest to declare for this publication.

ACKNOWLEDGEMENTS

Declared none.

REFERENCES

[1]   Magnani R, Sabin K, Saidel T, Heckathorn D. Review of sampling hard-to-reach and hidden populations for HIV surveillance. AIDS 2005; 19 (Suppl. 2): S67-72.
[http://dx.doi.org/10.1097/01.aids.0000172879.20628.e1] [PMID: 15930843]

[2]   Heckathorn DD. Respondent-driven sampling: a new approach to the study of hidden populations. Soc Probl 1997; 174-99.
[http://dx.doi.org/10.2307/3096941]

[3]   Lansky A, Drake A, Wejnert C, Pham H, Cribbin M, Heckathorn DD. Assessing the assumptions of respondent-driven sampling in the national HIV Behavioral Surveillance System among injecting drug users. Open AIDS J 2012; 6: 77-82.

[http://dx.doi.org/10.2174/1874613601206010077] [PMID: 23049656]

[4]   Semaan S. Time-space sampling and respondent-driven sampling with hard-to-reach populations Methodol Innov Online 2010; 5(2): 60-75. Available from: http://www.pbs.plym.ac.uk /mi/pdf/05-0- -10/7.%20Semaan%20English%20(formatted).pdf

[5]   Goel S, Salganik MJ. Respondent-driven sampling as Markov chain Monte Carlo. Stat Med 2009; 28(17): 2202-29.
[http://dx.doi.org/10.1002/sim.3613] [PMID: 19572381]

[6]   McCreesh N, Frost SD, Seeley J, *et al.* Evaluation of respondent-driven sampling. Epidemiology 2012; 23(1): 138-47.
[http://dx.doi.org/10.1097/EDE.0b013e31823ac17c] [PMID: 22157309]

[7]   Schonlau M, Liebau E. Respondent-driven sampling. Stata J 2012; 12(1): 72-93.

[8]   Salganik MJ. Variance estimation, design effects, and sample size calculations for respondent-driven sampling. J Urban Health : Bull New York Acad Med 2006; 83(6 Suppl): i98-112.
[http://dx.doi.org/10.1007/s11524-006-9106-x]

[9]   Wylie JL, Jolly AM. Understanding recruitment: outcomes associated with alternate methods for seed selection in respondent driven sampling. BMC Med Res Methodol 2013; 13: 93.
[http://dx.doi.org/10.1186/1471-2288-13-93] [PMID: 23865487]

[10]   Lu X, Malmros J, Liljeros F, Britton T. Respondent-driven sampling on directed networks. Electron J Stat 2013; 7: 292-322.
[http://dx.doi.org/10.1214/13-EJS772]

[11]   Malekinejad M, Johnston LG, Kendall C, Kerr LR, Rifkin MR, Rutherford GW. Using respondent-driven sampling methodology for HIV biological and behavioral surveillance in international settings: a systematic review. AIDS Behav 2008; 12(4) (Suppl.): S105-30.
[http://dx.doi.org/10.1007/s10461-008-9421-1] [PMID: 18561018]

[12]   Johnston LG, Malekinejad M, Kendall C, Iuppa IM, Rutherford GW. Implementation challenges to using respondent-driven sampling methodology for HIV biological and behavioral surveillance: field experiences in international settings. AIDS Behav 2008; 12(4) (Suppl.): S131-41.
[http://dx.doi.org/10.1007/s10461-008-9413-1] [PMID: 18535901]

[13]   Johnston LG, Chen YH, Silva-Santisteban A, Raymond HF. An empirical examination of respondent driven sampling design effects among HIV risk groups from studies conducted around the world. AIDS Behav 2013; 17(6): 2202-10.
[http://dx.doi.org/10.1007/s10461-012-0394-8] [PMID: 23297082]

[14]   McCreesh N, Johnston LG, Copas A, *et al.* Evaluation of the role of location and distance in recruitment in respondent-driven sampling. Int J Health Geogr 2011; 10: 56.
[http://dx.doi.org/10.1186/1476-072X-10-56] [PMID: 22008416]

[15]   Jenness SM, Neaigus A, Wendel T, Gelpi-Acosta C, Hagan H. Spatial recruitment bias in respondent-driven sampling: implications for HIV prevalence estimation in Urban heterosexuals. AIDS Behav 2013.
[http://dx.doi.org/10.1007/s10461-013-0640-8] [PMID: 24122043]

[16]   Tiffany JS. Respondent-driven sampling in participatory research contexts: participant-driven

recruitment. J Urban Health 2006; 83(6) (Suppl.): i113-24.
[http://dx.doi.org/10.1007/s11524-006-9107-9] [PMID: 16933100]

[17]   Paz-Bailey G, Miller W, Shiraishi RW, Jacobson JO, Abimbola TO, Chen SY. Reaching men who
        have sex with men: a comparison of respondent-driven sampling and time-location sampling in
        Guatemala City. AIDS Behav 2013; 17(9): 3081-90.
        [http://dx.doi.org/10.1007/s10461-013-0589-7] [PMID: 23963498]

[18]   Wejnert C. Social network analysis with respondent-driven sampling data: A study of racial
        integration on campus. Soc Networks 2010; 32(2): 112-24.
        [http://dx.doi.org/10.1016/j.socnet.2009.09.002] [PMID: 20383316]

[19]   Semaan S, Santibanez S, Garfein RS, Heckathorn DD, Des Jarlais DC. Ethical and regulatory
        considerations in HIV prevention studies employing respondent-driven sampling. Int J Drug Policy
        2009; 20(1): 14-27.
        [http://dx.doi.org/10.1016/j.drugpo.2007.12.006] [PMID: 18243679]

[20]   DeJong J, Mahfoud Z, Khoury D, Barbir F, Afifi RA. Ethical considerations in HIV/AIDS
        biobehavioral surveys that use respondent-driven sampling: illustrations from Lebanon. Am J Public
        Health 2009; 99(9): 1562-7.
        [http://dx.doi.org/10.2105/AJPH.2008.144832] [PMID: 19608961]

[21]   Rudolph AE, Latkin C, Crawford ND, Jones KC, Fuller CM. Does respondent driven sampling alter
        the social network composition and health-seeking behaviors of illicit drug users followed
        prospectively? PLoS One 2011; 6(5): e19615.
        [http://dx.doi.org/10.1371/journal.pone.0019615] [PMID: 21573122]

[22]   MacKellar D, Valleroy L, Karon J, Lemp G, Janssen R. The Young Men's Survey: methods for
        estimating HIV seroprevalence and risk factors among young men who have sex with men Public
        health rep: (Washington, DC : 1974) 1996; 111(Suppl 1): 138-44.

[23]   Wejnert C, Heckathorn DD. Web-based network sampling efficiency and efficacy of respondent-
        driven sampling for online research. Sociol Methods Res 2008; 37(1): 105-34.
        [http://dx.doi.org/10.1177/0049124108318333]

[24]   Karon JM, Wejnert C. Statistical methods for the analysis of time-location sampling data. J Urban
        Health 2012; 89(3): 565-86.
        [http://dx.doi.org/10.1007/s11524-012-9676-8]

[25]   Ferreira LO, de Oliveira ES, Raymond HF, Chen SY, McFarland W. Use of time-location sampling
        for systematic behavioral surveillance of truck drivers in Brazil. AIDS Behav 2008; 12(4) (Suppl.):
        S32-8.
        [http://dx.doi.org/10.1007/s10461-008-9386-0] [PMID: 18392673]

[26]   Wei C, McFarland W, Colfax GN, Fuqua V, Raymond HF. Reaching black men who have sex with
        men: a comparison between respondent-driven sampling and time-location sampling. Sex Transm
        Infect 2012; 88(8): 622-6.
        [http://dx.doi.org/10.1136/sextrans-2012-050619] [PMID: 22750886]

[27]   Kendall C, Kerr LR, Gondim RC, *et al.* An empirical comparison of respondent-driven sampling, time
        location sampling, and snowball sampling for behavioral surveillance in men who have sex with men,
        Fortaleza, Brazil. AIDS Behav 2008; 12(4) (Suppl.): S97-S104.

[http://dx.doi.org/10.1007/s10461-008-9390-4] [PMID: 18389357]

[28]   Johnston LG, Sabin K, Prybylski D. Update for sampling most-at-risk and hidden populations for HIV biological and behavioral surveillance. jHASE 2010; 2(1): 2.

CHAPTER 24

Recent Researches on HIV/AIDS

Ghobad Moradi[1,*] and **Soda Neamatzade[2]**

[1] *Social Determinants of Health Research Center, Kurdistan University of Medical Sciences, Sanandaj, Iran*

[2] *Kurdistan University of Medical Sciences, Sanandaj, Iran*

Abstract: Despite the publication of many papers on the HIV/AIDS field, the central topics and subjects of research is not clearly determined yet. Therefore, in this chapter we aimed to present the information that may be guide researchers in the field of HIV/AIDS. In order to find the most common studied topics we searched for the related keywords in PubMed and Science-direct. This chapter presents the results of a review of all articles that were published in these databases.

Moreover, we selected the top three journals and studied their most recent issues. All articles published in these journals were classified in view of their subjects, so that to identify and determine the current important topics in the field of HIV/AIDS all over the world; additionally, we tried to list about two percent of all articles which contained HIV/AIDS as their keywords and have been published in PubMed so far. Overall, 4.2% of all articles which were published in Science-direct-indexed journals contained HIV/AIDS as keywords in their titles. The most common and important studied topics include the followings: epidemiology and social topics, cure and antiretroviral therapy, co-morbidity in HIV/AIDS, virology and serology, and HIV/AIDS and cancer.

Epidemiology of HIV/AIDS is still the most frequent topic of research. Most of the reviewed studies were carried out in this field; however, as we found HIV/AIDS treatment planning was also among the most important studied topics. In addition, according to our findings, clinical trials have been increasingly utilized as a research method in the last 10 years.

* Correspondence to Ghobad Moradi: Department of Epidemiology and Biostatistics, Kurdistan University of Medical Sciences (MUK), Sanandaj, Iran, P.O.Bax:66177-13446, Sanandaj, Iran; Tel: (+98) 8716131366; Fax: (+98) 8716664674; E-mail: moradi_gh@yahoo.com

SeyedAhmad SeyedAlinaghi (Ed.)

Keywords: AIDS, Research, Database, HIV, PubMed.

1. INTRODUCTION

Thirty years is not a long time in the history of adisease. However, the past three decades have seen the most intensive investigations and research in to HIV/AIDS compared to any disease known to mankind [1, 2]. New articles are published daily on HIV and AIDS. The most common topics include HIV/AIDS news, antiretroviral therapy (ART), awareness, preventive measures, treatment options, and co-infections such as tuberculosis in HIV [2, 3]. Each step forward in the advance against HIV brings us to a crossroad, a point where a decision isneeded about the direction in which to proceed. ART is well established as an important tool for treatment and prevention; however, it is very likely that the provision of ART for 34 million people is unsustainable in the long term. In 30 years we have gone from warnings of the black plague, even in reputable publications, to advocating thereal possibility of eradication [1]. According to WHO reports on 2013, ischemic heart disease, stroke, lower respiratory infections, chronic obstructive lung disease, diarrhea and HIV/AIDS have remained the top major causes of deaths during the past decade. HIV/AIDS is the sixth cause of death in the world up to now; the disease is ranked differently in different countries with disparate incomes. The graphs show that in low-income countries HIV/AIDS is more important and is the second cause of death while in high-income countries HIV/AIDS is not among the 10 top causes of death [4].

Conducting a research always begins with a statement of a problem. Finding a problem therefore is not difficult, but identifying one for the purpose of research is not always easy. One of the most important primary tasks of research is to identify and clearly define the problem you wish to study [5]. Despite all the available resources, the appropriate areas to research for researchers have not been determined [5 - 7]. Therefore, we aim to present the information that may be useful for active researchers in the area of HIV/AIDS in the following section.

2. METHODS

There are many important databases of medical science such as PubMed, SCIENCEDIRECT, OVID, SPRINGER, and ISI. We screened PubMed and

Science-direct for our search. Thus this reportis based on a review of all articles that were published in these databases from November 2003 to November 2013. We carried out this review by searching AIDS OR HIV as keywords. The results, then, were classified based on time, place, method, type of article, and important subjects. The collected information was organized into tables. In addition, we studied ISI-indexed journals which were selected based on subject and the relevance to our searching terms. Afterward, they were classified based on their recent impact factor. We found top 10 journals that are focused on HIV/AIDS subject. We selected the top three journals and studied the most recent issues. All articles published in these journals were sorted according to subject in order to conclude the current important topics in the field all over the world. Besides, we searched AIDS or HIV in these databases, then studied the most recent 100 articles that were sorted by publication time, and classified these articles based on the subject to find the most important topics too. Our search results are presented in tables in results section.

3. RESULTS

Some tables are presented below which were designed to indicate the current most common topics of study about HIV/AIDS. Studying this information may help scholars to find a problem to start a research. All results were obtained in November 2013(Table **1**).

Table 1. The frequency of HIV/AIDS related articles published in journals indexed in PubMed and Elsevier databases in the last five and 10 years, from beginning up to now and in-press articles in different databases.

No.	Keywords	Database	Total search result	Articles published in last 10 years	Articles published in last 5 years
1	HIV	PubMed	261,958	125,973	67,928
2	HIV	Elsevier	232,404	138,558	84889
3	AIDS	PubMed	216,382	74,943	38,418
4	AIDS	Elsevier	280,206	126,835	76,500

We searched title field for the keywords of HIVand AIDS in PubMed database and we found 13839 articles from which 100 most recent articles were studied and then classified into common groups onthe their subject. The search results are presented in Table **2**.

Table 2. Classification of 100 HIV/AIDS-related studies based on the frequency of topics published in PubMed-indexed journals and in-press publications in the last 10 years.

NO.	Subject	Frequency of Articles, % (N) (among 100 recent articles)
1	Evidence and epidemiology of HIV/AIDS in MSM	20% (n=20)
2	HIV/AIDS Treatment	19% (n=19)
3	Knowledge and attitude toward HIV/AIDS and the effect of training	19% (n=19)
5	Co-morbidity in HIV/AIDS patients	10% (n=10)
6	Study of virology and hematology	10% (n=10)
7	HIV/AIDS co-infections	7% (n=7)
8	Case reports of HIV/AIDS	5% (n=5)
9	Social support for HIV/AIDS patients	5% (n=5)
10	Cost analysis of HIV/AIDS programs and care	3% (n=3)
11	Prevention and public health in HIV/AIDS	2% (n=2)

We searched the title field of Science-direct database for HIV and AIDS keywords and we found a total of 22138 articles from which 100 most recent articles were studied and then classified into common groups based on their subject. The search results are presented in Table **3**.

Table 3. Classification of 100 HIV/AIDS-related studies based on the frequency of topics published in Elsevier database-indexed journals and in-press publications during last 10 years.

NO.	Subject	Frequency of studies % (N) (among 100 recent articles)
1	Epidemiology of HIV/AIDS	22% (n=22)
2	Treatment of HIV/AIDS patients	15% (n=15)
3	Co-infection in HIV/AIDS patients	11% (n=11)
4	HIV/AIDS Co-morbidity	10% (n=8)
5	Social support for HIV/AIDS patients	8% (n=8)
6	Knowledge and attitude toward HIV/AIDS	8% (n=8)
7	Women and HIV/AIDS	6% (n=6)
8	Nutrition of HIV/AIDS patients	5% (n=5)

(Table 3) contd.....

NO.	Subject	Frequency of studies % (N) (among 100 recent articles)
9	Prevention of HIV/AIDS	5% (n=5)
10	HIV/AIDS and cancer	5% (n=5)
11	Quality of life in HIV/AIDS patients	5% (n=5)

Some important topics in WHO website:

- Immunization and HIV/AIDS
- Infant feeding and HIV
- Sexual and reproductive health and HIV
- Sexually transmitted and reproductive tract infections

Table 4. Frequency of HIV/AIDS-related articles classified based on type of study which were published during last 10 years in PubMed and Science-direct indexed journals.

NO.	Study type	Key words			
		HIV		AIDS	
		Pubmed	Elsevier	Pubmed	Elsevier
1	Clinical trials	8,716	9,241	5,264	3,113
2	Evaluation Studies	2,158	59,283	1,491	3,807
3	Case reports	6,429	67,83	4,277	2,654
4	Review	14,816	14,492	9,439	13,598
5	Systematic Reviews	3,065	1,227	2,155	1,235

We also searched HIV or AIDS keywords in PubMed and Science-direct databases, and then we classified them based on the type of study (Table **4**).

Table 5. Presents ISI journals which publish HIV/AIDS- related articles; they were searched using their ISSN to find their information and especially their impact factor, and then they were sorted in a table to be accessed easily. Thomson Reuter/ISI Web of Science List: Science (January 2013).

NO.	TITLE	PUBLISHER	ISSN	E-ISSN	COUNTRY	LANGUAGE	IF
1	AIDS	LIPPINCOTT WILLIAMS and WILKINS	0269-9370	1473-5571	UNITED STATES	English	6.40
2	AIDS and behavior	SPRINGER/PLENUM PUBLISHERS	1090-7165	1573-3254	UNITED STATES	English	2.979

(Table 5) contd.....

NO.	TITLE	PUBLISHER	ISSN	E-ISSN	COUNTRY	LANGUAGE	IF
3	AIDS CARE-PSYCHOLOGICAL AND SOCIO-MEDICAL ASPECTS OF AIDS/HIV	ROUTLEDGE JOURNALS, TAYLOR and FRANCIS LTD	0954-0121	1360-0451	ENGLAND	English	1.834
4	AIDS EDUCATION AND PREVENTION	GUILFORD PUBLICATIONS INC	0899-9546	1943-2755	UNITED STATES	English	1.484
5	AIDS PATIENT CARE AND STDS	MARY ANN LIEBERT INC	1087-2914	1557-7449	UNITED STATES	English	3.090
6	AIDS RESEARCH AND HUMAN RETROVIRUSES	MARY ANN LIEBERT INC	0889-2229	1931-8405	UNITED STATES	English	2.705
7	AIDS REVIEWS	PERMANYER PUBL	1139-6121	1698-6997	SPAIN	English	4.075
8	HIV MEDICINE	WILEY-BLACKWELL	1464-2662	1468-1293	England	English	3.155
9	HIV CLINICAL TRIALS	THOMAS LAND PUBLISHERS, INC	1528-4336	1945-5771	UNITED STATES	English	2.3

Table 6. Two recent issues of top three journals with high IF (December 2013).

NO.	JOURNAL NAME	SUBJECT OF ARTICLES	NUMBER OF ARTICLE (%) which studied the subject
1	AIDS	Epidemiology and social topics	21%
		Cure and antiretroviral therapy	17%
		Co-morbidity in HIV/AIDS	17%
		Virology and serology studies	17%
		HIV/AIDS and cancer	10%
		Other	18%
2	AIDS REWIEV	Genetic studies	33%
		HIV drug resistance	25%
		Epidemiology of HIV infections	25%
		Co-morbidity in HIV/AIDS	16%
		Other	1%
3	HIV MEDICINE	Treatment and antiretroviral therapy	46%
		Epidemiology and social topics	20%
		Co-infections in HIV	12%
		Co-morbidity in HIV	10%
		Other	12%

We searched ISI journals which publish HIV/AIDS-related articles (Table **5**) and then three ISI journals with the highest impact factor (IF) had been chosen and their two recent issues were studied then were sorted them by subject of articles. The results of the search are presented in Table **6**.

4. DISCUSSION

We searched the keywords HIV and AIDS to find the total number of articles according to subject area in HIV/AIDS. The total number of articles published in PubMed-indexed journals up to December 2013 was 23,401,237. Also, we found that 0.92 % of all articles indexed in PubMed contained HIV as a word in their titles. Similarly for HIV 1.12% and overall about 2% of all articles which have been published in PubMed had HIV or AIDS in their keywords [1].

We found that 12,082,291 articles have been published up to December 2013 and Science-direct indexed journals;the articles with HIV or AIDS keywords included 2.3% and 1.9% of all articles, respectively. In general,4.2% of all articles which were published in Science-direct indexed journals contained HIV or AIDS as keywords in their titles [2].

Epidemiology of HIV/AIDS is still the most important research topic [3, 4]. Most of studies are carried out in this area, however as we found in our E-search, knowledge and attitudes toward HIV/AIDS and treatment planning are also among the most important studies areas. In addition to review articles, clinical trials also comprised a large number of researches in the last 10 years, as the total frequency of clinical trials has increased [3].

Haghdoost *et al.* conducted a search in Iran which resembles our study [8]. According to the results that were obtained on their search on HIV/AIDS fields, it was concluded that the top research topics were about epidemiology of AIDS, prevention and efforts to prevent disease transmission. In fact the highest priority was assigned to research in preventive dimensions which call for training about the content of disease, transmission, and preventive interventions [8]. The most important priorities of researches on HIV/AIDS were preventive activities and development of national strategies. Since the high risk groups are the most affected people, special strategies should be included in the national strategy for the target groups. The second priority was assigned to research on HIV/AIDS national and international planning especially in the national administrative organization, health and legal system. The third priority was assigned to immunology subjects to find new drugs and treatment and finally to diagnose co-morbidity of HIV/AIDS [4, 8].

According to the results, HIV epidemic is one of the world's greatest health, political, economic, and scientific challenges. For some countries, particularly in sub-Saharan Africa, a large proportion of the population is infected with HIV and lack of resources for prevention and treatment poses a substantial threat. In Germany, in contrast and due to the solidarity-based statutory health insurance system, people living with HIV and AIDS have full access to treatment and care; besides they tried to explain how to research in HIV/AIDS field [9, 10].

5. SUGGESTION

We suggest to review more databases such as Springer, ISI, Ovid *etc.* to complete this information.

CONFLICT OF INTEREST

The authors confirm that they have no conflict of interest to declare for this publication.

ACKNOWLEDGEMENTS

Declared none.

REFERENCES

[1]   PubMed data base website. Available at: http://www.ncbi.nlm.nih.gov/PubMed. [Last access date: August 2014];

[2]   Science direct data base website. Available at: http://www.sceincedirect.com. [Last access date: August 2014];

[3]   Official journal of the international AIDS society. Available at: http://www.aidsonline.com. [Last access date: August 2014];

[4]   AIDS Reviews journal. Available at: http:// www.aidsreviews.com. [Last access date: August 2014];

[5]   HIV medicine journal. Available at: http://onlinelibrary.wiley.com/journal/10.1111/(ISSN)1468-1293. [Last access date: August 2014];

[6]   Joint United Nations Programme on HIV/ AIDS, a partnership of UNICEF, UNDP, UNFPA, UNDCP, ILO, UNESCO, WHO, World Bank. Available at: http://www.unaids.org. [Last access date: August 2014];

[7]   World Health Organization Department of HIV/AIDS. Available at: http://www.who.int. [Last access date: August 2014];

[8]   Haghdoost A, Sadeghi M, Nasirian M, Mirzazadeh A, Navadeh S. Research priorities in the field of HIV and AIDS in Iran. J Res Med Sci 2012; 17(5): 481-6.
        [PMID: 23626616]

[9]   Fisher AA, Foreit JR, Laing J, Stoeckel J, Townsend J. Designing HIV/AIDS intervention studies An operations research handbook. New York: Population Council 2002; p. 141. (USAID Award No. HRN-A-00-97-00012-00)

[10]   Kapiriri L, Martin DK. Successful priority setting in low and middle income countries: a framework for evaluation. Health Care Anal 2010; 18(2): 129-47.
        [http://dx.doi.org/10.1007/s10728-009-0115-2] [PMID: 19288200]

SUBJECT INDEX

A

Accountability 304, 305, 312

Advocacy 193, 263, 266

AFB 106, 110

Aging i, 158, 162, 230-233

AIDS 3, 4, 27, 44, 45, 49, 53, 56, 60, 67, 69, 81, 90, 92, 114, 136, 139, 140, 143, 148, 167, 169, 186, 208, 212, 215, 228, 253, 272, 274, 275, 313, 315, 325-333

Anal intercourse 21

Antiretroviral i, ii, 10, 12, 13, 16, 21, 23, 25, 27, 78, 87, 90, 96, 98, 103, 104, 106, 109, 116, 136, 141, 148, 149, 151, 152, 169, 170, 184, 186, 189, 200, 201, 203, 206, 207, 218, 219, 239, 242, 249, 274, 282, 283, 285, 288, 293, 295, 302, 307, 325, 326, 330

Antiviral therapy 44, 103, 137

Apoptosis 56, 58, 60, 63, 65, 66, 73, 74, 79, 80, 82, 83, 86, 88, 95, 98, 100, 118, 154, 232

Assessment 255, 257, 259, 260, 262, 280, 289, 311, 313

ATM 56, 73

B

Behavior and attitude 200, 212, 213

Bias 13, 322

Bio Behaviors 234

Breast feeding 27, 31, 32, 34, 35, 37, 38, 170, 248

C

Cardiovascular disorders 223, 224, 227

Caspase 56, 61, 66, 74, 232

CCR5 36, 68, 75, 77, 79, 82, 83, 85, 88, 89, 99, 122, 126, 132, 190, 202

CD4 cell 32, 50, 115, 133, 148, 153, 155, 157, 159, 160, 163, 176, 178, 231, 233

CD4 cells 31, 58, 79, 108, 119, 151, 169, 215, 223

CD4 concentration 27, 31

Clinical trial 25, 30, 40, 153, 178

Co-infection i, 11, 15, 20, 34, 49, 83, 92, 106, 108, 113, 114, 139, 140, 142, 151, 157, 160, 163, 173, 174, 223, 225, 227, 228, 230, 328

Committees 268, 269, 271, 273, 298

Communities 113, 166, 237, 249, 258, 263, 266, 269, 275, 290, 294, 295, 300, 304

Community involvement i, 244, 245, 251, 255, 281, 297

Council 257, 260, 261, 268, 269, 273, 301, 333

Counseling 27, 38, 45, 51, 134, 173, 200, 201, 203, 204, 206, 207, 217, 221, 229, 237, 244, 272, 274, 275, 281, 283, 295, 303, 305, 308

CRF 4

CXCR4 68, 75, 77, 79, 83, 88, 89, 95, 122, 137, 202

Cytokines 32, 61, 75, 82, 86, 95, 131, 144, 225

D

Database 5, 9, 23, 92, 97, 102, 219, 241, 326-328

DBS 297, 299, 300

Decentralization 280, 291

Delivery 11, 19, 20, 26, 27, 40, 44, 46, 53, 80, 158, 164, 167, 174, 269, 279, 280,

www.ingramcontent.com/pod-product-compliance
Lightning Source LLC
Chambersburg PA
CBHW041724210326
41598CB00008B/774